THE CLIMACTERIC
AN UPDATE

THE CLIMACTERIC
AN UPDATE

Proceedings of the fourth Jan Palfijn Symposium, European Conference on the Menopause, held in Antwerp, Belgium, on September 1–2, 1983, under the auspices of 'De Vereniging voor Nederlandstalige gynecologen van België' and 'The International Menopause Society'.

Edited by
H. and B. van Herendael, F. E. Riphagen, L. Goessens and H. van der Pas

MTP PRESS LIMITED
a member of the KLUWER ACADEMIC PUBLISHERS GROUP
LANCASTER / BOSTON / THE HAGUE / DORDRECHT

Published in the UK and Europe by
MTP Press Limited
Falcon House
Lancaster, England

British Library Cataloguing in Publication Data

Jan Palfijn Symposium (*4th : 1983 : Antwerp*)
The climacteric.
1. Menopause
I. Title II. Herendael, H. Van
III. Vereniging voor Nederlandstalige
IV. International Menopause Society
612'.665 RG186
ISBN-13:978-94-010-8973-9 e-ISBN-13:978-94-009-5608-7
DOI: 10.100/978-94-009-5608-7

Published in the USA by
MTP Press
A division of Kluwer Boston Inc
190 Old Derby Street
Hingham, MA 02043, USA

Library of Congress Cataloging in Publication Data

European Conference on Menopause (4th : 1983 : Antwerp, Belgium)
The climacteric—an update.

Bibliography: p.
Includes index.
1. Menopause—Congresses. I. Herendael, H. van. II. Vereniging voor Nederlandstalige Gynecologen van België. III International Menopause Society. IV. Title. [DNLM: 1. Climacteric—congresses. 2. Menopause—congresses WP 580 E89c 1983]
RG186.E97 1983 612'.665 84-11266

Softcover reprint of the hardcover 1st edition 1984

Contents

Contributors

G. L. Adessi
INSERM, U. 198,
Route de Dole,
25000 Besançon,
France

G. Agnani
Service de Gynécologie la Merè et l'Enfant,
Pr. Colette,
25000 Besançon, France

J. J. Amy
Department of Obstetrics and Gynaecology,
Vrije Universiteit Brussel,
Laarbeeklaan 101,
1090 Brussel,
Belgium

M. Baraldi
Department of Obstetrics and Gynaecology,
University of Modena,
Instituto Di Clinica Ostetrica e Ginecologica,
Via del Pozzo 71,
41100 Modena, Italy

F. Barbieri
Department of Obstetrics and Gynaecology,
University of Modena,
Instituto Di Clinica Ostetrica e Ginecologica,
Via del Pozzo 71,
41100 Modena, Italy

A. Basdevant
Department of Nutrition and Metabolism,
Hôpital de l'Hôtel-Dieu,
Place du Parvis Notre-Dame,
75181 Paris Cedex 04, France

D. Bekaert
Vereniging van Nederlandstalige Gynecologen van België,
Tulpenstraat 11,
8320 Brugge, Belgium

P. Belforte
Ospedale Ostetrico Ginecologico, 'Sant'Anna',
Corso Spezia 60,
10126 Torino, Italy

P. A. Beranek
Department of Chemical Pathology,
St. Mary's Hospital Medical School,
London W2 1PG, UK

E. W. Bergink
Organon International B. V.,
Scientific Development Group,
P. O. Box 20,
5340 BH Oss, The Netherlands

R. C. Bonney
Department of Chemical Pathology,
St. Mary's Hospital Medical School,
London W2 1PG, UK

J. Bonte
Department of Obstetrics and Gynaecology,
Akademisch Ziekenhuis, Katholieke Universiteit Leuven,
Kapucijnenvoer,
3000 Leuven, Belgium

V. Boraldi
General Laboratory of Clinical Pathology,
University of Modena,
41100 Modena, Italy

M. Brincat
Department of Gynaecology,
Dulwich Hospital,
London SE22, UK

J. Van Broeckhoven
Department of Gynaecology and Obstetrics,
Akademisch Ziekenhuis Middelheim OCMW,
Lindendreef 1,
2000 Antwerpen, Belgium

Ph. Buytaert
Department of Obstetrics and Gynaecology,
University of Antwerp,
Akademisch Ziekenhuis Antwerpen,
Wilrijkstraat 10,
2520 Edegem, Belgium

C. Campagnoli
Sezione di Ginecologia Endocrinologica,
Ospedale Sant'Anna – U. S. L. 1–23,
Corso Spezia 60,
10126 Torino, Italy

L. D. Cardozo
Department of Gynaecology,
Dulwich Hospital,
London SE22, UK

D. J. Cooper
Computer Unit,
King's College Hospital Medical School,
London SE5, UK

J. Dequeker
Arthritis and Metabolic Bone Disease Research Unit,
Katholieke Universiteit Leuven,
Universitair Ziekenhuis Pellenberg,
Weligerveld 1,
3041 Pellenberg, Belgium

M. Dhont
Department of Gynaecology,
Ghent State University,
De Pintelaan 135,
9000 Gent, Belgium

F. Facchinetti
Department of Obstetrics and Gynaecology,
University of Modena,
Instituto Di Clinica Obstetrica e Ginecologica,
Via del Pozzo 71,
41100 Modena, Italy

J. Ferin
Department of Obstetrics and Gynaecology,
Université Catholique de Louvain,
Cliniques Universitaires Saint-Luc,
Avenue Hippocrate 10,
1200 Bruxelles, Belgium

E. J. Folkerd
Department of Chemical Pathology,
St. Mary's Hospital Medical School,
London W2 1PG, UK

R. D. Gambrell, Jr.
Department of Endocrinology,
Medical College of Georgia,
Augusta, GA 30912, USA

A. R. Genazzani
University of Modena,
Instituto Di Clinica Ostetrica e Ginecologica,
Policlinico,
Via del Pozzo 71,
41100 Modena, Italy

P. Geusens
Arthritis and Metabolic Bone Disease Research Unit,
Katholieke Universiteit Leuven,
Universitair Ziekenhuis Pellenberg,
Weligerveld 1,
3041 Pellenberg, Belgium

D. M. F. Gibb
Department of Gynaecology,
Dulwich Hospital,
London SE22, UK

L. Goessens
VZW Jan Palfijn,
Gelaagstraat 82,
2648 Steendorp, Belgium

E. V. van Hall
University of Leiden,
Academisch Ziekenhuis Leiden,
Rijnsburgerweg 10,
2333 AA Leiden, The Netherlands

A. A. Haspels
Department of Obstetrics and Gynaecology,
Academisch Ziekenhuis Utrecht,
Catharijnesingel 101,
3500 CG Utrecht,
The Netherlands

B. van Herendael
Department of Gynaecology and Obstetrics,
OCMW Jan Palfijn,
Lange Bremstraat 70,
2060 Merksem (Antwerpen),
Belgium

H. van Herendael
Department of Gynaecology and Obstetrics,
OCMW Jan Palfijn,
Lange Bremstraat 70,
2060 Merksem (Antwerpen),
Belgium

P. Ide
Academisch Ziekenhuis St Rafael,
Gasthuisberg,
Herestraat 49,
3000 Leuven, Belgium

V. H. T. James
Department of Chemical Pathology,
St. Mary's Hospital Medical School (University of London),
London W2 1PG, UK

P. A. van Keep
International Menopause Society,
8 avenue Don Bosco,
1150 Brussels, Belgium

P. R. Koninckx
Department of Obstetrics and Gynaecology,
Department of Developmental Biology,
University Hospital St. Rafael,
Gasthuisberg,
3000 Leuven, Belgium

U. Larsson-Cohn
Department of Obstetrics and Gynaecology and Internal Medicine,
University Hospital,
S-581 85 Linköping, Sweden

C. Lauritzen
Klinikum der Universität Ulm,
Zentrum für Gynäkologie und
Geburtshilfe,
Postfach 3880,
7900 Ulm, West Germany

B. de Lignières
Department of Reproductive
Endocrinology,
Hôpital Necker,
149 rue de Sèvres,
75730 Paris, France

M. -A. Limouzin-Lamothe
Service du Pr. R. Taurelle,
Hôpital Boucicaut,
Paris, France

J. de Maeyer
VZW Jan Palfijn,
Belgiëlei 184,
2018 Antwerpen, Belgium

A. L. Magos
Department of Gynaecology,
Dulwich Hospital,
London SE22, UK

P. Mauvais-Jarvis
Department of Reproductive
Endocrinology,
Hôpital Necker,
149 rue de Sèvres,
75730 Paris, France

F. Meier
Klinikum der Universität Ulm,
Zentrum für Gynäkologie und
Geburtshilfe,
Postfach 3880,
7900 Ulm, West Germany

P. Nijs
Department of Obstetrics and
Gynaecology,
Catholic University of Leuven KUL,
University Hospital St Rafael,
Gasthuisberg,
3000 Leuven, Belgium

M. Notelovitz
Center for Climacteric Studies,
University of Florida,
The Professional Center,
901 NW 8th Avenue, Suite B-1,
Gainesville, Fl 32601, USA

H. van der Pas
VZW Jan Palfijn,
de Merodelei 141,
2300 Turnhout, Belgium

A. Petitjean
Service d'Anatomopathologie,
Pr. Oppermann,
25000 Besançon, France

O. Prost
INSERM, U.198,
Route de Dole,
25000 Besançon, France

M. J. Reed
Department of Chemical Pathology,
St. Mary's Hospital Medical School,
London W2 1PG, UK

F. E. Riphagen
International Health Foundation,
8 avenue Don Bosco,
1150 Brussels, Belgium

A. Sandri
Ospedale Ostetrico Ginecologico
'Sant'Anna',
Corso Spezia 60,
10126 Torino, Italy

R. Serreyn
Department of Gynaecology,
Ghent State University,
De Pintelaan 135,
9000 Gent, Belgium

L. Severne
Information Office,
International Health Foundation,
43 rue de Namur,
1000 Brussels, Belgium

R. Sitruk-Ware
Department of Reproductive Endocrinology,
Hôpital Necker,
149 rue de Sèvres,
75730 Paris, France

J. C. Stevenson
Royal Postgraduate Medical School,
Hammersmith Hospital,
Ducane Road,
London W12 0HS, UK

J. W. W. Studd
Department of Gynaecology,
Dulwich Hospital,
London SE22, UK

J. H. H. Thijssen
Department of Endocrinology,
University Hospital,
Catharijnesingel 101,
Utrecht, The Netherlands

S. M. Tuck
Department of Gynaecology,
Dulwich Hospital,
London SE22, UK

W. H. Utian
Department of Reproductive Biology,
Case Western Reserve University,
Department of Obstetrics and Gynaecology,
The Mount Sinai Medical Center,
University Circle,
Cleveland, OH 44106, USA

F. Uyttenbroeck
Sint Camilluskliniek UIA,
Dienst voor Gynaecologie en Verloskunde,
Lockaertstraat 10,
2000 Antwerpen, Belgium

D. Vandekerckhove
Department of Gynaecology,
Ghent State University,
De Pintelaan 135,
9000 Gent, Belgium

I. Vergote
Department of Obstetrics and Gynaecology,
University of Antwerp,
Akademisch Ziekenhuis Antwerpen,
Wilrijkstraat 10,
2520 Edegem, Belgium

A. Verstraeten
Arthritis and Metabolic Bone Disease Research Unit,
Katholieke Universiteit Leuven,
Universitair Ziekenhuis Pellenberg,
Weligerveld 1,
3041 Pellenberg, Belgium

A. Volpe
Department of Obstetrics and Gynaecology,
University of Modena,
Instituto Di Clinica Ostetrica e Ginecologica,
Policlinico,
Via del Pozzo 71,
41100 Modena, Italy

R. Walckiers
VZW Jan Palfijn,
Parklaan 55,
2700 Sint-Niklaas, Belgium

L. Wallentin
Department of Obstetrics and Gynaecology and Internal Medicine,
University Hospital,
S-581 85 Linköping, Sweden

S. Wesel
Unité Gynéco-obstétricale,
Hôpital de Braine-Waterloo,
Rue Wayez 35,
1420 Braine-l'Alleud, Belgium

E. Zirilli
General Laboratory of Clinical Pathology,
University of Modena,
41100 Modena, Italy

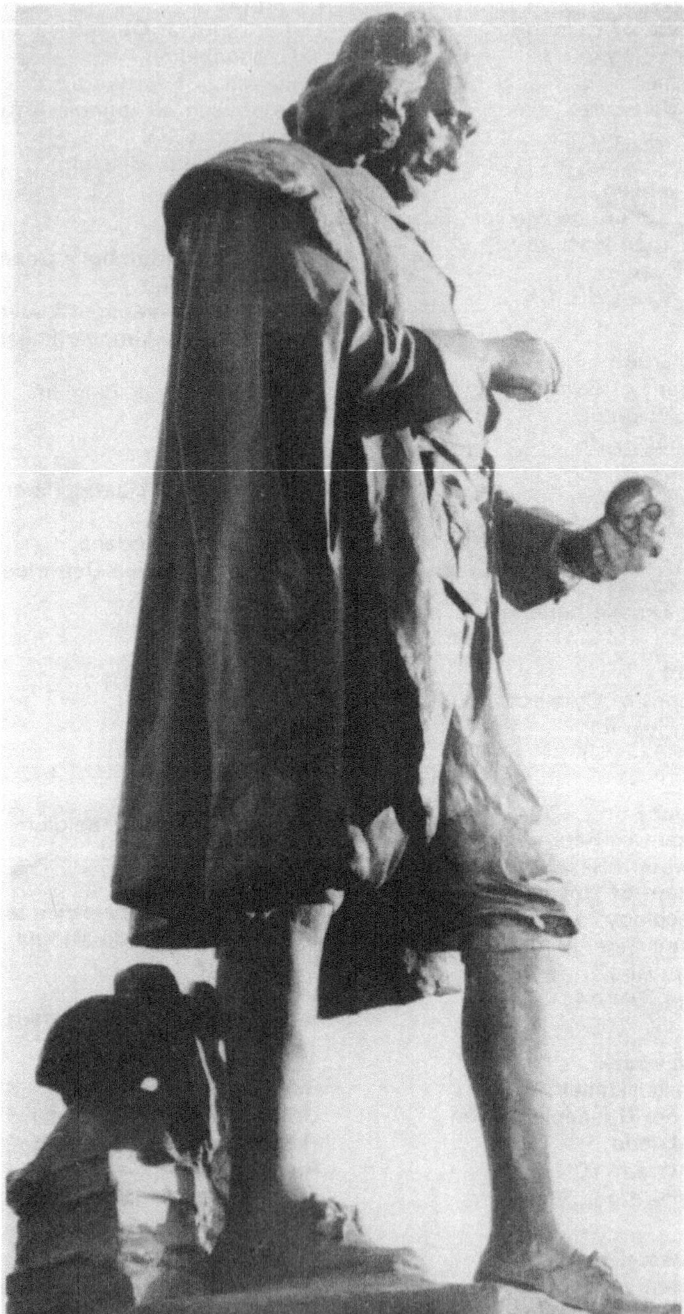

JAN PALFIJN

Preface

THE JAN PALFIJN SYMPOSIA

In 1979 the Department of Obstetrics and Gynaecology of the Jan Palfijn Hospital in Merksem, Antwerp, celebrated its 25th Anniversary. To mark the occasion, the first symposium was organized, the theme chosen being hysteroscopy. Thanks to the cooperation of specialists from both within and outside Belgium the event attracted such a large attendance that it was decided to follow up this first venture with others.

In the light of the experience gained from the first symposium, we established the Jan Palfijn Foundation for Gynaecological and Obstetrical Didactics, the reasons for this being budgetary and, in particular, organizational. This approach made it possible to attract the cooperation of enthusiastic fellow workers from outside the hospital on a permanent or ad hoc basis and hence to reach a much wider group of experts in all fields, both at home and abroad.

In 1981 the second symposium was held at the Jan Palfijn Hospital, the topic being echography in obstetrics and gynaecology. Almost all of the Belgian universities were represented and papers were presented by confreres from practically all of the EEC countries.

When the third symposium was held, in 1982, again on hysteroscopy, the speakers and audience could literally hardly be squeezed into the Jan Palfijn Hospital's facilities.

The fourth symposium was accordingly organized in the modern, luxurious facilities of the new administration building of the Antwerp Provincial Authority.

The theme of first choice proved to be the menopause because, for many reasons, there seemed to be an important need for a complete review of the syndrome involved. First, the growing awareness in modern society has brought with it a desire for information, explanation and, where appropriate, treatment of somatic and psychological symptoms that are not necessarily pathological as such. Secondly, only in recent years has a scientific approach been adopted towards the menopause and specific menopause clinics been established in numerous large centres.

The findings deriving from research and experience can now be accurately quantified and valuable guidelines can thus be provided as regards general handling and specific therapy.

During this fourth Jan Palfijn symposium every aspect of the menopausal syndrome was, without exception, introduced and discussed by eminent specialists. In addition to speakers from Belgium and other European countries, the organizing committee was also able to arrange for specialists from the United States and South Africa to take part.

The interest shown was exceptional and the large number of participants as well as the very high quality of the scientific presentations, will undoubtedly encourage the members of the Jan Palfijn Foundation to continue their efforts.

I personally felt a great sense of honour and tremendous satisfaction that Professor Jacques Ferin, one of the pioneers of hormone therapy in gynaecology, should undertake to act as honorary chairman of the fourth Jan Palfijn symposium.

Dr. H. van Herendael

Chapter 1

Introduction to hormonal therapy in the perimenopause

J. Ferin

Oestrogen therapy, and later on oestrogen–progestogen sequential therapy, of the climacteric syndrome in the menopause and postmenopause has been given to a growing number of patients over the last few decades, notwithstanding the fact that the many problems that this therapy brings along are far from being solved.

From the beginning on, it seemed that this treatment should be reserved to women with oestrogen deprivation, more specifically those women in whom a progestogen challenge test of 8 to 10 days does not produce a withdrawal bleeding. But later on questions rose on the following issues:

(1) Can the treatment be given to patients with obesity, hypertension, disturbances of plasmalipids, genital disease and, especially, with pancreatitis or diabetes?
(2) What should the duration of the therapy be? Until the production of androgen precursors within the adrenal cortex declines, until the age of sixty, or until some point later in life?

To these questions definite answers still have to be given.

The choice of the oestrogen compound is important. Several C17 alkylated steroids, like ethinyloestradiol, have a considerable and long-lasting impact on the liver. New sex steroid derivatives as tibolone (OD14) are being synthesized. These substances have lost their oestrogenic, progestogenic and androgenic potency, and remain only active as an anabolic targetting on bone tissue.

On the other hand, it is wrong and useless to keep oestrogenic substances with a totally different non-sex-steroid chemical structure such as diethylstilboestrol and dienoestrol in the therapeutic arsenal.

The choice of the progestogen compound also poses a problem, because certain progestogens exert, more than others, a lowering influence on the plasma HDL (high density lipoprotein).

Though oral administration is most widely used, pharmacologists have also held on to the older ways of administration such as the percutaneous and vaginal methods, which ensure a bypass of the first passive hepatic passage.

The major difficulty with these ways of administration remains in the maintenance of constant plasma levels. Finding the lowest dose producing the desired effect, as the adequate one, is not easy.

Once more, that adequate dose varies with the choice of the oestrogen preparation and the way of administration. Administered daily, effective doses for preventing the loss of bone tissue should be in the order of 0.01 mg for ethinyloestradiol, 0.625 mg for conjugated equine oestrogen and 6–8 mg for oestriol, while, when applied vaginally, a dose lower than 0.5 mg oestriol is able to produce an oestrogenic cytological picture, resembling that of the preovulatory period.

In this brief introduction, the main points and problems concerning hormone therapy in the perimenopause are outlined. The majority of them will be discussed more elaborately during the sessions to come.

On the other hand, the risk of developing an adenocarcinoma of the endometrium is greatly reduced by the use of sequential therapy.

As far as breast cancer is concerned, the risk encountered by patients treated with oestrogen, or better sequential therapy, remains difficult to estimate. Also, the choice, in order to reduce the risk for breast cancer, of either sequential or oestrogen therapy, in women who have had a hysterectomy, is controversial.

Chapter 2

Menopause: The beginning of a curable disease or a lucky phenomenon?

P. R. Koninckx

INTRODUCTION

Menopause is a word which seems full of contradictions.

The endocrinology of the perimenopause and the consequences of oestrogen deprivation are well known. It is true, also, that the benefits and risks of hormonal replacement therapy are relatively well established. Yet an enormous gap exists between medical knowledge and common medical practice: the number of women, in Belgium at least, receiving some kind of hormone replacement therapy is still very small.

It is widely accepted that the postmenopausal ovary secretes relatively large amounts of androgens[1]. Yet the postmenopausal ovary is generally regarded as a useless organ and is often removed at the same time as hysterectomy is performed. 'Prevention of ovarian cancer' seems to provide a good argument for most surgeons who elect to remove the ovary.

Socially, attitudes towards the climacteric can be positive or negative according to cultural circumstances[2]. Although the impression prevails that the menopause is the beginning of getting old, one tends to forget that by many women the menopause is welcomed with relief as the end of the fertile period, as the end of distressing menstrual periods.

The incidence of osteoporosis, and its consequences for morbidity, are well known[3-5]. Yet the general preventive effort of society is minimal when compared, for example, to cancer screening programs or prevention of road accidents and accidents at the work place.

Therefore, in this second Jan Palfijn Lecture, I would like to discuss the communication gap which exists between medical research, medical practice and social attitudes towards the menopause.

IS THE CLIMACTERIC A NATURAL PHENOMENON OR A DISEASE OCCURRING IN ALL WOMEN?

The medical profession's attitude towards the climacteric varies according to the way it is looked upon, either as a natural phenomenon or as a disease which occurs in all women.

Traditionally, the idea of a natural phenomenon prevails, since the menopause occurs in all women, generally between the ages of 45 and 55, since the climacteric condition is not life threatening, and since in any case no therapy was available up to a few decades ago. It is therefore logical that the general attitude towards the climacteric is extremely conservative: the menopause is inevitable, the climacteric is – at least to some extent – a bad time where hot flushes and night sweats must be endured but where the symptoms will subside spontaneously. It suffices that the woman is strong. A new equilibrium will be found, if necessary medical help can temporarily be given to overcome this 'difficult time'. The long-term consequences of the menopause, such as atrophy of secondary sex characteristics, osteoporosis and cardiovascular accidents, are considered to be the consequences of increasing age and thus almost inevitably by definition a woman of 70 with a hip fracture will say 'I broke my leg' but never 'I am suffering from the menopause'.

The words 'natural' and 'normal' are often misused: a clear distinction should be made between these words and the mean established for a given population. Dental caries will occur in every man and woman, but will never become 'normal' or 'natural'. Similarly the fact that the menopause occurs in every woman is no argument in favour of it being, therefore, a 'natural condition'. Our mean life expectancy has gradually extended further and further beyond the age at which the menopause occurs. The woman outlives her ovaries. Therefore I favour the view that the climacteric is a syndrome – a disease – a hormonal deficiency occurring in all women.

Why should we have such a different attitude towards ovarian hormone deficiency in comparison to our attitude to mild maturity onset diabetes, to mild hypothyroidism or to mild adrenal insufficiency?

THE CLIMACTERIC SYNDROME: THE FAILURE OF AN ENDOCRINE ORGAN

The endocrine and the physical consequences of the diminished ovarian steroid hormone secretion are well known[6,7]. Briefly, the situation in the postmenopause is characterized by the virtual absence of progesterone, by a low oestrogen concentration – mainly derived from peripheral conversion of testosterone and androstenedione into oestrone – and an almost normal androgen concentration. The physical consequences are, usually, a brief period of vasomotor instability, atrophy of secondary sex characteristics, bone loss and increased risk of cardiovascular accidents.

The psychological consequences of the climacteric[8,9], in contrast to the physical consequences, are much less understood. It is extremely difficult, if not impossible, to define exactly the consequences for the brain of oestrogen and progesterone deficiency, of the changed oestrogen–progesterone–androgen balance, or of a tonic versus a cyclic hormonal pattern. How much of the observed changes in mood, dynamism, general feeling of well-being, libido, etc. must be attributed solely to the hormonal changes and how much must be explained by the social background, by the general prevailing attitudes towards the climacteric, by the feeling of becoming older? How much of the psychological changes occurring during the climacteric can and must be explained as a consequence of physical problems, i.e. hormone deprivation, night sweats and the accompanying lack of sleep?

The consequences of the climacteric for the skin are even less understood[7]. Although it has been demonstrated that after the menopause the skin becomes thinner, the real question is: what makes a woman good-looking? How is it that women (and men) of the same age can look relatively younger or older than their chronological age? How much of the postmenopausal psychology can be explained by the woman looking in the mirror and seeing herself as less attractive?

The challenge to answer these questions is still with us.

The emphasis I want to make by these unproven, but difficult to disprove, postulations is that the physical and psychological impact of sex hormone deficiency – beginning at the menopause – could be much more far-reaching than one is generally willing to believe or to accept. Because of the general attitude of considering the climacteric as a natural phenomenon, a tendency exists therefore to minimize the physical and psychological impact of sex steroid hormone deficiency and to accept only 'proven' facts. Scientific honesty requires, however, that all hypotheses and postulations, as long as they are not disproved, should at least be given the benefit of doubt.

HORMONE REPLACEMENT THERAPY

Risks and benefits

The physical risks and benefits of postmenopausal oestrogen treatment are to-day beginning to be clearly delineated. It is no exaggeration to say that the physical consequences of the climacteric can be adequately treated or prevented, except maybe in relation to the increase in cardiovascular accidents. Put at its simplest, the risk of hormone replacement therapy can be summarized as follows: if relatively high doses of oestrogen alone are given an increased incidence of endometrial adenocarcinoma can be expected. If low doses of oestrogen alone, or higher doses of oestrogen sequentially combined with a progestogen are administered, there seems to be almost no risk at all. The latter treatment will, moreover, lower the risks of endometrial adenocarcinoma and breast carcinoma[10–12].

Briefly, hormone replacement therapy can adequately cure or prevent the physical consequences of the climacteric, with the additional advantage of decreasing the incidence of endometrial and breast cancer. The treatment can, therefore, be given without risk.

Since it is impossible to delineate exactly what are the psychological consequences of ovarian steroid hormone deficiency, it is logical to expect that no clear answers are available as far as risks and benefits of hormone replacement therapy in this area are concerned. What does seem to be beyond doubt, however, is that the therapy will result in an improved libido and sexual response, and will have a 'mental tonic' effect.

Contraindications

The list of contraindications is fairly long. To my mind, many of these so-called relative contraindications result from conservatism in medical thinking. It is indeed difficult to understand, that a condition which is not an indication for surgical or medicamental castration before the menopause, could constitute a contraindication for hormone replacement therapy. This double thinking can best be illustrated: a growing fibroid before menopause is considered to be an indication for hysterectomy; the same growing fibroid would be a contraindication for hormone replacement therapy; why should it not be an indication for hysterectomy *and* hormonal replacement therapy?

Methodological limitations of hormone replacement therapy

If the postmenopause is considered as an endocrine deficiency due to the reduced functioning of the ovary, the logical approach would be to replace ovarian hormone secretion as exactly as possible. Because of the cyclical nature of ovarian secretion, a daily administration of different doses of hormones would be required. Obviously, implants and monthly injections do not meet this criterion. Oral ingestion, on the contrary, has two major drawbacks: 'natural' 17β-oestradiol and progesterone is poorly resorbed and rapidly metabolized in the liver. Therefore synthetic steroids, or very high doses of the natural ones, have to be used. Moreover, since all hormones taken by mouth have to pass the liver before reaching the peripheral circulation, supraphysiological liver concentrations are the obligatory counterpart of physiological concentrations in the target tissues. A supplementary difficulty arises when the individual resorption and metabolism is taken into account.

Ideal replacement therapy is thus obviously not yet available[13-15].

THE IMPACT OF THE CLIMACTERIC UPON SOCIETY

All women sooner or later will become postmenopausal. Most men live with a woman. All children have a mother. For centuries society has learned to live with the climacteric and to change attitudes to it is almost akin to changing society. The minimal statement one could make about the climacteric would be that after going through a more or less difficult stage in their lives women find a new equilibrium. The word 'new' implies that the postmenopausal equilibrium is different from the premenopausal, maybe better, possibly worse, but at least different. Since society functions as a coalition of men and women, of young and old, of parents and children, the impact of this 'new equilibrium' should not be underestimated. To change dramatically attitudes to the menopause could be as impactful in changing society as the introduction of contraception has proved to be over the last half century.

Not only the psychological aspects of the climacteric but also the physical aspects have a great effect on individual members of society. With increasing life expectancy, the problem of bone fractures as a result of osteoporosis will become more and more common. The individual suffering, the anxiety of those who are close to the patient, the energy spent in treatment, re-education, and new social arrangements are all aspects which can be seen to present difficulties in this regard.

MENOPAUSE: THE BEGINNING OF A CURABLE DISEASE OR A LUCKY PHENOMENON?

The strength of our conservative thinking, of our acceptance of nature, can be seen when the question is asked as to whether the climacteric is in any way a lucky phenomenon. If one should make a list of the benefits of the menopause, it would be a very short list indeed. In fact, I do not see a single advantage, a single piece of 'luck', except that conception is no longer possible, and that possibly existing menstrual discomfort ceases. If, on the other hand, we were able to control the rate at which ovarian follicles start to grow, we might be able to determine freely the age at which menopause occurs. We can easily imagine the excitement of the debate which would be held if we had to decide for young girls whether the age at which their menopause should occur would be set for them at age 40, 50, 60, 70 or even later. We all agree, I think, that in that case, the onset of the menopause should be postponed for as long as possible and the main question could even become whether we should induce the menopause at all.

We thus have the medical conviction that the menopause occurs too early and that, if possible, it should be postponed. If, on the other hand, we know that the risks of hormone replacement therapy in comparison to those of continuing menstrual cycles and a postponed menopause are very small or negligible, it seems confusing to observe current medical practice. It is strange to relate the general lay opinion with their fears, their acceptance of the climacteric and their resistance to hormone replacement therapy to the overall conviction that the menopause occurs too early.

CONCLUSION

It would seem obvious, therefore, that education of both the public and the medical profession on the subject of the climacteric and its treatment is of crucial importance, in order to fill the gaps between research knowledge, medical practice and public opinion. Either the menopause has to be accepted as a lucky phenomenon, or as the beginning of a disease for which adequate therapy is readily available. Research should be stimulated in order to improve existing therapies and to develop new ones. Ideally, one should aim at some kind of artificial ovary which regulates cyclical steroid hormone secretion and ensures proper physiological levels of oestrogens, progestogens and androgens in the female body.

References

1. James, V. H. T., Folkerd, E. J., Bonney, R. C., Beranek, P. A. and Reed, M. J. Factors influencing oestrogen production and metabolism in postmenopausal women with endocrine cancer. This volume, Chapter 5
2. van Keep, P. A. The climacteric in different cultural contexts. This volume, Chapter 3
3. Dequeker, J., Geusens, P. and Verstraeten, A. Osteoporosis and its treatment. This volume, Chapter 17
4. Notelovitz, M. Early diagnosis of osteoporosis. This volume, Chapter 18
5. Stevenson, J. C. Interrelation of oestrogen and the major calcium regulating hormones. This volume, Chapter 19
6. Thijssen, J. H. H. Steroid hormone receptors and their changes in the perimenopause. This volume, Chapter 6
7. Utian, W. H. Problems of the untreated menopause. This volume, Chapter 11
8. Nijs, P. The perimenopausal woman: guidance and treatment. This volume, Chapter 12
9. Severne, L. The view of the woman. This volume, Chapter 4
10. Gambrell, R. D., Jr. Benefits of progestogen therapy in the postmenopause. This volume, Chapter 24
11. Lauritzen, C. and Meier, F. Risks of endometrial and mammary cancer morbidity and mortality in long-term oestrogen treatment. This volume, Chapter 20
12. Limouzin-Lamothe, M.-A. Cardiovascular impact of therapy and risks. This volume, Chapter 21

13. Studd, J. W. W., Cordozo, L. D., Gibb, D. M. F., Tuck, S. M., Magos, A. L., Brincat, M. and Cooper, D. J. Hormone implants in women following hysterectomy and bilateral salpingo-oophorectomy. This volume, Chapter 16
14. Campagnoli, C., Sandri, A. and Belforte, P. Oral oestrogen treatment of the climacteric and the postmenopausal period. This volume, Chapter 13
15. Sitruk-Ware, R., Basdevant, A., de Lignières, B. and Mauvais-Jarvis, P. Percutaneous oestrogen therapy. This volume, Chapter 14

Chapter 3

The climacteric in different cultural contexts

P. A. van Keep

INTRODUCTION

When Mrs. X reaches the age of fifty, she begins to experience symptoms. Gradually these begin to bother her, to the point where they interfere with her lifestyle. She goes to her doctor, who, after confirming the climacteric as the possible cause of her problems, treats her with hormones.

This is a common story, something that happens all over the world, all the time, it seems. Or is it? When we look closer at this case history, we will discover that it is based on a number of preconceived ideas, stereotypes that hardly find their bases in reality. Let us examine the various aspects of this case history somewhat closer to see how typical is the situation of this Mrs. X.

The menopause as such is a universal phenomenon. Women everywhere will experience the relative deficiency of oestrogens in the postmenopause. The typical metabolic changes due to this will be the same everywhere, although different patterns of nutrition, differences in body weight and fat may lead to differences in morbidity. There may also be differences in women's tolerance for discomfort and, whereas an atrophic vaginitis may be brought to the attention of the doctor by some women, it might be a complaint other women would not even dare to talk about. A mild vaginal wall atrophy which would lead 'only' to dyspareunia will not be noticed in a culture where sexual intercourse after the menopause no longer takes place. However, the real difference in the experiencing of climacteric complaints is to be found in the non-genital complaints and symptoms. It is on this aspect that this paper concentrates.

CULTURE

The culture of a given society may be regarded as an organized unity which attributes meanings to reality, thus giving each natural phenomenon a particular place and significance. The meaning and impact of any phenomenon will depend on the significance attributed to it and will therefore differ from culture to culture and, by the same token, from subculture to subculture.

Some examples will clarify this: menarche, pregnancy and childbirth have a different significance in different cultures. In the traditional society, dependent on agriculture, the value of fertility is, because of the resulting children, much greater than in the modern society where the bearing of children is no longer a necessity for survival. It will be clear that the end of the fertile period has a different cultural meaning attached to it in both societies. Hence the symptoms that accompany the menopause may be different[1].

It seems reasonable to put forward the following hypothesis. Climacteric symptoms and complaints are due to hormonal and social changes at the end of the fertile period. It will depend on the (sub)culture to which a woman belongs, to what degree such symptoms are experienced as unpleasant – as complaints – or as signs only.

The literature should give us some clue about the validity of this hypothesis. Yet all research in this field is complicated by the heterogeneity of the syndrome. Even in the seemingly most homogeneous group of women there is a wide variety of ways to go through the climacteric. It is impossible to predict with sufficient certainty which woman will go through an easy and which woman through a difficult climacteric.

Many studies, particularly older ones, are based on clinical impressions or surveys of women attending out-patient clinics. However, to obtain reliable data on the total population concerned, non-biased samples, including the non-symptomatic, and consequently non-help-seeking women, must be studied. An alternative is to study all women in a certain population who are in the right age bracket, for instance 45 to 55. Jaszmann's study in 1967 is an example of this[2].

There are few or no data on how many months or years climacteric symptoms last. McKinlay and Jefferys reported that of those women who were at least five years into the postmenopause, 82% had had flushes during more than one year and 6% for more than five years[3]. Thompson *et al.* found that of their patients who were still having flushes, 17% had been having them for over one year, 50% for 3 to 5 years and 19% for more than 5 years. Of those respondents who had previously suffered from hot flushes which had now stopped, 15% reported having had them for more than 1 year; 25% for 2 to 5 years and 19% for more than 5 years[4]. No such data are available for other cultures than the UK.

Roughly 20% of all women sail through the climacteric without extragenital symptoms at all. Eighty percent will during some period experience such symptoms and half of these will ask for medical help (Table 1)[5].

The most detailed study into the climacteric syndrome has been done by Jaszmann *et al.*[2]. A questionnaire was sent to all women between the ages of 50 and 60 in the city of Ede (The Netherlands). Of the 6628 women in the target group, 71% responded.

Jaszmann presumed that if climacteric symptoms are analysed on the basis of the menstrual status of the respondent, climacteric complaints should be rarely mentioned by women who are still menstruating regularly, relatively frequently by women who are having an increasingly irregular menstrual pattern and less often again by women who are in the postmenopause. In other words: a typical climacteric complaint should have a peak in its occurrence in one of these menstrual age groups. He found three different patterns:

(1) A number of complaints showed the highest incidence in the group of perimenopausal women, i.e. women who have an increasingly irrregular menstrual pattern but who will have had

Table 1 Answers to the question: 'Have you at any time asked for medical help or advice about the problems of the menopause?'

	Country				
	West Germany	*Italy*	*Great Britain*	*France*	*Belgium*
Number of respondents	400	400	400	400	400
Yes (%)	51	46	30	40	40
No (%)	48	52	60	48	60
No information (%)	1	2	10	12	—

Source: International Health Foundation (1969)

at least one menstruation in the last twelve months. These complaints were: fatigue, headache, irritability, dizziness, and depressed feelings.

(2) A second group of complaints had a peak in the early postmenopause: hot flushes, pains in the muscles and joints and bones, perspiration and tingling sensations of the extremities.

(3) A third group of complaints do not show a peak in any of these menstrual age groups. These complaints are therefore probably not complaints associated with the menopause but are associated with ageing in general : insomnia, shortness of breath, palpitations and mental imbalance.

Marcha Flint studied women of the Rajput caste in India. She found that very few women had any problems with the menopause, other than menstrual cycle changes; there were no depressions, no dizziness, no incapacitation nor any of the symptoms usually associated with the climacteric syndrome[6]. She explains this, also on the basis of the work of other anthropologists, as follows: in cultures where women increase in status after the menopause, because they are no longer contaminated with menstrual blood, the menopause is associated with less troubles or no troubles at all. In cultures where women decrease in status, the menopause will be more difficult. This explanation – contamination with menstrual blood – is not accepted by Wilbush, who points out that also in cultures where the concept of pollution by menstrual blood is absent, e.g. South of Sahara, an increase in status of women in the postmenopause is observed. However, Wilbush does not give any data on climacteric complaints in those cultures[7].

Practically all epidemiological studies on the incidence of climacteric complaints have been done in women living in North American and West European societies and little work has been reported from comparable studies in developing countries. Yet recently some interesting studies have appeared.

Sharma studied 405 married women between the ages of 40 and 55 living with their husbands in Varanasi City in India[8]. Interestingly enough the incidence of climacteric complaints was more or less the same as that found in Western European samples of this size. This is at variance with the findings of Flint. Sharma's sample was urban, middle class women of at least college education level. Are these women so westernized that their climacteric also resembles that of western women?

Moore interviewed women in the jungle of Zimbabwe, Africa. All these women were illiterate. A total of 43% were experiencing symptoms, attributed to imbalance of the autonomic nervous system, such as hot flushes, sweat, palpitations and dyspepsia. 58% were experiencing 'psychogenic' symptoms such as insomnia, depression, anxiety, irritability, fear of ageing, poor memory and reduced libido, and 42% were experiencing metabolic symptoms: dyspepsia, vaginal dryness, hair or skin changes, headache, backache, joint pains and urinary problems[9].

In cooperation with Dr Agoestina we carried out a study in Bandung in Indonesia in 1982. A questionnaire was completed by 1025 women. This was the first time that such a study had been done in Indonesia. The age at menopause was found to be 48–49 years. Here, too, there was not much difference in the incidence of climacteric complaints compared to those in the West. There were a few striking features, however. Unlike in European studies we found that the hot flush was not the most typical symptom. Bouts of transpiration ranked as the major complaint. A second observation was that the period of transition from a regular menstrual pattern via an irregular pattern to complete amenorrhoea was shorter than is observed in Western Europe. Relatively many women continue to have regular menstruations until suddenly the menopause occurs and the postmenopause sets in[10].

SUBCULTURES

By no means is the distribution of climacteric complaints the same in all groups in one society. In 1974 we were able to demonstrate that various social factors influenced the severity of the climacteric syndrome. Women of the lower socio-economic group had a higher score on the index of climacteric complaints than women of the higher socio-economic group. Women who still had a maternal rôle, i.e. still had young children at home, had a lower score than women whose children had already left home. Women surrounded by friends and acquaintances had a lower score than women who were less well integrated[1]. Liesbeth Severne later published the results of the IHF survey done in Belgium in 1974 in which the influence of a job on the climacteric syndrome was studied. It was interesting to note that the score on the circulatory index did not differ much in the various socio-economic groups but that the difference was mainly found in the score on the index of nervous complaints[11]. This suggests that the changes in the autonomic nervous system are less influenced by psychosocial factors than the secondary climacteric complaints, such as irritability, nervousness, etc. In the same study it was found that the influence of having a job was different in the two socio-economic classes studied. Women in the higher socio-economic group who had a job had less climacteric complaints than those who were only housewives. In the lower socio-economic group the situation was reversed: there women who had a job had more complaints than those who were not working[11].

The influence of having a job on the incidence and severity of the climacteric symptoms and complaints could not be found in the above-mentioned study in Bandung. The incidence of climacteric complaints was the same in women who were working or those who were not. The maternal rôle which, to a certain extent, seems to protect women from climacteric symptoms was also significant in this study. Even women who only had grandchildren at home had less complaints than those who were not surrounded by children[10].

SEEKING HELP

Jaszmann has suggested to distinguish between climacteric *symptoms* and climacteric *complaints*, climacteric complaints being still acceptable to the patient. When symptoms become complaints the woman is likely to ask for medical help (at least when she knows that such help is available). That not all women at climacteric age are aware about the availability of medical treatment for the menopause became clear in our comparative study in 1969[5]. Particularly in the UK women were relatively often not aware that medical treatment existed and consequently 'endured what supposedly could not be cured', as Wendy Cooper says. It is clear that many women will, before they are brave enough to go and ask for medical help, check with other women around them whether their complaints justify a visit to a doctor. Presumably also the health insurance system in the various countries will influence help-seeking behaviour but it is surprising that, at least in 1969, when the financial consequences of a visit to a doctor in England were much smaller than for example, in France or Belgium so few women in England asked for medical help in comparison with these other countries.

THE DOCTOR'S ATTITUDE

Hardly any research has been done with regard to the attitude of the doctor towards a patient who presents herself with climacteric complaints. The often quoted study of Marion Crawford makes us fear for the worst[12]. She found that practically all medical students regarded a woman of about 50 who had vague complaints when presenting herself to her doctor as needing no further attention. This was typical of the attitude of the medical profession at the time, an attitude which has spun off to the students. I wonder whether in most medical schools any meaningful time is spent discussing the climacteric and hormone therapy. The same thing can be said of the training of the gynaecologist. Few universities on the Continent have a special menopause clinic and if the head of the department is not specially interested in the subject, his or her pupils will not be encouraged to listen sympathetically to the woman, to hear her complaints and explore their cause, let alone to treat her with hormones. This is reflected in the drugs that women in this age use, as can be seen from Table 2.

CONCLUSION

Back to Mrs. X, the woman with which this paper began. The story has to be rewritten and should read as follows: When women approach the age of fifty, 80% of them begin to experience climacteric symptoms or complaints. About half of these go and see their doctor. The other

Table 2

Country (age range)	*Women interviewed*	*% Taking tranquillizers*	*% Taking medicaments for menopause*	*% Taking oestrogens/ hormones*
West Germany (40–59)	295	20.0	10.2	4.8
Italy (45–55)	176	23.9	20.5	2.3
France (45–55)	135	24.4	18.5	1.5
Belgium (46–55)	243	27.2	9.5	4.9

Source: International Health Foundation (1975)

half will not; either because they can live with these symptoms or they are afraid to ask for medical help, or they do not know that medical help exists. Of those who go to the doctor some are lucky. They find that their doctor takes their problems seriously, is willing to listen to them, willing to treat them or to refer to a specialist. Again, if she is lucky, she will be treated with hormones. But unfortunately a vast majority will still be sent home with a prescription for a psycho-active drug.

References

1. van Keep, P. A. and Kellerhals, J. M. (1974). The impact of socio-cultural factors on symptom formation. *Psychother. Psychosom.*, **23**, 251
2. Jaszmann, L. (1973). Epidemiology of climacteric and post-climacteric complaints, In van Keep, P. A. and Lauritzen, C, (eds) *Frontiers of Hormone Res.*, Vol. 2, *Ageing and Estrogens* pp. 22–34. (Basel: Karger)
3. McKinlay, S. M. and Jefferys, M. (1974). The menopausal syndrome. *Br. J. Prev. Soc. Med (UK)*, **28**, 108
4. Thompson, B., Hart, S.A. and Durno, D. (1973). Menopausal age and symptomatology in a general practice. *J. Biosoc. Sci.*, **5**, 71
5. International Health Foundation (1970). *The menopause study of the attitudes of women in Belgium, France, Great Britain, Italy and West Germany*. (Geneva: International Health Foundation)
6. Flint, M. (1975). The menopause: reward or punishment. *Psychomatics*, **16**, 161
7. Wilbush, J. (1980). The female climacteric. *Ph. D. Thesis*. (Oxford University)
8. Sharma, V. K. and Saxena, M. S. L. (1981). Climacteric symptoms; a study in the Indian context. *Maturitas*, **3**, 1
9. Moore, B. (1981). Climacteric symptoms in our African community. *Maturitas*, **3**, 25
10. van Keep, P. A. and Agoestina, T.: The climacteric in Bandung, Indonesia. (To be published)
11. Severne, L. (1979). Psycho-social aspects of the menopause. In Haspels, A. A. and Musaph, H. (eds) *Psychosomatics in the Peri-menopause*, pp. 101–120. (Lancaster: MTP)
12. Crawford, M. (1970). What happens at 'the change'. *New Society*, Oct. 29th., p. 771

Chapter 4

The view of the woman

L. Severne

INTRODUCTION

The life circumstances of women at any age – and certainly around 50 – are various and do not fit into simple stereotype patterns. Thus whenever we speak about *the* climacteric woman, we should bear this in mind: she does not exist. Nevertheless we can draw a fairly general picture in which many women will be able to recognize themselves at least to some degree.

In medical and psychological literature – even nowadays – the perimenopause is described as a time of loss, a time when women are confronted with existential crises, having to redefine themselves, facing an uncertain future in which they might expect to go steadily downhill.

Surveys of the International Health Foundation conducted in several European countries in 1969 and 1974 showed that many women believed this to be so but also that cultural factors have a major influence on their opinions.

Today a survey would without doubt reflect a much less negative attitude towards the menopause. An important change has been taking place in that more women have been playing a significant role in society, professionally and politically.

This emancipation has brought its own problems, and although their causes are readily identified, solutions are not always easy to find. Women in their fifties today are in more than one sense a 'middle generation' and often feel caught between the old ways or models and the new opportunities and values.

During the premenopause and the perimenopause, a time when other signs of ageing are also evident, the fear of physical decline and a loss of attractiveness are often amplified. We live in a society which is geared to young values and to productivity. Although textbooks always mention complaints like hot flushes, those in contact with women have found them to be much more worried about symptoms like the 'Tatt-syndrome' (Tired all the time), about unreasonable fears, lack of enthusiasm for work, hobbies and sex, or about forgetfulness, inner tension, nervousness, sleep and weight problems. Not to mention very common mastodynia or premenstrual problems in premenopause; muscle stiffness, pains in the joints, paraesthesia, and later, urinary and genital tract complaints. These are problems which often take women entirely by surprise and which they do not associate with the climacteric, usually due to lack of information.

Not surprisingly a number of women at this time suffer from a feeling of loss of control over their own bodies and their own lives, which may be further aggravated by other events occurring independently.

Approaching or passing through the middle years implies for the majority of women a considerable risk of changes in the professional and/or the family sphere, which not only demand a series of adaptations, but which may reactivate dormant problems or arouse a host of ambivalent feelings. At this point women have to reassess their priorities in life, to give new meaning to the parental and partner roles, to redefine their self-image and to come to terms with their changed environment.

It is in this sense of closing the door on one period of life and heading for another, of reassessment and redefinition, that middle age can be regarded as a period of potential crisis. Not because the stressful events (even 'happy' events such as a promotion, a move, marriage or a birth can carry their load of mixed feelings and of stress) which may occur, are necessarily much more numerous or difficult to deal with than those which occur in other phases of life. But essentially because at middle age everyone leaves behind what many consider as their most constructive and productive period, without clearly seeing what lies ahead. The life perspective has changed.

Whether or not middle age deserves its reputation as a 'dangerous passage', it is fallacious to use biological changes as a convenient peg for climacteric problems. Studies show that the relationship between life events, stress, and symptoms at the climacteric is complex and depends both on the nature of the event, its significance and on the type of symptoms (somatic or psychological). Cooke and Greene (1981) for instance, did not find an increase in the amount of stressful changes in life, but a greater stress-response, which might be due to a higher vulnerability to stress.

They note also an additive or rather multiplicative effect of stress, especially in the case of stress arising from the departure of significant people from the social field, which is not surprising since in most cases this involves bereavement and often also the deprivation of material and emotional support.

VULNERABILITY FACTORS

Why should women at this time of life be more vulnerable? The hormonal imbalance around the menopause certainly plays a role, but knowledge is lacking about the exact mental effects of the hormones involved and their complicated interactions. Oestrogen treatment can bring a relief here, but is not always sufficient.

Ignorance can exacerbate both anxiety and symptoms. Many women feel that their healthy body betrays them in the perimenopause. However, the discomforts come often less from her body than from the anxious concern a woman feels about it. That is why it is essential to give simple, realistic information, not provoking anxiety, about possible climacteric reactions. Equally important is the need to stress the normality of such reactions (in the sense that many women have them, and that they do not mean that one is becoming crazy or less fit to cope with life), and above all to point out that periods of change can be viewed as offering new possibilities for development. This may imply being off-balance for a time, having less self-confidence, until one stands on firm ground once again and the new situation is as secure or comfortable as the one left behind.

Finally, numerous studies show that those who feel powerless, as if their lives were controlled not from within, but entirely by outside events, are particularly vulnerable in times of change. Not surprisingly the fair (or weaker?) sex appears to be more at risk. Older women, especially in the lower socio-economic categories, not only freqently score high in feelings of lack of confidence and loss of self-esteem, but have in fact an insufficient hold on the material aspects of their lives. In other words the impact of 'the change' and that of other events which may occur in and after mid-life, is related to the social position of women in our society; this has also been illustrated by a survey by the International Health Foundation in Belgium.

UNPREPARED FOR CHANGE

In order to understand better the difficulties that women in their fifties today are encountering, it is necessary to recall the typical background of such women. Most were brought up to become good wives and mothers and, as girls, were denied the possibilities for further education or an independent life. In a man's world such a woman would be appreciated for playing the delicate, feminine role. This meant both to be on show and to be self-effacing, ('sois belle et tais-toi'), to be likeable while keeping a safe distance, to be caring, intuitive, non-aggressive, non-competitive, and helpless, yet competent in well-defined fields, etc.

It meant foregoing (or feeling guilty about) activities or goals which could threaten close relationships, these being the main source of a woman's feeling of identity and self-esteem. It also could mean the inhibition of any overt expression of feelings of frustration, anger or aggression. Safe 'masculine' outlets such as sports were not encouraged in past generations of women. The price has been high in psychosomatic ailments and depression.

Nancy Chodorow (1972), who gave a new impetus to psychoanalytic theory on the development of girls has said: 'Girls have been socialized to use more oblique forms of aggression such as verbal injury and interpersonal rejection. Having learned *not to risk* the precarious heterosexual sources of love (father/husband) they tend to direct anger or aggression towards people whose return-anger will not be catastrophic to self-esteem – that means: other females'. This may also help one to understand the ambivalent relationship between mothers and daughters, the often manifested rejection or lack of trust in other women and the ensuing social isolation.

However, times are changing fast and simplistic stereotypes are becoming less and less valid in everyday life. The changing norms constitute a challenge to women in mid-life to explore and develop qualities and capacities left dormant. This may be a frustration for women who feel that it is too late, or who lack the necessary self-confidence and social skills to cope with them. During unsettling periods of change – and certainly with respect to the life changes women have been so badly prepared for – support may be necessary.

SELF-HELP FOR WOMEN IN MID-LIFE

One of the important breakthroughs has been in the creation of self-help groups for climacteric women.* Often mistrusted by the medical profession, such groups nevertheless seem to function well.

In a recent survey, comparing members with non-members of VIDO (self-help groups of middle-aged women in the Netherlands) 25% of the members said they felt less depressive than before joining and had learned to bring their problems into perspective; 20% felt more self-confident. Few differences were found with regard to the pattern of medical consultations, a slight tendency being noted for higher than average medical consultations amongst members. The motivations expressed for becoming a member were often the lack of a supportive doctor, the possibility to meet other women and to compare how they coped, to verify one's 'normality', and also the fear of doing something or going somewhere alone.

In fact, the possibility of exploring formerly unexpressed feelings, of finding in a congenial atmosphere an outlet for problems in the family or frustrations about missed opportunities, have been for many women the first step towards a more rewarding and autonomous life.

THE DOCTOR'S ROLE

Traditionally, it is to her doctor that a climacteric woman will first turn for help. For many (s)he has been her true support and best friend through sometimes troubled times. For others, the relationship with the doctor has proved to be unsatisfactory. In my encounters with middle-aged women the subject of doctors was so often raised spontaneously that I did a small survey amongst more than 700 Belgian women throughout the country, in the age group 45–58, in order to have a better idea of their experiences and expectations.

In this sample the majority (60%) said that they would prefer to consult a gynaecologist for their specific feminine ailments, whereas 30% preferred to see their GP for these. However, the last medical visit they had had was in 61% to the GP and in 39% to the gynaecologist.

* Note. In Belgium self-help groups called VIM (Vrouwen In de Middenleeftijd) exist in several cities. The addresses can be obtained at the IHF Information Office for Belgium, Naamsestraat 43, 1000 Brussels, T. 02/512 40 17.

The younger age group went more frequently to the latter, the older more to general practitioners. More than one-third of the women wished the doctor would take more time for examination so as to arrive at a better based diagnosis and a clearer picture of the situation. Only half of the women said that their doctors readily gave information concerning his findings or concerning the treatment. Whereas 50% of the women did not think it appropriate to consult the physician on other than medical subjects, 36% said they would like to do so. Of these, 44% said they would like to be able to talk about family problems, 40% about sexual problems and only 28% about professional and work problems. Since there is clearly a reluctance to discuss work problems spontaneously, perhaps the doctor might more often take the initiative here.

On the whole it seemed that the women interviewed were fairly satisfied, and that they trusted their doctors. Treatment compliance (67%) seemed to confirm this. Nevertheless 20% had difficulties with the instructions concerning medication, could not follow the explanations, or complained that their doctor didn't try to explain anything.

Climacteric women, just as women consulting for contraception or pregnancy, are basically healthy adults, looking for *information*, *reassurance* that all is well – medically speaking – and for *relief* of their problems. The newer generations are looking for a doctor who will listen with interest and who can conceive of a relationship with the patient as a joint effort to find the best solutions in each individual case. Being associated with the treatment, in the choice between different possibilities, in the discussion of the pros and cons, will increase the woman's positive feelings of awareness of herself and of control over her own life.

Women appreciate a doctor who is able to, or who at least tries to, understand their problems and they think this is more likely to be the case with female doctors whom they consider to be generally more considerate and conscientious. Male gynaecologists more often give them the feeling that they are not being seen as a whole person but rather as an assembly of some more or less interesting parts. Strongly expressed is the wish to be treated respectfully, with discretion and tact, *not* as a number. Having to wait for a long time without explanation or without an excuse before the consultation begins, the unsolicited presence of other persons, having to wait, undressed, in a cabin or – even worse – on the gynaecological chair, is greatly resented. A thorough, gentle and patient examination during which the doctor communicates what (s)he is looking for and what (s)he sees; precise information in the dossier (or a very good memory concerning former complaints, treatment, or life situation); the feeling that the doctor is open minded, will tell the truth, take the time to answer all questions or admit when (s)he is not sure and refer to a specialist, all this is of course important and will enhance confidence.

Climacteric women are often described as 'problem patients'. This is in part at least due to the fact that the medical profession is not immune to the prevailing ideas and values of our society and this also has an impact on the information or advice on climacteric problems and the treatment women receive. Some examples:

- Mention is still made in many texts that around the menopause a woman's breasts will tend to sag and decrease in size, when a walk on any beach today shows often quite the contrary to be the case (curiously enough the possibility of acquiring bigger breasts is never mentioned!).
- There are doctors who refuse to prescribe oestrogens for climacteric or postmenopausal complaints to an otherwise healthy woman, explaining that 'they cause cancer' or 'nature must take its course' meanwhile hooking her on tranquillizers or sedatives. A survey amongst GPs in Ede, The Netherlands, showed that 60% prescribed psycho-active drugs to climacteric women having only a very vague idea of the origin or the seriousness of their problems. The experience of the menopause clinic at the Academic Hospital in Utrecht is that about half of the cases referred to this clinic were suffering from ailments due to causes other than the climacteric, such as diabetes, thyroid dysfunction, cancer, hypertension, etc, Too often a thorough examination and tests are omitted and women are dismissed with the implicit message 'you are bound to have some complaints; what else can you expect at your age?'
- The 'empty nest' syndrome which continues to be used as a convenient explanation for some women's climacteric problems can usually be disregarded since it is known that the departure of children in normal circumstances, is welcomed by most mothers today. On the contrary the disorganization and frequent confrontations brought about by teenagers using home as a convenient lodging-house, can be a source of tension and resentment.

- The advice is often given to women under stress or combining a job with the running of a household to give up the job when overworked. To date, surveys show that full-time home-makers generally have more climacteric complaints than professional women. And why not suggest that the husband take a larger share in the running of the household or help to find assistance for the care of a handicapped child or parent or a sick partner?

Large scale surveys such as the one recently completed by the German women's magazine *Brigitte* (1983) show an astonishing discrepancy between the doctor's perception of the attention and care he gives to his patients, and the women's perception of the care received. Often communication is bad between the two parties. Doctors are unaware of the number of patients who do understand insufficiently their diagnosis or the treatment, and who do not comply with the prescribed treatment. This is – once again – in particular the problem of the less-educated patient, the one who has a greater risk of being affected by climacteric symptoms and who will – because of the greater social gap between her and her doctor – often receive less attention and fewer explanations.

Much remains to be done, but I am optimistic for the future. The new generations of middle-aged women will have different and more positive models to follow. Women yesterday were taught to hide and to dislike their bodies, to fear the menopause and to reject the idea of ageing. Today they are learning to be more at ease with their bodies and with themselves, they are discovering the new opportunities available and making use of the better medical care which will enable them to take the ageing process in their stride.

Bibliography

Ballinger, S., Cobbin, D., Krivanek, J. and Saunders, D. (1979). Life stresses and depression in the menopause. *Maturitas*, **1**, 191

Bardwick, J. M. and Douvan, E. (1972). Ambivalence: The socialization of women. In Gornick, V. and Moran, B. K. (eds) *Women in Sexist Society*, pp. 225–242. (New York: The New American Library, Mentor Book 1351)

Bart, P. (1971). The sociology of depressive disorders. In Roman, P. and Trice, H. (eds) *Current Perspectives in Psychiatric Sociology* (USA: Science House)

Beck, A. T. and Rush, A. J. (1975). A cognitive model of anxiety formation and anxiety resolution. In Sarason, I. D. and Spieberger, C. D. (eds) *Stress and Anxiety* (Washington: Hemisphere Publishing Co.)

Beljon, J. A. S., Geelen, K. R. J. and Maas, J. M. A.G. (1983). *Vidogroepen, leden en niet leden vergeleken*. Instituut voor sociaal-wetenschappelijk onderzoek, Projektgroep Zelfhulp Tilburg (Tilburg: Katholieke Hogeschool)

Schneider, S. (1983). Umfrage Frauenärtze. *Brigitte*, **10**, 100; **11**, 119; **12**, 169 (Hamburg: Brigitte)

Brown, G. W and Harris, T. (1978). *Social Origins of Depression*. (London: Tavistock)

Catron, L., Chiriboga, D. A. and Krystal, S. (1980). Divorce at midlife: psychic dangers of the liminal period. I. Empirical considerations. *Maturitas*, **2**, 131

Chessler, P. (1972). *Women and Madness* (New York: Doubleday and Cie)

Chodorow, N. (1972). Being and doing : a cross-cultural examination of the socialization of males and females. In Gornick, V. and Moran, B. K. (eds) *Women in Sexist Society*, pp. 259–292. (New York: The New American Library, Mentor Book 1351)

Cobb, S. (1976). Social support as a moderator of life stress. *Psychosom. Med.*, **38**, 300

Cooke, D. J. and Greene, J. G. (1981). Type of life events in relation to symptoms at the climacteric. *Psychosom. Res.*, **25**, 5

Dege, K. and Gretzinger, J. (1982). Attitudes towards menopause of women, their husbands and their children. In Voda, A. M., Dinnerstein, M. and O'Donnel, S. R. (eds) *Changing Perspectives on Menopause*, pp. 60–70. (Austin: University of Texas Press)

Dowling, C. (1982). *"The Cinderella Complex"; Women's Hidden Fear of Independence.* (Glasgow: Fontana)

Ensink, B. (1977). *De Klachten tijdens de overgangsperiode in relatie tot de sexerol en enkele persoonlijkheidseigenschappen*. (Amsterdam: Vrije Universiteit)

Ensink, B. (1980). *De sociale determinanten van klachten tijdens de overgang*. Projektgroep climacteriële klachten, Vakgroep klinische psychologie (Leiden: Rijksuniversiteit)

Freidin, R. B., Goldman, L. and Cecil, R. R. (1980). Patient–physician concordance in problem identification in the primary care setting. *Ann Intern. Med.*, **93**, 490

Frick-Bruder, V. (1981). Die Frau und die Frauenheilkunde. *Sexualmedizin*, **7**, 263

Friedan, B. (1965). *The Feminine Mystique*. (Middlesex, (UK): Penguin)

Gerdes, L. C. (1980). Vulnerability and resilience in climacteric women. *S. Afr. Med. J.*, **58**, 763.

Girardi, M. R. (1982). Das erwartet Ihre patientin. *Sexualmedizin*, **11a**, 528.

Hailes, J. (1981). Ingrained male view of menopause hurts credibility of clinics. Communication at the *Third International Congress on the Menopause*, Ostend, Belgium

International Health Foundation (1973). *The Mature Woman*. (Geneva: International Health Foundation)

International Health Foundation (1977). *De overgangsjaren: een onderzoek in België by 922 vrouwen tussen 45 en 55 jaar*. (Brussels: International Health Foundation)

International Health Foundation. *Vrouw en arts*, Research of the information office of the International Health Foundation, Belgium. (To be published)

Judd, H. L. (1981). Hormone replacement discussed in patient groups. *Obstet. Gynecol. News*, **16**, 23

Kaufert, P. A. (1980). The perimenopausal woman and her use of health services. *Maturitas*, **2**, 191

Ley, P., Pike, L. A., Whitworth, M. A. and Woodward, R. (1979). Patient information; effects of source, context of communication and difficulty level on the success of health education communications concerning contraception and the menopause. *Health Educ. J.*, **38**, 47

Meyboom-de Jong, B. (1981). Hoe ervaren vrouwen het vaginaal onderzoek, een explorerende studie. *Medisch Contact*, **51**, 1577

Olivier, C. (1980). *Les enfants de Jocaste*. (Paris: Denoel-Gonthier)

Projektgroep Climacteriële Klachten (1979). *De sociale determinante van – en de ziektedrempel bij overgangsklachten – Eindrapport onderzoek onder de Ede'se vrouwen*. Deel I, Vakgroep klinische psychologie van de Rijksuniversiteit Leiden, 1979

Roberts, H. and Barrett, M. (1981). Women's opinions on menopause devalued in medical community. *Obstet. Gynecol. News*, **16**, 20

Rossi, A. S. (1972). Family development in a changing world. *Am. J. Psychiat.*, **128**, 47

Serverne-van Loon, L. (1981). De middenjaren. In Mertens, J. (ed.) *Welzijnsgids*. Noden, 1.A, 1.7. (Antwerpen: Van Loghum Slaterus)

Severne-van Loon, L. (1982). Psychological aspects of the menopause. In Voda, A. M., Dinnerstein, M. and O'Donnel, S. R. (eds) *Changing Perspectives on Menopause*, pp. 238–248. (Austin: University of Texas Press)

Sheehy, G. (1977). *Passages – Predictable Crises of Adult Life*. (New York: Bantam Books)

Sheehy, G. (1982). *Pathfinders – Overcoming the Crises of Adult Life*. (New York: Bantam Books)

Vido & VIM-groepen (1983). Vrouwen helpen zichzelf. In *Heden en toekomst van vrouwen boven de vijftig*, pp. 97–103. (Brussels: International Health Foundation)

Vrouwengroep Vrouw en Huisarts (1981). *Huisarts en overgang*, Subfaculteit geneeskunde (Amsterdam: Vrije Universiteit)

Chapter 5

Factors influencing oestrogen production and metabolism in postmenopausal women with endocrine cancer

V. H. T. James, E. J. Folkerd, R. C. Bonney,
P. A. Beranek and M. J. Reed

INTRODUCTION

The role which steroid hormones play in the development and maintenance of human cancer is a problem which has attracted the attention of research investigators for many years. Oestrogens have come under particular scrutiny, since there is a good deal of indirect evidence that altered oestrogen production may be protective in some situations (e.g. the diminished risk of female breast cancer conferred by earlier castration) and disadvantageous in others (e,g, the enhanced risk of endometrial cancer attributable to increased oestrogen exposure in women bearing oestrogen-secreting tumours). Furthermore, in the last decade or so, studies of cellular receptors have clearly delineated the importance of oestrogens amongst other hormones in the maintenance of tumour growth. It is therefore entirely logical to investigate oestrogen metabolism in detail in the hope and expectation that some metabolic abnormality exists in women who are predisposed to these types of endocrine cancer, which may be revealed by careful biochemical examination. As a group, postmenopausal women are particularly important in this context, not only because of the increased incidence of breast and endometrial cancer at and around the menopause, but because it is at this time that major changes occur in the endocrine milieu which may relate directly to the risk of developing cancer.

So far though, there is very little unequivocal evidence for any consistent abnormality in oestrogen metabolism in postmenopausal women with breast or endometrial cancer[1].

Unfortunately, the minute amount of oestrogen produced poses major methodological problems of measurement, but even with recent techniques, neither oestrogen excretion, nor plasma levels are obviously abnormal, provided that due attention is paid to obtaining proper controls.

However, these findings by no means rule out the possibility that the tissues of women with breast or endometrial cancer have, or have had at some time, abnormal exposure to oestrogen.

An attempt to indicate in a relatively simple way some facets of this complicated problem is shown in Figure 1. It seems likely that target tissue exposure to hormone is an important factor to consider. The concentration of steroid in the tissue is influenced by at least two considerations, tissue metabolism and plasma steroid concentration.

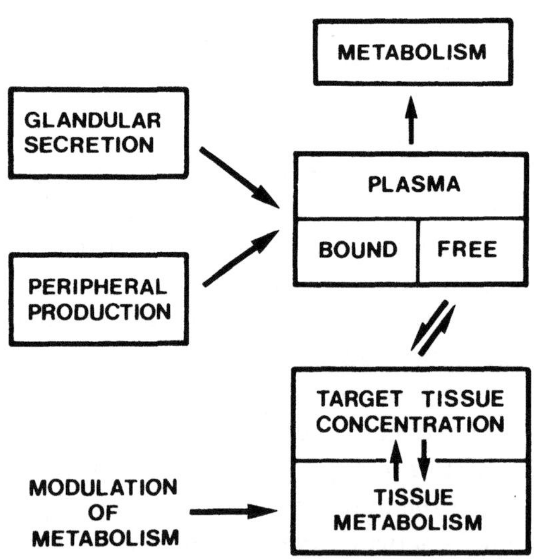

Figure 1 The major aspects of hormone metabolism which may influence the tissue exposure of target organs such as breast or uterus

Modulation of tissue metabolism is therefore highly relevant, and the effect of progesterone on 17β-oestradiol dehydrogenase activity in endometrial tissues is an important example[2]. The plasma steroid concentration will influence tissue exposure, but the physical state of the plasma steroid is very important. There is good evidence that for some steroids at least, it is the unbound fraction which is biologically significant[3].

Thus, measurement of just the total steroid concentration without regard to binding effects may be misleading. Plasma levels are the reflection of the balance between overall production and metabolism. Both these factors can therefore influence the plasma concentration.

In this review some of the recent work we have carried out to investigate oestrogen production and metabolism in relation to endocrine cancers is presented. Several different approaches to this problem have been used including isotopic tracer studies, measurements of the distribution and concentrations of oestrogens in plasma and *in vitro* methods, using adipose, breast and endometrial tissues.

The problem of tissue metabolism can be investigated by examining the rate at which oestrogen is cleared from the blood into the tissues, using a radio tracer technique to measure the metabolic clearance rate[4,5]. The results of such a study in a series of women with endometrial cancer, or endometrial hyperplasia, a condition which predisposes to cancer, showed that both oestrone and oestradiol were cleared from the body at a higher rate than in normal postmenopausal women[5]. Clearance rates for oestradiol in postmenopausal women with breast cancer are compared with those in women with endometrial cancer and normal women in Figure 2. In 3 of 4 subjects studied so far with breast cancer the metabolic clearance rate for oestradiol was at the upper limit of normal range or significantly higher than in normal women. Kirschner[6] found similarly elevated clearance rates in women with this condition.

Thus, these cancer patients appear to remove, or utilize oestrogens more rapidly than do healthy women. Factors that influence clearance rates are not fully understood, but binding to plasma proteins[7] and weight[5] can both affect clearance rates.

Thus, one of the consequences of obesity, which is a major risk factor for endometrial and breast cancer, is enhanced oestrogen clearance, but the mechanism by which this occurs is not clear. Recently metabolic clearability has been equated with biological availability[8] and increased clearance rates may reflect increased tissue exposure to

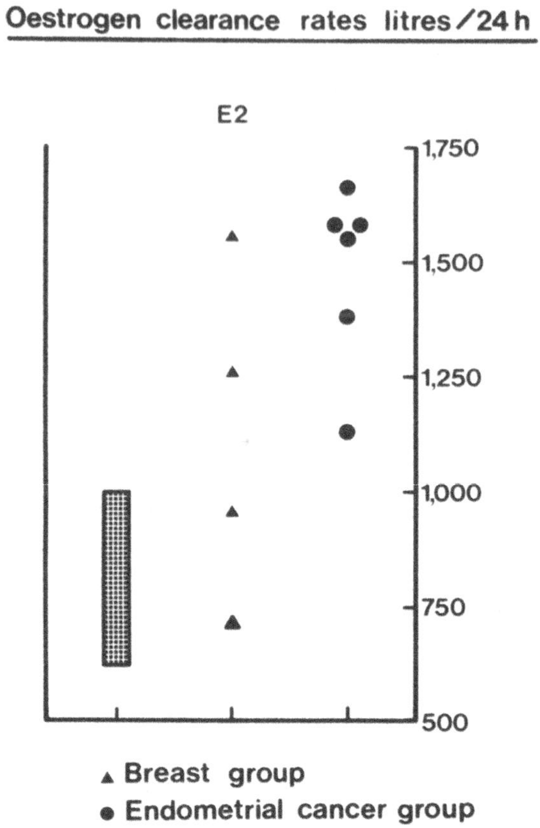

Figure 2 Metabolic clearance rates of oestradiol in postmenopausal women with breast or endometrial cancer. The range for normal postmenopausal women is indicated by the shaded bar[59]

oestrogens, but further studies are required to confirm this relationship.

The clearance measurements previously discussed were also used to calculate oestrogen production rates in these patients. Siiteri and MacDonald[9] have already reported that the production of oestrone is increased in some endometrial cancer patients, but it is now known that this is a weight-related phenomenon[10,11].

However, as most of the available evidence suggests that it is oestradiol rather than oestrone which is biologically important[12] the significance of oestrone may be more that it is a prehormone for oestradiol. However, although we have studied a number of women with endrocrine cancer, oestradiol production was not greatly increased, and only one woman had a clearly increased production rate[5].

The normal production rate of oestradiol, taken together with the considerably increased clearance rate of this steroid, directs attention to the fundamental question of tissue exposure. Total plasma concentrations of oestrogens have not been found to be consistently different from normal in either endometrial[13] or breast cancer patients[14], although increased levels[15,17] have been reported. A highly significant correlation with ideal body weight was found, both for oestrone and oestradiol in breast cancer patients, again emphasizing the importance of body weight[5].

Oestrogens circulate in blood bound to plasma proteins, notably sex hormone binding globulin and albumin, and the biological activity of the steroid is thought to be associated with either the unbound fraction[3] or the non-sex-hormone binding globulin fraction, that is, free plus albumin bound[18].

Measurement of the free fraction showed that it was elevated in patients with breast disease, and even when careful matching for weight was made a significant difference was still detected[5].

However, the binding capacity of the globulin was normal suggesting that something in the plasma of the cancer patients inhibits the protein binding. So far insufficient data have been obtained to say whether the non-sex-hormone binding globulin fraction is also increased, although the concentration of this fraction is much greater than that of free oestradiol. Siiteri[19] has suggested that altered binding to plasma protein may be due to plasma lipids. A highly significant relationship between lipid intake and the incidence of breast cancer on a geographical basis has been demonstrated by Wynder[20].

Thus various factors which have been implicated as risk factors may also be involved in changes in binding globulin concentration, namely, obesity, nutrition, thyroid function and androgens, and the common factor may be the increased presentation of unbound or biologically available oestradiol to the tissues, which is reflected by the enhanced rate of clearance.

Although studies of steroid production, clearance and binding are important, it is likely that a better insight into steroid metabolism will come from studies at the tissue level. Currently, little is known about the factors which influence steroid hormone activity at, or in, the cell, and details of tissue steroid concentration and tissue metabolism are still not clear.

Peripheral steroid production is a particularly important aspect, since it can produce local tissue concentrations of hormone independently of the overall plasma level, and so peripheral production and local modulation represent a microendocrine system to which local tissues may be exposed and may respond. In this regard, modulation of aromatase and dehydrogenase activity are potentially critical control points. In endometrial tissue, progesterone is an important factor, since it induces dehydrogenase and by increasing back conversion into oestrone, effectively diminishes tissue exposure to oestradiol. There may well be other factors, of which we are unaware. Thus, studies of the mechanism of aromatization and the factors mediating oestrone – oestradiol conversion are central to an understanding of the problem of tissue exposure to oestrogen, and to the design of potentially useful therapeutic measures which involve removal of oestrogen exposure.

Several tissues are capable of aromatization, including adipose tissue[21], liver[22], skin[23], fibroblasts[24], muscle[25] and neural tissue[26]. Adipose tissue is particularly important because of the relatively large amounts present in the body. In addition, interest is directed towards adipose tissue by the relationship of cancer to obesity, and the dietary factors previously discussed. In women, aromatization increases with age and body weight when studied by *in vivo* techniques[10,27], but the cause is unknown. It has been claimed that adipose tissue from women with endometrial cancer is more efficient than normal tissue from control subjects in converting androgens into oestrogens[28,29], but this has not been confirmed by *in vivo* methods by us[11], or by others[10,30]. We have therefore examined adipose tissue *in vitro* to establish the effects of age and weight on aromatization, and also to try to define the factors which influence the conversion of oestrone to oestradiol. The method employed has been to obtain abdominal or breast adipose tissue at surgery and to study the conversion of radiolabelled androgens or oestrone to their products. Details of the techniques used have been described elsewhere[31,32]. We have measured the aromatization of androstenedione to oestrone in adipose tissue and could find no correlation with the weight of the tissue donor[32], and therefore it would appear that the increased efficiency of conversion observed *in vivo*[10] in heavier women is not because the tissues are relatively more efficient but is probably a reflection of the larger mass present in heavier women.

Our results have shown that aromatization varies with age[32], reaching a peak at the time of the menopause and subsequently declining. This is not entirely similar to the *in vivo* situation since the increased activity is not maintained in the older women.

There have been reports[28,29] that oestrone formation is increased in adipose tissue from women with endometrial cancer or hyperplasia. Although it is an attractive hypothesis that cancer patients have a more effective aromatization capability, it seems likely that this observation is restricted to very obese women. Forney *et al.*[29] were unable to demonstrate an alteration in oestrone formation in cancer patients who had less than 25 kg total body fat mass. In a similar study[32] we have also been unable to show any marked difference in aromatase activity between adipose tissue taken from controls, and from women with endometrial cancer. All the cancer patients in this study had less than 17 kg total body fat mass.

The mechanism of control of aromatization in gonadal tissue clearly involves follicle stimulating hormone (FSH)[33,34]. If this were true for adipose tissue, the high gonadotrophin levels in menopausal women could account for the increased efficiency seen *in vivo*[27]. However, we have found no receptors for FSH in adipose tissue, nor in tissue taken from younger women with gonadal failure, in whom FSH levels are obviously greatly increased[35].

Recently, Simpson and his colleagues in Dallas, USA[36], reported that stromal cells from adipose tissue are sensitive to dexamethasone and increase their aromatization when they are treated with this glucocorticoid. We have studied this phenomenon using explants of adipose tissue taken at surgery and kept in culture for short periods of time. We have preferred to work with cortisol since this is the natural glucocorticoid.

Some of the results from this study are shown in Figure 3. In agreement with Simpson's results[36], we found that dexamethasone was capable of inducing aromatase activity in adipose tissue. At these relatively short induction times, cortisol will also induce aromatase but only in relatively high concentrations (> 500 nmol/l). In contrast, none of the other hormones studied were able to induce the enzyme.

Equating *in vitro* and *in vivo* studies is difficult, but assuming it is only the free fraction of plasma cortisol that is available to the cell, one would not expect the tissue to be exposed to concentrations of cortisol much in excess of 100 nmol/l. Even at these very low concentrations though, we have found that it is possible to induce aromatase activity *in vitro*, provided the incubation period is long enough and the medium

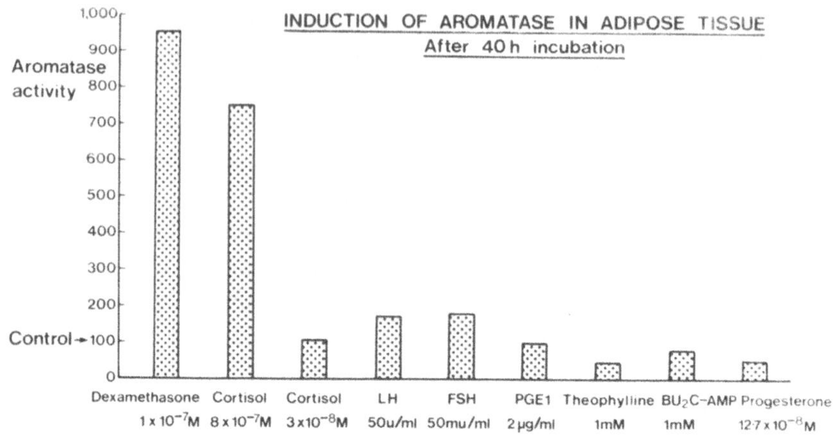

Figure 3 The effect on aromatase activity in human adipose tissue of the inclusion of various substances in the supporting medium. Fresh adipose tissue slices were incubated in flasks containing 5 ml medium 199 containing penicillin G (100 U/ml), streptomycin sulphate (100 μg/ml) and fetal calf serum (10%). Five hundred mg of tissue was added to each flask and allowed to float. The gas phase was air. Various substances, as indicated above, were added to the flasks which were sealed and incubated at 37°C for 40 h. After incubation the tissue was resuspended in 0.1 mol/l phosphate buffer and aromatase activity measured as described previously[32]. Results are expressed as percentage of the control activity, i.e. that attained in the absence of media additions = 100%

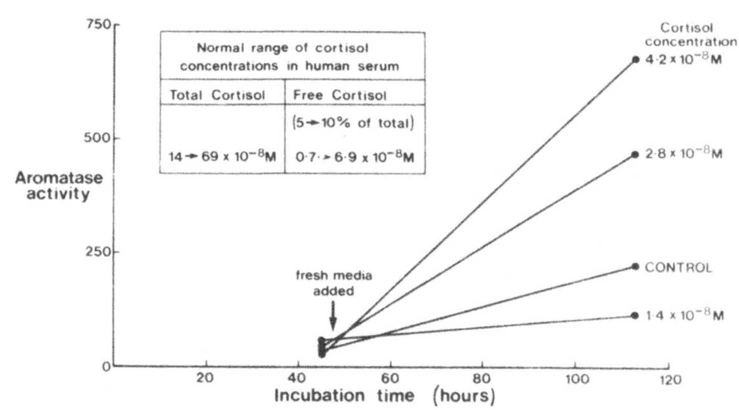

Figure 4 The effect of low cortisol concentrations on aromatase activity in human adipose tissue maintained in tissue culture for up to 112 h. The experimental procedure was as described for Figure 3. The medium was replaced after 48 h in each flask and aromatase activity measured after a total of 112 h at 37°C. Aromatase activity is expressed as pg oestrone/0.5 g tissue/3 h

is replaced as shown in Figure 4. Thus, since these are truly physiological concentrations, these data suggest that this may be an important mechanism for controlling aromatase activity *in vivo*.

If this hypothesis is correct, then it might be reasonable to assume that there may be some relationship between aromatase activity measured in human adipose tissue and plasma concentrations of cortisol. An obvious clinical example in which one might expect to find induction of aromatase is Cushing's syndrome, since in this condition the tissues are exposed to elevated concentrations of cortisol. We have obtained abdominal adipose tissue from two women with Cushing's syndrome.

The aromatase activity was measured in the tissue and is shown in Table 1 with the results obtained using adipose tissue from a group of control women measured under the same conditions. There appears to be an increase in aromatase activity in the patients with Cushing's syndrome, although not as pronounced as might have been expected from the *in vitro* studies.

Another indication that this may be a physiological mechanism is shown in Figure 5, in which we have compared, in a number of subjects, the free serum cortisol concentrations with the aromatase activity, and there is a significant correlation ($r = 0.67$, $p < 0.02$).

These data then suggest that a possible physiological mechanism of controlling peripheral aromatization lies in glucocorticoid activation, and tissue exposure to cortisol, e.g. in times of prolonged stress, there may well be sufficient cortisol to induce aromatase activity and thus increase the oestrogen production within peripheral tissues.

The next stage of oestrogen production, conversion of oestrone into oestradiol, requires dehydrogenase. We know something about the control of this enzyme system, at least in endometrial tissue. Progesterone induces dehydrogenase activity[2] and this increases the

Table 1 Comparison of aromatase activity *in vitro* in adipose tissue from normal women and women with Cushing's syndrome

	Normal women	*Women with Cushing's syndrome*
Number of subjects	17	2
Age range (years)	28–88	27–35
Aromatase activity (pg oestrone/mg protein/3 h) range	ND*31.9	19.7–24.1
Mean	12.7	21.9

* Not detectable

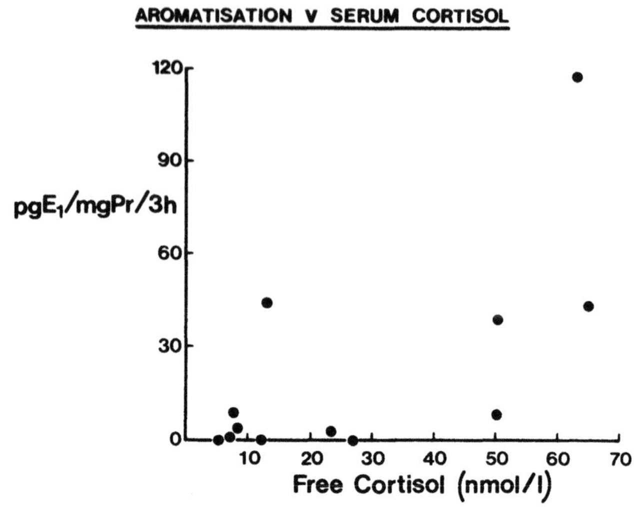

Figure 5 Correlation between aromatase activity in adipose tissue and the free cortisol concentration in the serum of the tissue donor. The unbound fraction of cortisol was measured in an equilibrium dialysis system by a method similar to that descriibed in reference 60. A Dianorm dialysis machine[61] was used. In the dialyser, two half cells are separated by a semipermeable membrane. Undiluted serum (1 ml) and saline (1 ml) were introduced into the two half cells. The dialysis cells were kept at 37°C and rotated at 12 rpm for 4 h to allow the cell contents to equilibrate. After this time an aliquot of the unbound cortisol was estimated by radioimmunoassay

metabolism of oestradiol to oestrone and other products. This diminishes the biological effect of oestradiol. These observations have led to the concept that treatment with oestradiol for replacement therapy is best combined with progesterone to diminish the risk of endometrial neoplasia. Apart from the endometrium though, other tissues are potential sources of dehydrogenase, but in contrast to the fairly extensive studies of endometrial tissue, much less is known about them.

The adipose tissue from abdomen or breast is potentially an important site of oestradiol formation and invites further study.

In postmenopausal women the reduction of oestrone produced by the aromatization of androstenedione could be an important source of intracellular oestradiol. To study such oestradiol production we have used similar methods to those employed for studying aromatase activity, that is, removal of tissue at surgery and study of the conversion of isotopically labelled precursor, in this case oestrone, into oestradiol. *In vivo* the reaction catalysed by 17β-hydroxysteroid dehydrogenase is reversible. The direction of metabolism in the tissue will depend on intracellular oestrogen concentrations and the availability of cofactors for the reaction.

Our results have shown that *in vitro*, in the presence of NADPH, human adipose tissue, whether taken from abdomen or breast, was able to convert oestrone into oestradiol[31]. In contrast to aromatase, there was a positive correlation between 17β-hydroxysteroid dehydrogenase activity in breast adipose tissue and the total body weight of the tissue donor as shown in Figure 6 ($r = 0.72$, $p < 0.01$ cancer patients; $r = 0.42$, NS normal patients).

In addition, a similar relationship exists with age, as was found for aromatase. Although the number of observations was relatively small, it was in the perimenopausal women that the enzyme activity reached a peak.

The conversion to oestradiol is inhibited by progesterone in a competitive manner[31], and so it is possible that as progesterone secretion diminishes towards the menopause, inhibition is removed. The mechanism of action is not clear and further studies are needed to determine the concentration of progesterone in adipose tissue and the nature of the inhibitory process.

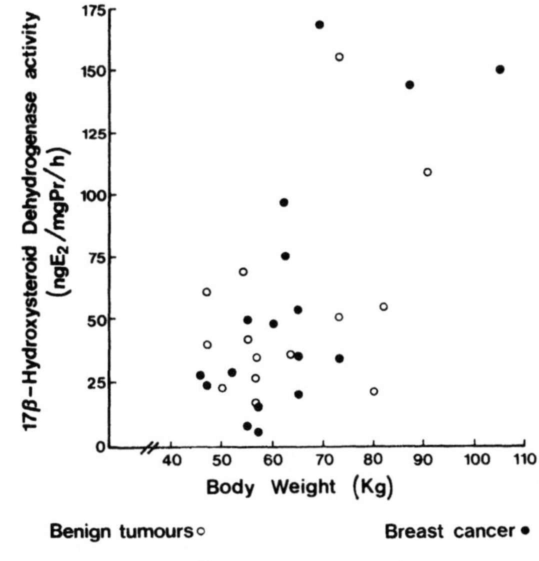

Figure 6 Correlation between 17β-hydroxysteroid dehydrogenase activity in human breast fat and the total body weight of the tissue donor. (●) Women with breast cancer. (o) Women with benign tumours or undergoing reductive mammoplasty

So far, we have been unable to demonstrate enhanced activity in tissue from patients with endometrial cancer[31]. In summary, as shown in Figure 7, specimens of fat taken from abdomen or breast show different activities in oestrogen production, but no significant differences emerge in the cancer tissues. However, it is clear that an active mechanism for local production of oestrogen exists in these tissues, and we do not know whether tissue concentrations are altered from normal.

This requires a further step forward in techniques, both to measure perhaps intracellular concentrations of steroids, and to seek indicators of oestrogen activity.

For the last part of this review, the possible role which androgens play in female endocrine cancer will be considered.

In postmenopausal women, the adrenal gland assumes the major role in steroid production, and as previously discussed, is indirectly the main source of oestrogen, arising from androstenedione[9]. The adrenal also secretes dehydroepiandrosterone (DHA) and its sulphate (DHAS), for which no clearly defined biological function has so far been found. Nevertheless, there is a lot of experimental evidence,

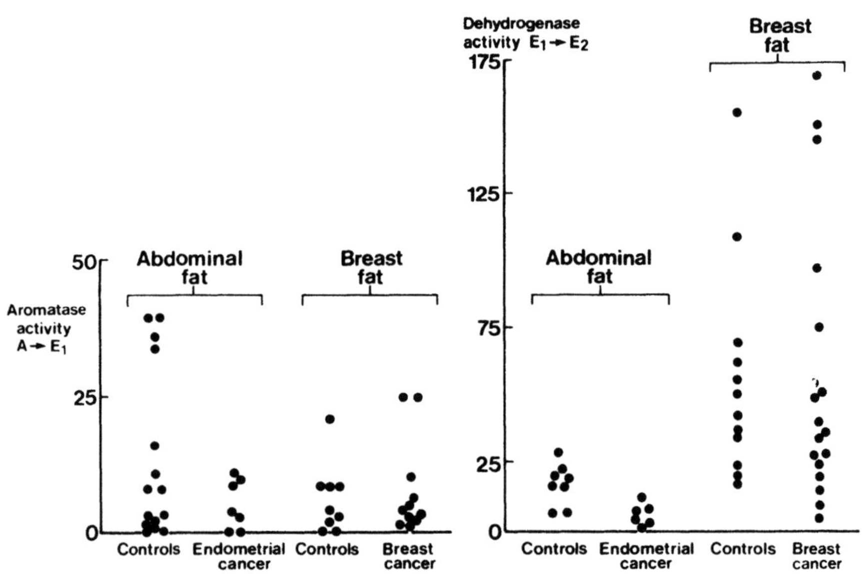

Figure 7 Comparison of the activity of aromatase and 17β-hydroxysteroid dehydrogenase in abdominal and breast fat in normal women and women with cancer. Aromatase activity is expressed as pg oestrone/mg protein/3h and 17β-hydroxysteroid dehydrogenase activity is expressed as ng oestradiol/mg protein/h

although much of it is conflicting, which suggests that androgens are somehow involved in the aetiology or progression of breast and endometrial cancer[1].

Measurement of urinary steroid excretion suggested that diminished androgen secretion is an unfavourable factor[37]. However, both normal[38] and subnormal[39] plasma levels of DHAS have been reported. In premenopausal women with breast cancer, plasma DHA levels have been reported as subnormal[40].

In postmenopausal patients, however, when 24 hour profiles were measured, both DHA and DHAS plasma levels were increased. Our data are similar: in postmenopausal women aged over 55 years with breast cancer, plasma DHAS levels were found to be higher than in control patients. Carlström *et al.*[41] have also found elevated plasma levels in postmenopausal women with endometrial cancer. Plasma levels of DHAS are also elevated in a number of conditions which are risk factors for endocrine cancers, e.g. obesity[42], hypertension[43,44], polycystic ovarian disease[45] and oestrogen therapy[46]. If these findings are accepted, they imply either increased steroid production, or diminished clearance, or both.

There is supporting evidence for some degree of adrenal hyperfunction in both breast cancer patients[15,47], and in women with endometrial cancer[48]. If either the production or metabolism of DHA and DHAS is altered in cancer patients, what role could these steroids play? Possibilities include conversion into oestrogen, conversion into some other biologically active steroid or modulation of tissue activity.

Conversion of DHAS into oestrogen is an attractive possibility since it is still not possible to define the origin of all the oestrogen produced in postmenopausal women with cancer[5,6]. However, the evidence is controversial with some groups finding evidence of increased oestrogen excretion after administration of DHAS[49] while others did not[50]. Evidence of biological activity has also been reported in immature subjects after administration of DHAS[49,51]. We have infused DHAS and examined the changes in plasma oestrogen levels, but as shown in Figure 8, there was no apparent change in plasma oestrogen levels, in contrast to our findings after infusion of androstenedione[52].

So, unless cancer patients behave differently, DHAS does not seem to be a significant oestrogen precursor, at least in short-term studies. However, DHA is a potential precursor for another steroid – androstenediol – and as also shown in Figure 8 infusion of a physiological dose of DHAS rapidly increases the plasma level of this steroid.

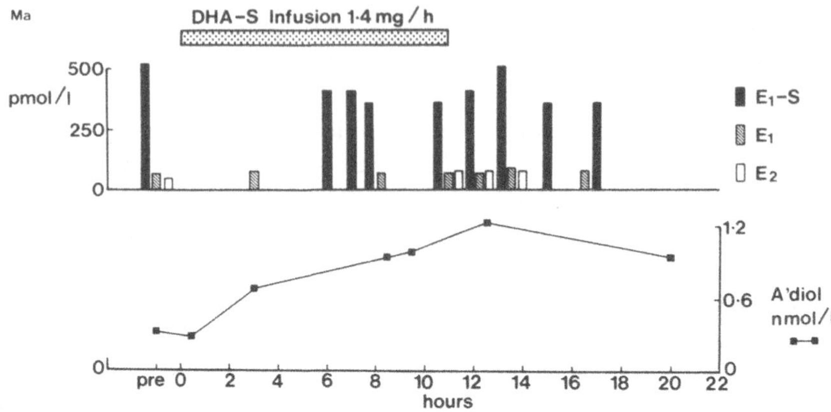

Figure 8 Plasma levels of oestrone (E1), oestrone sulphate (E1S), oestradiol (E2) and androstenediol (A'diol) during and after infusion of dehydroepiandrosterone sulphate (DHA-S) in a postmenopausal woman after treatment for 1 week with dexamethasone (2 mg/day)

Recently, both Thijssen[53] and Adams[54] have drawn attention to the potentially important role of this steroid in breast cancer. In addition to acting in some tissues as an androgen, it also has well-documented oestrogenic activity, and thus elevated DHAS levels in women with breast cancer may result in elevated plasma or tissue levels of androstenediol.

In a preliminary study we have not so far found any significant differences from normal, but this interesting steroid hormone obviously merits further study.

Finally, there is the possibility that DHA, DHAS or androstenediol may influence oestrogen action by inhibiting oestradiol metabolism, or potentiating oestradiol action. Metabolism of oestradiol to oestrone for example is diminished in breast tumour tissue[55,56]. Furthermore, our own studies *in vivo* have suggested that DHAS may directly, or through a metabolite, inhibit the deactivation of oestradiol[57]. Further studies were therefore carried out to investigate the possibility that androgens may influence oestrogen metabolism. As shown in Figure 9, all three steroids DHA, DHAS and androstenediol are efficient inhibitors of oestradiol dehydrogenase. These results are in agreement with the observation that, if androstenediol is administered to rats simultaneously with oestradiol the plasma and nuclear receptor levels of oestradiol were increased above the levels found for oestradiol alone[58].

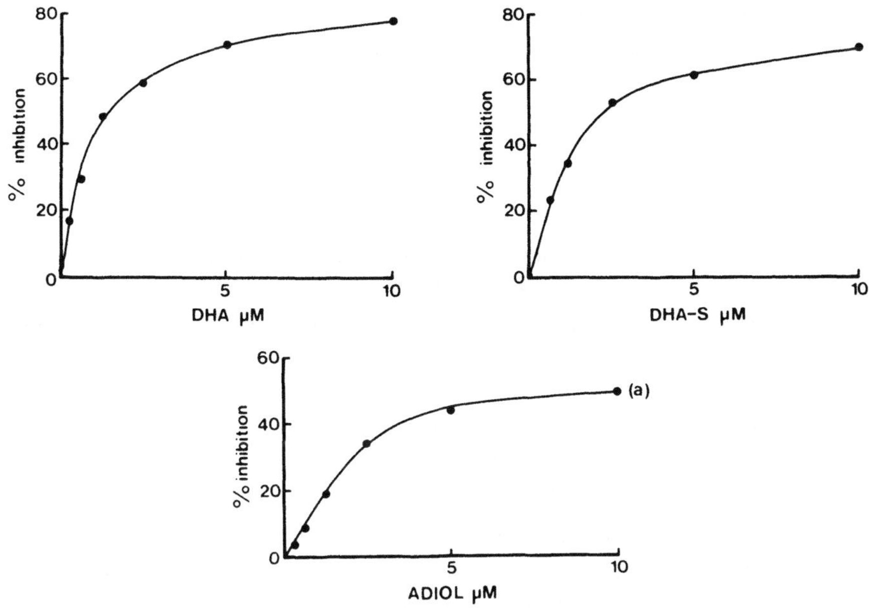

Figure 9 Inhibition of 17β-hydroxysteroid dehydrogenase activity ($E_2 \rightarrow E_1$) in endometrium by various concentrations of DHA, DHA-S and ADIOL in the presence of 2.9 μmol/l oestradiol. Enzyme activity was measured by an isotope ratio technique and the results expressed as percentage inhibition of control activity

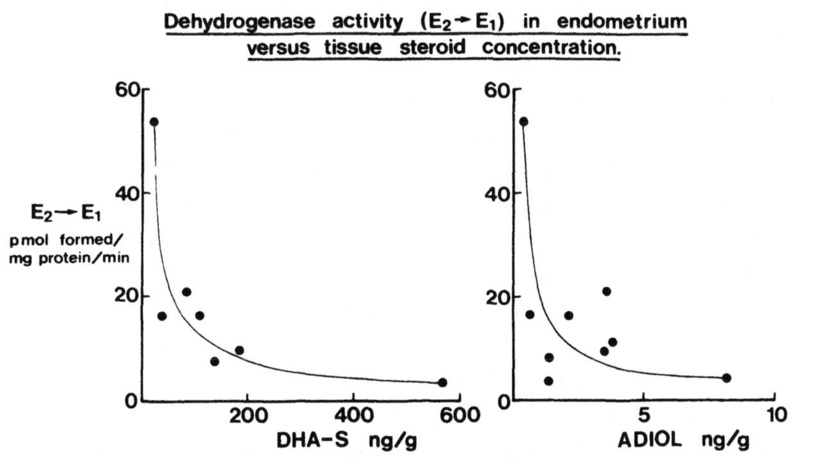

Figure 10 Correlation between 17β-hydroxysteroid dehydrogenase activity and concentrations of DHA-S and ADIOL in endometrium. The metabolism of oestradiol was measured using an isotope ratio technique and the results expressed as pmol of oestrone formed per mg protein per min. Tissue steroid concentrations were measured by radioimmunoassay following ether extraction and thin layer chromatography and the results were expressed as ng of steroid per g tissue wet weight

In further support of a role for this steroid, there is an association of higher tissue levels of DHAS and androstenediol with lower conversion of oestradiol into oestrone, as shown in Figure 10.

CONCLUSION

Many major cancer risk factors are now known – particularly obesity, nutrition, lipid intake, stress and possibly inadequate or abnormal ovarian function. Lipid intake is remarkably well correlated with breast cancer incidence.

Major steroid endocrine abnormalities seem to be enhanced oestrogen metabolism, increased free oestrogen concentration, altered adrenal androgen status. On the other hand, oestrogen production and total plasma oestrogen levels are not consistently abnormal. It is accepted by most investigators that the role of oestrogen is as a co-carcinogen, acting on a tissue which has already been exposed to various factors, such as a virus, radiation, chemical and others, which have initiated the cancer. It is possible that a further important event is increased tissue concentration of oestradiol which then stimulates the abnormal tissue further. In postmenopausal women, this peripheral production is particularly significant. Figure 11 suggests how these apparently unrelated risk factors may act, through directly or indirectly altering the tissue exposure to oestradiol. Thus, enhanced ovarian or adrenal activity produces an increase in the production of androgen substrate, and hence an increase in tissue oestrogen concentration produced by peripheral metabolism. This process is enhanced by the action of cortisol. Adrenal androgens may also act by inhibition of oestradiol dehydrogenase, but also through conversion into androstenediol, an oestrogenic metabolite.

Siiteri[19] has pointed out the possible significance of protein binding, and these factors may therefore also enhance tissue exposure to oestrogen. Thus, the overall effect of several risk factors may be to alter the intracellular levels of oestrogen.

Classical studies of the role of oestrogens in female endocrine cancer have leaned heavily and necessarily towards investigation of initially, urinary excretion, as an index of production, then plasma concentrations, and more recently production rates. However, the local tissue environment is only partly determined by the presentation of plasma hormones; intracellular production, protein binding and metabolism

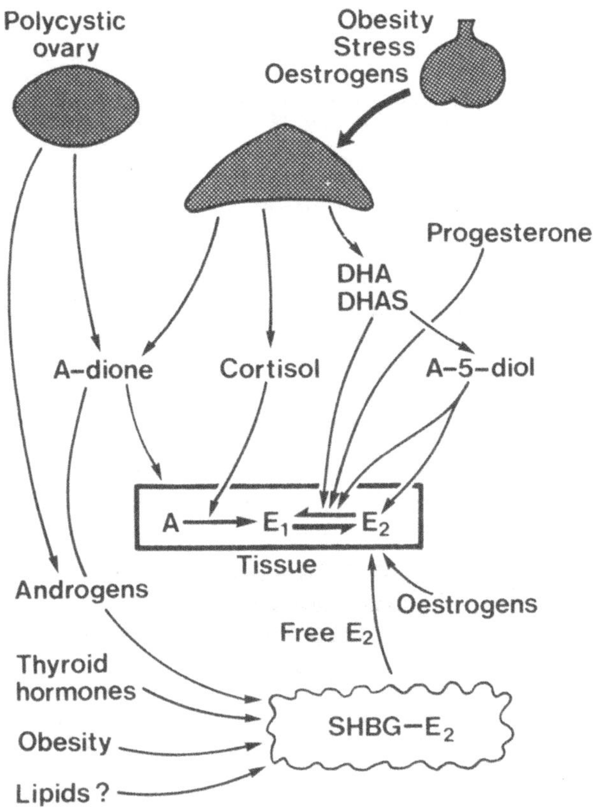

Figure 11 Composite diagram incorporating various suggested points of action of steroid hormones and other risk factors in modulating tissue concentration of oestrogen. (See text for further details and relevant references)

may individually or collectively be of far greater significance in determining tissue exposure. As yet, laboratory and clinical techniques to study these factors are imperfect, but a better understanding of them is essential if we are to design improved preventive and therapeutic methods.

Acknowledgements

The work described in this paper was supported by the Cancer Research Campaign. This article was previously published in *Journal of Endocrinological Investigation*, **5**, 335 (1982) and is reprinted with permission of the editor.

References

1. James, V. H. T. and Reed, M. J. (1980). Steroid hormones and human cancer. In Iacobelli, S., King, R. J. B., Lindner, H. R. and Lippman, M. E. (eds) *Hormones and Cancer*, pp. 471–487. (New York: Raven Press)
2. Tseng, L. and Gurpide, E. (1975). Induction of human endometrial estradiol dehydrogenase by progestins. *Endocrinology*, **97**, 825
3. Anderson, D. C. (1974). Sex-hormone-binding globulin. *Clin. Edocrinol. (Oxf.)*, **3**, 69
4. Longcope, C. (1978). The significance of steroid production by peripheral tissue. In Scholler, R. (ed.) *Endocrinology of the ovary*, pp. 23–35 (Paris: Editions Sepe)
5. James, V. H. T., Reed, M. J. and Folkerd, E. J. (1981). Studies of oestrogen metabolism in postmenopausal women with cancer. *J. Steroid Biochem.*, **15**, 235
6. Kirschner, M. A., Cohen, F. B. and Ryan, C. (1978) Androgen–oestrogen production rates in postmenopausal women with breast cancer. *Cancer Res.*, **38**, 4029
7. Vermeulen, A., Verdonck, L., van der Straeten, M. and Orie, N. (1969). Capacity of the testosterone-binding globulin in human plasma and influence of specific binding of testosterone on its metabolic clearance rate. *J. Clin. Endocrinol. Metab.*, **29**, 1470
8. Siiteri, P. K., Hammond, G. L. and Nisker, J. A. (1981). Increased availability of serum estrogens in breast cancer: a new hypothesis. In Pike, M. C., Siiteri, P. K. and Welsch, C. W. (eds) Banbury Report No. 8, *Hormones and Cancer*, pp. 87–101. (Cold Spring Harbour Laboratory)
9. Siiteri, P. K. and MacDonald, P. C. (1973). Role of extra-glandular estrogen in human endocrinology. In Greep, R. O. and Astwood, E. B. (eds) *Handbook of Physiology*, Vol. 2, pp. 615–629. (Washington D.C.: American Physiological Society)
10. MacDonald, P. C., Edman, C. D., Hemsell, D. L., Porter, J. C. and Siiteri, P. K. (1978). Effect of obesity on conversion of plasma androstenedione to estrone in women with and without endometrial cancer. *Am. J. Obstet. Gynecol.*, **130**, 448
11. Reed, M. J., Hutton, J. D., Baxendale, P. M., James, V. H. T., Jacobs, H. S. and Fisher, R. P. (1979). The conversion of androstenedione to oestrone and production of oestrone in women with endometrial cancer. *J. Steroid Biochem.*, **11**, 905
12. Thijssen, J. H. H., Wiegerinck, M. A. H. M. and Poortman, J. (1978). Estrone at the cellular level in target tissues *in vivo* in postmenopausal women. *J. Steroid Biochem.*, **9**, 893
13. Judd, H. L., Davidson, B. J., Frumar, A. M., Shamonki, I. M., Lagasse, L. D. and Ballon, S. C. (1980). Serum androgens and estrogens in postmenopausal women with and without endometrial cancer. *Am. J. Obstet. Gynecol.*, **136**, 859
14. McFadyen, I. J., Prescott, R. J., Groom, G. V., Forrest, A. P. M., Golder, M. P., Fahmy, D. R. and Griffiths, K. (1976). Circulating hormone concentrations in women with breast cancer. *Lancet*, **1**, 1100
15. Drafta, D., Schindler, A. E., Milcu, S. M., Keller, E., Stroe, E., Horodniceanu, E. and Balanescu, I. (1980). Plasma hormones in pre- and postmenopausal breast cancer. *J. Steroid Biochem.*, **13**, 793
16. Benjamin, F. and Deutsch, S. (1976). Plasma levels of fractionated estrogens and pituitary hormones in endometrial carcinoma. *Am. J. Obstet. Gynecol.*, **126**, 638
17. Moore, J. W., Clark, G.M. G., Bulbrook, R. D., Hayward, J. L., Murai, J. T.,

Hammond, G. L. and Siiteri, P. K. (1982). Serum concentrations of total and non-protein-bound oestradiol in patients with breast cancer and in normal controls. *Int. J. Cancer*, **29**, 17
18. Pardridge, W. M., Mietus, L. J., Frumar, A. M., Davidson, B. J. and Judd, H. L. (1980). Effects of human serum on transport of testosterone and estradiol into rat brain. *Am. J. Physiol.*, **239**, E 103
19. Siiteri, P. K. (1981). Extraglandular oestrogen formation and serum binding of oestradiol: relationship to cancer. *J. Endocrinol.*, **89** (Suppl.), 119 P
20. Wynder, E. L. (1980). Dietary factors related to breast cancer. *Cancer*, **46**, 899
21. Nimrod, A. and Ryan, K. J. (1975). Aromatization of androgens by human abdominal and breast fat tissue. *J. Clin. Endocrinol. Metab.*, **40**, 367
22. Smuk, M. and Schwers, J. (1977). Aromatization of androstenedione by human adult liver *in vitro*. *J. Clin. Endocrinol. Metab.*, **45**, 1009
23. Schindler, A. E. (1975). Steroid metabolism of fetal tissues II Conversion of androstenedione to estrone. *Am. J. Obstet. Gynecol.*, **123**, 265
24. Schweikert, H. U., Milewich, L. and Wilson, J. D. (1976). Aromatization of androstenedione by cultured human fibroblasts. *J. Clin. Endocrinol. Metab.*, **43**, 785
25. Longcope, C., Pratt, J. H., Schneider, S. H. and Fineberg, S. E. (1978). Aromatization of androgens by muscle and adipose tissue *in vivo*. *J. Clin. Endocrinol. Metab.*, **46**, 146
26. Naftolin, F., Ryan, K. J. and Petro, Z. (1971). Aromatization of androstenedione by the diencephalon. *J. Clin. Endocrinol. Metab.*, **33**, 368
27. Hemsell, D. L., Grodin, J. M., Brenner, P. F., Siiteri, P. K. and MacDonald, P. C. (1974). Plasma precursors of estrogen. II Correlation of the extent of conversion of plasma androstenedione to estrone with age. *J. Clin. Endocrinol. Metab.*, **38**, 476
28. Schindler, A. E., Ebert, A. and Friedrich, E. (1972). Conversion of androstenedione to estrone by human fat tissue. *J. Clin. Endrocrinol. Metab.*, **35**, 627
29. Forney, J. P., Milewich, L., Chen, G. T., Garlock, J. L., Schwartz, B..E., Edman, C. D. and MacDonald, P. C. (1981). Aromatization of androstenedione to estrone by human adipose tissue *in vitro*. Correlation with adipose tissue mass, age and endometrial neoplasia. *J. Clin. Endocrinol. Metab.*, **53**, 192
30. Rizkallah, T. H., Tovell, H. M. M. and Kelly, W. G. (1975). Production of oestrone and fractional conversion of circulating androstenedione to oestrone in women with endometrial carcinoma. *J. Clin. Endocrinol. Metab.*, **40**, 1045
31. Folkerd, E. J. and James, V. H. T. (1982). Studies on the activity of 17β-hydroxysteroid dehydrogenase in human adipose tissue. *J. Steroid Biochem.*, **16**, 539
32. Folkerd, E. J., Reed, M. J. and James, V. H. T. (1982). Oestrogen production in adipose tissue from normal women and women with endometrial cancer *in vitro*. *J. Steroid Biochem.*, **16**, 297
33. Erickson, G. F., Hsueh, A. J. W., Quigley, M. E., Rebar, R. W. and Yen, S. S. C. (1979). Functional studies of aromatase activity in human granulosa cells from normal and polycystic ovaries. *J. Clin. Endocrinol. Metab.*, **49**, 514
34. Moon, Y. S., Tsang, B. K., Simpson, C. and Armstrong, D. T. (1978). 17β-Estradiol biosynthesis in cultured granulosa and thecal cells of human ovarian follicles: stimulation by follicle-stimulating hormone. *J. Clin. Endocrinol. Metab.*, **47**, 263
35. Folkerd, E. J., Jacobs, H. S., van der Spuy, Z. and James, V. H. T. (1982). Failure of FSH to influence aromatization in human adipose tissue. *Clin. Endocrinol. (Oxf.)*, **16**, 621

36. Simpson, E. R., Ackerman, G. E., Smith, M. E. and Mendelson, C. R. (1981). Estrogen formation in stromal cells of adipose tissue of women: Induction by glucocorticosteroids. *Proc. Natl. Acad. Sci. USA*, **78**, 5690
37. Bulbrook, R. D., Hayward, J. L. and Thomas, B. S. (1964). The relation between the urinary 17-hydroxycorticosteroids and 11-deoxy-17-oxosteroids and the fate of patients after mastectomy. *Lancet*, **1**, 945
38. Wang, D. Y. (1969). Plasma androgens in breast cancer. In Griffiths, K. and Cameron, E. H. D. (eds) *The Human Adrenal Gland in Relation to Breast Cancer*, pp. 71–79. (Caerphilly: Alpha Omega Alpha)
39. Rose, D. P., Stauber, P., Thiel, A., Crowley, J. J. and Milbrath, J. R. (1977). Plasma dehydroepiandrosterone sulphate, androstenedione and cortisol and urinary free cortisol excretion in breast cancer. *Eur. J. Cancer*, **13**, 43
40. Zumoff, B., Levin, J., Rosenfeld, R. S., Markham, M., Strain, G. W. and Fukushima, D. K. (1981). Abnormal-24hr-mean plasma concentrations of dehydroisoandrosterone and dehydroisoandrosterone sulphate in women with primary operable breast cancer. *Cancer Res.*, **41**, 3360
41. Carlström, K., Damber, M. G., Furuhjelm, M., Joelsson, I., Lunell, N. O. and von Schoultz, B. (1979). Serum levels of total dehydroepiandrosterone and total estrone in postmenopausal women with special regard to carcinoma of the uterine corpus. *Acta. Obstet. Gynecol. Scand.*, **58**, 179
42. Feher, T. and Halmy, L. (1975). Dehydroepiandrosterone and dehydroepiandrosterone sulfate dynamics in obesity. *Can. J. Biochem.*, **53**, 215
43. Shao, A., Nowaczynski, W., Kuchel, O. and Genest, J. (1970). Secretion rate of dehydroepiandrosterone and dehydroepiandrosterone sulphate in benign essential hypertension as compared to normal subjects. *Can. J. Biochem.*, **48**, 1308
44. Sekihara, H., Ohsawa, N. and Kosaka, K. (1975). Serum dehydroepiandrosterone sulphate and dehydroepiandrosterone levels in essential hypertension. *J. Clin. Endocrinol. Metab.*, **40**, 156
45. Yen, S. C. C., Chaney, C. and Judd, H. L. (1976). Functional aberrations of the hypothalamic pituitary system in the polycystic ovary syndrome: a consideration of the pathogenesis. In James, V. H. T., Serio, M. and Giusti, G. (eds) *The Endocrine Function of the Human Ovary*, pp. 373–385. (London: Academic Press)
46. Abraham, G. E. and Maroulis, G. B. (1975). Effect of exogenous estrogen on serum pregnenolone, cortisol and androgens in postmenopausal women. *Obstet. Gynecol.*, **45**, 271
47. Saez, S. (1979). Corticotrophin secretion in relation to breast cancer. In Stoll, B. A. (ed.) *Mammary Cancer and Neuroendocrine Therapy*, pp. 101–122. (London: Butterworth)
48. Sommers, C. S. and Meissner, W. A. (1957). Endocrine abnormalities accompanying human endometrial cancer. *Cancer*, **10**, 516
49. Mills, I. H., Tait, A. D. and Galley, J. (1969). Metabolism of dehydroepiandrosterone sulphate in a patient with 17-hydroxylase deficiency. *J. Endocrinol.*, **43**, xlix
50. Mancuso, S., Mancuso, F. P., Tillinger, K. G. and Diczfalusy, E. (1965). Lack of aromatization of circulating dehydroepiandrosterone and dehydroepiandrosterone sulphate in amenorrhoeic women stimulated with human gonadotrophins. *Acta Endocrinol.*, **49**, 248
51. Drucker, W. D., Blumberg, J. M. ., Gandy, H. M., David, R. R. and Verde, A. L. (1972). Biological activity of dehydroepiandrosterone sulphate in man. *J. Clin. Endocrinol. Metab.*, **35**, 48
52. James, V. H. T., Tunbridge, R. D. G., Wilson, G. A., Hutton, J. D., Jacobs, H. S.

and Rippon, A. G. (1978). Steroid profiling: A technique for exploring adrenocortical physiology. In James, V. H. T., Serio, M., Giusti, G. and Martini, L. (eds) *The Endocrine Function of the Human Adrenal Cortex,* pp. 179–192. (London: Academic Press)

53. Poortman, J. and Thijssen, J. H. H. (1978). The role of androgens in the aetiology of endometrial cancer: a hypothesis. In Brush, M. G., King, R. J. B. and Taylor, R. W. (eds) *Endometrial Cancer,* pp. 375–382. (London: Baillière Tyndall)
54. Adams, J. B., Archibald, L. and Clarke, C. (1978). Adrenal dehydroepiandrosterone and human mammary cancer. *Cancer Res.*, **38**, 4036.
55. Pollow, K., Boquoi, E., Baumann, J., Schmidt-Gollwitzer, M and Pollow, B. (1977). Comparison of the *in vitro* conversion of estradiol-17β to estrone of normal and neoplastic human breast tissue. *Mol. Cell. Endocrinol.*, **6**, 333
56. Geier, A., Horn, H., Levij, I. S. and Lichtshtein, E. (1975). The metabolism of ^{3}H-estradiol-17β in human breast cancer in organ culture. *Eur. J. Cancer*, **11**, 127
57. Reed, M. J., Noel, C. T., Johns, E. A., Jones, D. L. and James, V. H. T. (1982). Oestradiol production and factors that influence the interconversion of oestrone and oestradiol in postmenopausal women with endometrial hyperplasia, endometrial cancer or cirrhosis. In Fioretti, P., Martini, L., Melis, G. B. and Yen, S. S. C. (eds) *The Menopause: Clinical, Endocrinological and Patho-physiological Aspects*, pp. 325–330. (London: Academic Press)
58. Van Doorn, J. G., Valstar, E. and Poortman, J. (1981). Metabolic fate of intraperitoneally administered 5-androstene-3β, 17β-diol, estradiol-17β and their combination in the immature female rat. *J. Steroid Biochem.*, **14**, 657
59. Longcope, C. (1971). Metabolic clearance and blood production rates of estrogens in postmenopausal women. *Am. J. Obstet. Gynecol.*, **111**, 778
60. Clerico, A., Del Chicca, M. G., Zucchelli, G. C., Mariani, G. and Materazzi, F. (1978). Radioimmunological determination of free (diffusible) cortisol in an equilibrium dialysis system. *J. Nucl. Med. All. Sci.*, **22**, 5
61. Weder, H. G., Schildknecht, J. and Kesselring, P. (1971). A new equilibrium dialysing system. *Am. Lab.*, **10**, 15

Chapter 6

Steroid hormone receptors and their changes in the perimenopause

J. H. H. Thijssen

IINTRODUCTION

Steroid hormones are able to induce specific biological effects in many cells and cell systems in the body. Within one organ or cell system different cell populations may show divergent reactions towards the same stimulus and some cells will not react at all.

After the development of radioactive steroids with sufficiently high specific radioactivity, it became apparent that the target cells are able to concentrate the steroid under investigation[1]. Despite the qualitatively and quantitatively different reactions, all responding cells are able to concentrate the steroid because they contain an intracellular protein capable of binding specifically with a high affinity towards the stimulating steroid hormone. These binding proteins are called steroid receptors. They exist for five distinct classes of steroids: oestrogens, androgens, progestogens, glucocorticosteroids and mineralocorticosteroids.

MECHANISM OF ACTION OF STEROID HORMONES

The basic mechanism of action is supposed to be very similar for each of the five groups of steroids mentioned; the following steps can be distinguished.

Entry of the steroids into the cells

This entry very probably does not take place by active uptake; passive diffusion is thought to be the underlying process[2]. For the uptake of oestradiol by endometrial cells this diffusion step has been documented experimentally[3]. The question of the importance of protein binding of steroids in the blood for the uptake process has not been settled yet. Especially the role of high-affinity binders in plasma such as SHBG (for testosterone and oestradiol) and CBG (for cortisol) may be of relevance for these steroids.

Binding of steroids to specific receptors and transformation of the steroid–receptor complex

Only in those cells which contain the receptor for the steroid under investigation, will this substance bind to its specific receptor protein with high-affinity binding. This binding results in a rapid transformational change in the receptor molecule, making dissociation of the steroid–receptor complex much more difficult, the receptor becomes activated. For androgens, an additional metabolic transformation into the biologically more active DHT (dihydrotestosterone) before binding the receptor is necessary for a number of the biological effects.

Translocation of the activated complex to the nucleus

After the activation step the steroid–receptor complex can be translocated to the nucleus of the target cell. Within the nucleus the complex will bind to 'acceptor sites' on the nuclear chromatin. This binding will result in the formation of newly formed RNA molecules and ultimately in the production of specific mRNA[4].

Nuclear processing and final effects

The presence of the steroid–receptor complex in the nucleus is necessary during a certain prolonged period of time for biological effects[5]. These effects result from the translation of the mRNA at the ribosomes into specific proteins. The steroid–receptor complex in the nucleus very probably will ultimately dissociate and the receptor will undergo a process which is only partly understood, called 'nuclear processing'. Finally the receptor will re-enter the cytoplasm, the replenishment of the receptor, and will be available to start a new sequence of the events described[4].

The above-mentioned similarity in the mechanism of action of the five classes of steroids does not mean that all steroid interactions with their receptors in the cells are identical. Clear differences between classes have been described. Furthermore, not all steps have been documented extensively for all steroids. In particular for oestrogens and progesterone all steps described have been shown to be part of the intracellular handling of these steroids in target cells.

The dissimilarities of the final biological effects can not simply be explained by differences in the first steps in the mechanism of action. Most probably the nuclear handling, the binding of the complex to available unmasked acceptor sites on the chromatin and the transcription to mRNA are of more importance for the specificity of the effects[4]. All events described are not static processes but dynamic ones, the concentrations of both the steroid and its receptors in a cell are subject to variations in addition to the changes caused by their interactions.

OESTROGEN AND PROGESTERONE RECEPTORS

In the following part of this chapter attention will only be paid to the oestrogen and progesterone receptor concentrations in human tissues. These two steroid–receptor systems clearly show mutual interactions.

Stimulation of the target cells with *oestrogens* results initially in a decrease in the unoccupied receptor concentration in the cytoplasm with a concomitant increase in the nuclear receptors, due to translocation of the oestrogen–receptor complex. The presence of this complex in the nucleus is necessary during a period of about 12 hours to elicit the specific oestrogenic effects, which include an increase in both the oestrogen and progesterone receptor levels in the cytoplasm of the cells.

The interaction of *progestational substances* with the progesterone receptor results in a similar initial decrease and increase respectively in cytosol- and nuclear progesterone–receptor concentrations. One of the specific effects of this stimulation is the induction of the enzyme 17β-hydroxysteroid dehydrogenase, capable of converting oestradiol into the less active oestrone and vice versa. Within the cell the equilibrium of this reaction is in the direction of oestrone, which means that an increase in the enzyme will result in a decrease in the intracellular oestradiol concentration. In addition, under the influence of progestational substances the translocation of the oestrogen–receptor complex to the nucleus is diminished by a mechanism different from the enzyme induction just mentioned.

TISSUE CONCENTRATIONS OF RECEPTORS

The presence of unoccupied oestrogen and progesterone receptors has been demonstrated in the cytosol of a variety of human target tissues, including endometrium[6], myometrium[7], cervix[8], vagina[9,10] and mammary tumours[11]. The available systematic studies have shown that for endometrium[12] and myometrium[13] the levels of oestrogen receptors are directly dependent on the stage of the menstrual cycle. In both tissues the changes are very similar, cytosol levels of oestrogen receptors increase during the follicular phase of the cycle, induced by the enhanced oestrogen secretion of the growing follicle. The higher concentrations of oestradiol cause a rise in the translocation of the receptors to the nucleus and therefore occupied nuclear oestrogen receptors increase during the first part of the cycle.

As the effect of the interaction between oestradiol and its receptor the concentration of unoccupied progesterone receptors in the cytoplasm is also highest at the end of the follicular phase. During the last part of the follicular phase a positive correlation exists between plasma oestradiol and tissue progesterone receptor levels. After ovulation the diminished secretion of oestradiol and the increasing secretion of progesterone induce decreases of both receptors in the cytosol of the uterine tissues. The nuclear oestrogen receptors are also low because of the interaction of progesterone with the translocation of the oestrogen–receptor complex. The nuclear progesterone receptor level increases during the first days of the luteal phase. In Figure 1 a schematic representation is given of the changes in nuclear and total (= nuclear plus cytoplasmic) receptor concentrations in the human endometrium during the menstrual cycle.

The great changes in oestrogen receptor concentrations during the menstrual cycle have not been found for other tissues, the levels in the cervix[8] and the vagina[9,13] are comparable during the follicular and luteal phases of the cycle. For malignant mammary tumours some variations in oestrogen receptors have been described during the cycle but because of the large ranges of the measured concentrations, the

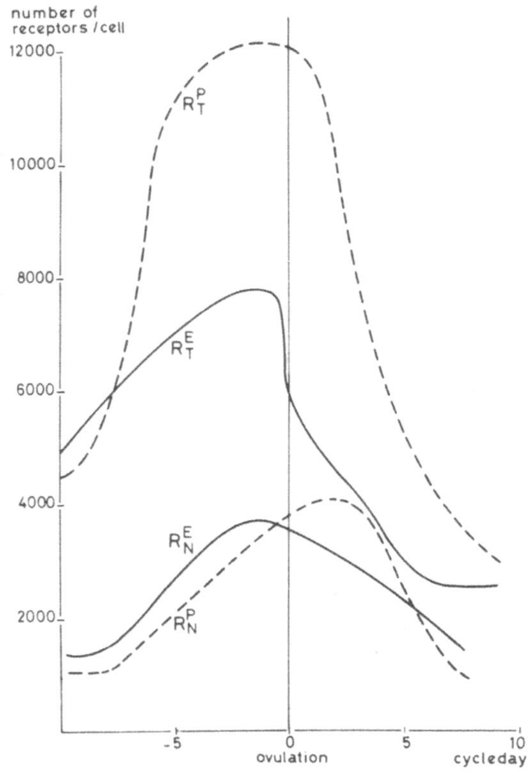

Figure 1 Schematic representation of the nuclear and total concentration of eostradiol and progesterone receptors in the human endometrium during the menstrual cycle. R^E_N and R^E_T means oestradiol receptors in the nucleus and total tissue R^P_N and R^P_T means progesterone receptors in nucleus and total tissue. The levels have been expressed as numbers of receptor sites per cell

differences were statistically not significant[14]. The progesterone receptors in the cervix follow the same pattern as in the uterus, highest levels were found in the late follicular phase. Vaginal tissue surprisingly gave completely different results: although generally the induction of progesterone receptors is considered to be a specific response of target tissues after oestrogen stimulation, no progesterone receptors could be demonstrated in the large majority of tissue samples studied[10,13]. Because the vagina clearly is an oestrogen target tissue, these findings indicate that progesterone receptor induction is not an obligatory reaction in all target cells.

After menopause the levels of oestrogen receptors do not change dramatically in the endometrium, myometrium and vagina; the concentrations measured are similar to those found during the early proliferative phase of the menstrual cycle. In the uterine tissues progesterone receptors were demonstrated in low concentrations, again comparable to those in the early proliferative phase of the cycle; only small numbers of tissues have been described as yet.

In contrast, in malignant breast tumours an increase in the oestrogen receptor levels has been shown following the menopause. Several studies have documented a higher percentage of tumours containing detectable receptor concentrations and also a higher mean receptor level per g of tumour[15]. For progesterone receptors there appeared to be no difference in the incidence of receptor-positive tumours and in the mean receptor concentration[16]. No real explanation is available for the increase in the oestradiol receptors at the much lower levels of oestradiol production after menopause. The suggestion that the observed differences in the tissue receptor are caused by the interaction of high ($>$ 300 pg/ml) levels of oestradiol in peripheral blood of premenopausal women during the processing of the tumour specimen in the laboratory, is not very likely the explanation of the lower receptor levels in tumours from premenopausal women.

A significant seasonal and/or (circa) annual variation has been reported for the oestrogen receptor content in the cytosol of breast tumours of postmenopausal women[17]. However, extensive statistical analysis performed on data from large populations of breast cancer patients did not support the existence of any periodicity in the oestrogen receptor concentration which was significant and consistent from year to year[18].

TISSUE CONCENTRATIONS OF OESTROGENS

From the mechanism of action of oestrogens as described, it is obvious that in addition to receptors the steroid itself is necessary to elicit biological effects in tissues. Hence knowledge of the concentration of oestrogens in target tissues, particularly in the nuclear compartment of the cells, will provide more accurate information on the steroid action than the determination of peripheral plasma levels. In order to obtain more information on the tissue uptake and concentration of oestrogens and on their subcellular distribution, two studies have been carried out in our laboratory:

(1) One using long-lasting ($>$10 hours) *infusions* of subphysio-

logical amounts of *³H-labelled oestrone, oestradiol or oestriol*, conditions chosen in an attempt to reach equilibrium of the infused tracers, implicating that the data obtained can be interpreted in terms of physiological phenomena.

(2) After development of an improved method for the quantitative extraction and *determination of oestrogens in tissues*, oestrone and oestradiol concentrations have been measured in the cytosol and in the nuclear fractions of normal uterine tissues obtained from women after a hysterectomy for benign pathology.

UPTAKE AND SUBCELLULAR DISTRIBUTION OF OESTROGENS IN TARGET TISSUES

After the infusions of radioactive oestrone, oestradiol or oestriol, total tissue radioactivity and the distribution of the infused steroid and its metabolites were measured specifically in three different subcellular fractions of endometrium, myometrium and vagina of normal postmenopausal women[19]. The three fractions studied consisted of steroids present in:

(a) Free (unconjugated) fraction in the high speed cytosol (CF);
(b) Receptor-bound fraction in the cytosol (CR);
(c) Total activity in the nuclear fraction (N).

The results have been expressed as the ratio of the radioactivity in total tissue or in a particular fraction to the plasma concentration of the unconjugated oestrogen, each time measured specifically as the steroid indicated. A ratio of 1 means that the amount of radioactivity in the tissue or a tissue fraction (in dpm/g tissue) equals the radioactivity level in plasma (in dpm/ml plasma).

Total tissue radioactivity after ^{3}H-oestrone infusions was very similar in the three tissues studied, the ratio was approximately 5; after labelled oestradiol and oestriol administrations the total tissue ratio was about 35 for endometrium, 20 for myometrium and 10 for the vagina.

Specific measurements of the steroids revealed that after oestrone infusions the mean tissue/plasma gradient for oestrone itself did not differ much from one; the oestradiol ratio, however, amounted to 15, 10 and 6 for endometrium, myometrium and vagina respectively. Higher tissue/plasma gradients for ^{3}H-oestradiol were found after labelled oestradiol infusions: the ratios were 33, 21 and 11 for endometrium, myometrium and vagina respectively. The mean ratio for oestrone after ^{3}H-oestradiol infusions amounted to 7, 4, and 6 for these tissues. After ^{3}H-oestriol administrations no detectable amounts of oestrone or oestradiol could be detected in either plasma or tissues, the tissue/plasma gradients could mainly be explained by the presence of the infused steroid. A metabolite of oestriol could be detected in smaller quantities, which was tentatively identified as 16α-hydroxyoestrone. The mean tissue/plasma gradient for this metabolite was calculated as 5 in endometrium, 2 in myometrium and 2 in vagina.

Measurement of the subcellular distribution of the radioactive compounds showed that 60–80% was accumulated in the nuclear fraction after the oestradiol and oestriol infusions. In this respect there were only minor differences between the three tissues studied. In contrast oestrone showed only a small accumulation from the plasma to the cytosol-free and receptor-bound fractions and almost no nuclear oestrone could be detected. The concentration of oestrogens in the CF fraction was very similar to the level of the unconjugated steroid in the plasma, the mean CF/plasma ratio was approximately one.

Our data show that continuous exposure of the studied target tissues to oestrone does not lead to an accumulation of this steroid in these tissues. Comparable exposure to oestradiol or to oestriol leads to a marked accumulation of radioactivity in the three tissues, with clear differences between them in their ability to concentrate these oestrogens. Evidently the supposed higher sensitivity of the vagina to oestrogenic stimulation is not associated with a higher accumulation of these oestrogens or their metabolites in this organ.

The findings of the subcellular and nuclear distribution show that there is a progressive increase in the ratio from the CF fraction to the CR and to nuclear fractions. These increases were only seen for oestradiol and oestriol, oestrone did not show a specific accumulation in any of the fractions studied.

SUBCELLULAR DISTRIBUTION OF OESTROGENS IN THE UTERUS DURING THE MENSTRUAL CYCLE

The availability of a method for the fractionation of tissues and for the quantitative extraction and measurement of oestrone and oestradiol enabled us to measure these steroids in subcellular fractions of normal uterine tissue, obtained during operations for myoma or for vaginal prolapse[20]. Immediately after hysterectomy parts of normal endometrium and myometrium were obtained and stored frozen at – 70°C until further processing. At the time of the operation a blood sample was taken for the measurement of plasma oestrone and oestradiol levels. Histology of the endometrium together with the course of the menstrual cycle and progesterone estimations in the plasma enabled us to divide the subjects studied into four groups according to the phase of the cycle.

The oestradiol concentration in total tissue showed large fluctuations over the cycle, the levels varied between 550 and 3500 pg/g endometrium and between 380 and 1700 pg/g myometrium at plasma concentrations varying from 40 to 110 pg/ml. Oestrone was present in smaller quantities, at mean plasma levels between 40 and 80 pg/ml the tissue concentrations were from 250 to 410 pg/g for the endometrium and 160 to 340 pg/g for myometrium. Oestradiol clearly was present in higher amounts in the endometrium than in the myometrium, except for the secretory phase of the cycle during which oestradiol and oestrone were very similar. The concentration of oestrone was lower in the myometrium at all stages of the cycle. In both tissues the levels of oestradiol and oestrone increased during the follicular phase, and the highest levels were found in the late proliferative phase. After ovulation much lower concentrations of oestradiol were seen with plasma oestradiol levels comparable to those found in the follicular phase.

The results obtained on the subcellular distribution of the steroids showed that before ovulation oestradiol was distributed over the cell compartments in a pattern highly comparable to that seen during the infusion experiments: a progressive increase in the concentration from the free fraction in the cytosol to the cytosol receptor bound to the nuclear fraction. The largest increases were seen during the late-proliferative phase of the cycle. The tissue/plasma gradient for endometrium at this stage reached a level of 1 for CF, 8 for CR and 25 for the N fraction. The myometrium showed a smaller gradient of 1 for CF, 4 for CR and 12 for N. All tissue/plasma gradients were lower for oestrone, they varied maximally from 0.7 to 2.8 in all fractions.

In the peri-ovulatory phase of the cycle there was a sharp drop in the oestradiol gradient in the CR and N fractions, both in the endometrium and in the myometrium. This decline in oestradiol was not accompanied by an increase or decrease in the oestrone concentrations.

These fairly rapid fluctuations in the subcellular oestradiol gradients cannot be explained by variations in the oestradiol receptor levels in the uterine tissues or by the induction of 17β-hydroxysteroid-dehydrogenase under the influence of the secretion of progesterone. It is more likely that the influence of progesterone on the nuclear translocation of the occupied oestradiol receptor plays an important role[21].

SUBCELLULAR OESTROGEN CONCENTRATIONS IN MALIGNANT MAMMARY TUMOURS

With the same method the total concentration and the subcellular distribution of oestradiol and oestrone were studied in a number of samples of normal breast tissue and in malignant mammary tumours. Surprisingly, total tissue concentrations were very similar in pre- and postmenopausal women, whereas plasma levels are largely different. Also the subcellular distribution of both oestrogens was comparable in both age groups. In addition, the intracellular distribution of the oestrogens was different from that in the uterine tissues: almost no accumulation of oestradiol was found in the nuclear fraction, in tumours of pre- and postmenopausal patients.

At the present time we are unable to explain in a simple way our results, which are in agreement with those reported by others. The large oestradiol gradients in tumours in postmenopausal women, not due to nuclear accumulation, are puzzling.

CONCLUSION

From the data discussed above a number of conclusions can be drawn:

- Results of measurements of steroid hormone receptors in oestrogen and progesterone target tissues have definitely increased our understanding of the processes going on in these tissues during and after stimulation by steroids;

- The concentration of oestrogen and progesterone receptors shows fluctuations during the menstrual cycle and also after menopause. These differences can largely be explained by the changes in the oestradiol and progesterone secretions by the ovary. No explanation is available for the increase in oestradiol receptors in malignant breast tumours following menopause;

- The low incidence of demonstrable receptors for progesterone in the human vagina demonstrates that induction of these receptors may not be an obligatory reaction to oestrogen stimulation by target cells;
- The specificity of the oestrogenic effects in different tissues cannot be explained by differences in the first steps in the mechanism of action. The interaction of the steroid–receptor complex with the chromatin and the processes thereafter are most probably of more importance;
- Measurements of oestrogens in subcellular compartments including the nuclear compartment show that the translocation of oestradiol together with its receptor to the nucleus of uterine cells is influenced by the progesterone secretion of the ovary;
- Although the steroid is supposed to travel in the cell in equimolar concentrations with its receptor, discrepancies are clearly visible between uterine and malignant breast tissue;
- The different behaviour of the oestrogens as far as their subcellular distribution is concerned, between uterine and breast tissue, cannot be explained at the present time.

References

1. Jensen, E. V. and Jacobson, H. I. (1962). Basic guides to the mechanism of estrogen action. *Recent Progr. Hormone Res.*, **18**, 387
2. Rao, G. S. (1981). Mode of entry of steroid and thyroid hormones into cells. *Mol. Cell. Endocrinol.*, **21**, 97
3. Müller, E. R. and Wotiz, H. H. (1979). Kinetics of estradiol entry into uterine cells. *Endocrinology*, **105**, 1107
4. Spelsberg, T. C., Littlefield, B. A., Seelke, R., Dani, G. M., Toyoda, H., Boyd-Leinen, P., Thrall, C. and Kon, O. L. (1983). Role of specific chromosomal proteins and DNA sequences in the nuclear binding sites for steroid receptors. *Recent Progr. Hormone Res.*, **39**, 463
5. Clark, J. H., Markaverich, B., Upchurch, S., Eriksson, H., Hardin, J. W. and Peck, E. J. (1980). Heterogeneity of estrogen binding sites: relationship to estrogen receptors and estrogen responses. *Recent Progr. Hormone Res.*, **36**, 89
6. Neumannova, M., Kauppila, A. and Vihko, R. (1983). Cytosol and nuclear estrogen and progestin receptors and 17β-hydroxysteroid dehydrogenase activity in normal and carcinomatous endometrium. *Obstet. Gynecol.*, **61**, 181
7. Schmidt-Gollwitzer, M., Eiletz, J., Genz, T. and Pollow, K. (1979). Determination of estradiol, estrone and progesterone in serum and myometrium: correlation with the content of sex steroid receptors and 17β-dehydroxysteroid dehydrogenase activity throughout the menstrual cycle. *J. Clin. Endocrinol. Metab.*, **49**, 370
8. Holt, J. A., Schumacher, G. F., Jacobson, H. I. and Swartz, D. P. (1979).

Estrogen and progestin binding and changes in secretions by human cervical tissues during the ovarian cycle. *Fertil. Steril.*, **32**, 170

9. Wiegerinck, M. A. H. M., Poortman, J., Agema, A. R. and Thijssen, J. H. H. (1980). Estrogen receptors in human vaginal tissue. *Maturitas*, **2**, 59
10. van Haaften, M., Wiegerinck, M. A. H. M., Poortman, J., Haspels, A. A. and Thijssen, J. H. H. (1982). Progesterone receptors in human oestrogen target tissues. *Maturitas*, **4**, 57
11. McGuire, W. L., Osborne, C. K., Clark, G. M. and Knight, W. A. (1982). Steroid hormone receptors and carcinoma of the breast. *Am. J. Physiol.*, **243**, E99
12. Schmidt-Gollwitzer, M., Genz, T., Schmidt-Gollwitzer, K., Pollow, B. and Pollow, K. (1978). Correlation between oestrogen and progesterone receptor levels, 17β-hydroxysteroid dehydrogenase activity and endometrial tissue levels of oestradiol, oestrone and progesterone in women. In Brush, M. G., King, R. J. B. and Tayor, R. W. (eds) *Endometrial Cancer*, pp. 227–241. (London: Baillière Tyndall)
13. Cao, Z. Y., Eppenberger, U., Roos, W., Torhorst, J. and Almendral, A. (1983). Cytosol estrogen and progesterone receptor levels measured in normal and pathological tissue of endometrium, endocervical mucosa and cervical vaginal portion. *Arch. Gynecol.*, **233**, 109
14. Heise, E. and Görlich, M. (1982). Estradiol receptor in human breast cancers throughout the menstrual cycle. *Oncology*, **39**, 340
15. Braunsberg, H., James, V. H. T., Jamieson, C., Desai, S., Carter, A. E. and Hulbert, M. (1974). Effect of age and menopausal status on estimates of oestrogen binding by human malignant breast tumours. *Br. Med. J.*, **4**, 745
16. Saez, S., Martin, P. M. and Chouvet, C. D. (1978). Estradiol and progesterone receptor levels in human breast adenocarcinoma in relation to plasma estrogen and progesterone levels. *Cancer Res.*, **38**, 3468
17. Hughes, A., Jacobson, H. I., Wagner, R. K. and Jungblut, P. W. (1976). Ovarian-independent fluctuations of estradiol receptor levels in mammalian tissues. *Mol. Cell. Endocrinol.*, **5**, 379
18. van Landeghem, A. A. J., Poortman, J., Faber, J. A. J. and Thijssen, J. H. H. (1981). Absence of seasonal variation of estrogen receptor levels in human breast cancer tissue. *Mol. Cell. Endocrinol.*, **23**, 265
19. Wiegerinck, M.A. H. M., Poortman, J., Donker, T. H. and Thijssen, J. H. H. (1983). *In vivo* uptake and subcellular distribution of tritium-labelled estrogens in human endometrium, myometrium and vagina. *J. Clin. Endocrinol. Metab.*, **56**, 76
20. Alsbach, G. P. J., Franck, E. R., Poortman, J. and Thijssen, J. H. H. (1983). Subcellular distribution of estradiol and estrone in human endometrium and myometrium during the menstrual cycle. *Contraception*, **27**, 409
21. MacDonald, R. G., Okulicz, W. C. and Leavitt, W. N. (1982). Progesterone-induced inactivation of nuclear estrogen receptor in the hamster uterus is mediated by acid phosphatase. *Biochem. Biophys. Res. Commun.*, **104**, 570

Chapter 7

Clinical significance of the binding between oestrogens and intra- and extracellular proteins

E. W. Bergink

The purpose of this study is to analyse whether the properties of oestrogens to interact with intra- and extracellular binding proteins can be linked to their clinical profile. At present different oestrogens are used for the treatment of oestrogen withdrawal symptoms. These compounds can be subdivided into different classes depending on structure and origin:

(1) Natural oestrogens
   (a) Human origin: oestriol and 17β-oestradiol and their ester derivatives
   (b) Equine origin: conjugated equine oestrogens composed of the 3-mono-sulphates, oestrone sulphate, equiline sulphate and 17α-dihydroequiline sulphate.

(2) Synthetic oestrogens
   (a) Steroids: ethinyloestradiol, mestranol, quinestrol
   (b) Non-steroidal compounds: diethylstilboestrol, dienoestrol.

Some of these compounds are directly active at the target cell level (e.g. oestriol, 17β-oestradiol, ethinyloestradiol, diethylstilboestrol) whereas others are precursors and require metabolic conversion prior to their interaction with the target cell (e.g. conjugated oestrogens and ester derivatives of oestriol and 17β-oestradiol must be hydrolysed and oestrone must be converted into 17β-oestradiol prior to interaction with receptor proteins in the target cell). The active compounds at the target cell level are: oestriol, 17β-oestradiol, equiline, ethinyloestradiol and the non-steroidal stilbene derivates. They can be classified as short-acting compounds (oestriol) or long-acting compounds (e.g. ethinyloestradiol) as will be discussed in this paper.

Oestrogen replacement therapy is used for relief of oestrogen withdrawal signs and symptoms (vasomotor instability, vaginal atrophy, urinary incontinence, osteoporosis) but this therapy may also have adverse effects (endometrial overstimulation and increased hepatic production of factors which will affect blood pressure and coagulation)[1]. It has been found that therapeutic effectiveness is not necessarily associated with adverse effects[2].

The comparative evaluation of different oestrogens has been reported in several studies and it was found that oestrogens can vary in their relative effectiveness to stimulate different target tissues[3]:

- Oestrogens that occur naturally in humans (e.g. oestriol and 17β-oestradiol) have the lowest potency in the hepatic system relative to their therapeutic effects[4-8], whereas ethinyloestradiol and conjugated oestrogens remain in plasma much longer than 17β-oestradiol and oestriol[3] and cause a rise in oestrogen-sensitive hepatic proteins when therapeutic doses have been ingested[4,6].

- Oestriol when administered in daily single doses of 2–8 mg has the capacity to relieve vasomotor instability and improve vaginal symptoms without endometrial overstimulation[9-14]. However, when oestriol is administered in multiple doses which give prolonged elevation of blood levels it produces the same effect on endometrium as other oestrogens[14,15].

- From animal studies it has been known for a long time that oestriol, in addition to having oestrogenic activity, may also have anti-oestrogenic activity[16]. Recently it was found this was also true in the human, namely oestriol lowered pregnancy zone protein levels in postmenopausal women[7] and inhibited the effect of 17β-oestradiol on LHRH dependent LH secretion in hypogonadal women[17].

- Studies in rats have shown that continuous administration of oestriol prior to the administration of the carcinogen DMBA significantly reduced tumour takes compared to animals treated continuously with 17β-oestradiol[18]. These results are not completely understood and cannot be explained on the basis of receptor binding studies[19]. However, recent information indicates that some of the pathophysiological effects of oestrogens may be due to formation of 16α-hydroxyoestrone which, in addition to its interaction with the oestrogen receptor, can also form covalent steroid–protein complexes through binding with the free amine groups of various proteins[20,21].

The clinical effectiveness of oestrogenic compounds depends on the following processes:

(1) Absorption and metabolism. These processes are strongly influenced by route of administration[16] and this aspect is particularly important when compounds are easily metabolized. For instance, oestriol is considered weaker than 17β-oestradiol when administered subcutaneously. When administered orally, oestriol is relatively more effective since it remains oestriol whereas 17β-oestradiol in the small bowel is mainly converted into oestrone[22]. Oestrone has to be reconverted into 17β-oestradiol in order to be active at the target cell level[23,24].

(2) Binding to plasma proteins.

(3) Binding to oestrogen receptor or oestrogen binding proteins in various target tissues.

In order to understand the mechanism by which oestrogens exert their therapeutic and adverse effects, the binding to binding sites in plasma and in various target tissues has been examined.

BINDING OF OESTROGEN TO PLASMA PROTEINS

Both natural and synthetic oestrogens interact with plasma proteins[25,26]. The major transport proteins for oestrogenic compounds are human serum albumin (HSA) and sex hormone binding globulin (SHBG); the distribution of a given compound between these carrier proteins and the non-protein-bound fraction strongly depends on the structure of the compound. The physiological rôle of the protein-bound and free fractions and especially the question whether steroid bound to serum albumin is available for biological activity is a matter of dispute. It has been found that 17β-oestradiol bound to albumin is transported into brain and uterus whereas 17β-oestradiol bound to sex hormone binding globulin is not[27].

The binding to plasma proteins in general and to SHBG in particular will also influence the metabolic clearance rate[28]. Following a single oral dose of various oestrogenic compounds different pharmacokinetic patterns have been found (Table 1). Plasma levels following administration of ethinyloestradiol (3 mg orally) show a discontinuity at 10 h which is due to the beginning of enterohepatic circulation and decline thereafter with a half-life of about 13 h[29]. It can be concluded that following oral administration of different oestrogenic compounds the appearance of peak levels and the half-life(s) of the active metabolite(s) varies considerably. Oestriol has a short half-life and disappears rapidly from the circulation whereas conjugated oestrogens, oestradiol esters and ethinyloestradiol remain longer in circulation[29–31]. The question is whether these differences in pharmacokinetic patterns can be explained on the basis of differences in plasma distribution.

We estimated the percentage of non-protein-bound oestriol, 17β-oestradiol and ethinyloestradiol *in vitro* following addition of a tracer amount of ^{3}H-oestriol, 17β-^{3}H-oestradiol and ^{3}H-ethinyloestradiol respectively in serum of women and in a solution containing human serum albumin (HSA) at a concentration normally present in serum (50 mg/ml) (Table 2). The percentages of free oestriol in native serum and in the solution containing only HSA were very similar as was the case when the percentages of free ethinyloestradiol were estimated.

Table 1 Pharmacokinetic patterns of various oestrogens; intervals between oral intake and maximal levels in plasma and the time needed for elimination of the active substance from plasma

Compound	*Peak level (time)*	*Time needed for elimination*	*Reference*
Oestriol (6 and 12 mg)	45 min	about 4–5 h	Englund *et al.*[33]
Conjugated equine oestrogens (10 mg)	3–5 h	at least 24 h	Bhavnani *et al.*[50]
Conjugated equine oestrogens (1.25 mg)	3–5 h	at least 24 h	Englund and Johansson[51]
Oestradiol-valeriate (2 mg)	3–8 h	at least 48 h	Englund and Johansson[52]

Table 2 Percentage of non-protein-bound ^{3}H-oestriol, 17β-^{3}H-oestradiol and ^{3}H-ethinyloestradiol added in tracer amount to native serum samples (fertile women) and a solution containing human serum albumin (50 mg/ml). The method used to determine the percentage free steroid is a precipitation technique[53]

	Percentage non-protein bound (Mean ± SD)		
	^{3}H-*oestriol*	17β-^{3}H-*oestradiol*	^{3}H-*ethinyloestradiol*
Native serum (n = 12)	13.8 ± 2.9	1.87 ± 0.2	1.01 ± 0.18
Human serum albumin (50 mg/ml)	14.0	2.67	0.95

The percentage of free 17β-oestradiol in native serum was lower than that in the HSA solution. These results confirm that the main carrier protein for oestriol and ethinyloestradiol is HSA[26] whereas 17β-oestradiol also binds to other carrier protein in native serum (most likely SHBG)[25].

The percentage non-protein-bound oestriol in native serum is much higher than that of 17β-oestradiol and ethinyloestradiol and this result may explain why oestriol is readily taken up by target cells[32] and rapidly removed from the circulation[33].

The pharmacodynamic profile of oestriol is that of a short-acting oestrogen; a similar profile can be derived from receptor binding studies as will be discussed in the next section.

BINDING OF OESTROGENS TO TISSUE SPECIFIC OESTROGEN BINDING PROTEINS

Current molecular models of steroid hormone action[34] suggest that the response of an oestrogenic compound is the result of its interaction with oestrogen receptors in different target cells. The initial step in the process of target cell activation is the binding of the oestrogen to the cytoplasmic oestrogen receptor. This complex undergoes an energy-dependent transformation (or activation) which enables its entry into the nucleus and its subsequent binding to chromatin[35]. As a result RNA polymerase actively increases[36] and new RNA species are transcribed; the final effect is a hormonal response which depends on the following aspects.

The biological stability of the cytoplasmic complex

The biological activity depends on the capacity of the oestrogen to form a complex sufficiently stable to be activated in the cytoplasm and translocated to the nucleus[35]. Under *in vivo* conditions it has been found that the initial binding and transformation steps are dynamic processes; occurring within 2 min at 37°C[37]. Bouton and Raynaud[38] have shown that binding affinity values estimated under non-equilibrium conditions reflect better differences in association rate constants than those estimated under equilibrium conditions. The comparative estimation of binding affinities under non-equilibrium conditions and equilibrium conditions has shown that short-acting oestrogens like oestriol and 11α-methoxyethinyloestradiol (and also epimestrol) compete more strongly with 17β-oestradiol under non-equilibrium conditions than under equilibrium conditions, whereas strong agonists such as ethinyloestradiol compete equally strongly under equilibrium and non-equilibrium conditions[19,38]. Stronger binding under non-equilibrium conditions suggests that oestriol forms complexes with the oestrogen receptor or competes with 17β-oestradiol for the formation of the receptor complex in the cytoplasm; though the stability of this complex is relatively low and insufficient for long-term oestrogenic responses. Full oestrogenic responses on early effects and weakly oestrogenic or even antagonistic responses on late effects[39] are typical of short-acting oestrogenic compounds such as oestriol. Recently Sasson and Notides[23] investigated the kinetics of the interaction between oestrogen receptor and 17β-oestradiol, oestriol and oestrone and showed that the binding of these compounds to the receptor was of a 'cooperative' nature, i.e. oestrogen binding shifts the equilibrium between inactive and active forms towards the active form. The low degree of cooperativity of the complex formation between oestriol and the oestrogen receptor and the inhibitory effect of oestriol on the cooperativity of the 17β-oestradiol–receptor complex formation can be correlated with the partial agonistic–antagonistic activities of oestriol observed *in vivo*. The biological response was not only correlated with the initial stability of the complex in the cytoplasm (which determines the capacity of the complex to be translocated to the nucleus) but also with the stability of the complex in the nucleus, as will now be discussed.

The stability of the nuclear complex

The stability of the oestrogen–receptor complex in the nucleus of the target cell has been determined *in vivo* in rat and mouse uteri and *in vitro* in human breast cancer cells.

Clark *et al.*[32] administered oestriol and 17β-oestradiol and a combination of the two to young female rats and measured the nuclear retention times of the nuclear receptor complexes. The complex formed after subcutaneous administration of oestriol (1 μg) or 17β-oestradiol (0.1 μg) plus oestriol (1 μg) was detectable for only 6 h, a period too short for proliferation of uterine cells[40] whereas the nuclear oestrogen–receptor complex resulting from a single injection of 17β-oestradiol (0.1 μg) was still detectable after 12 h.

A similar study was performed by Stern and Givner[41] who measured the time of residence of receptor complexes in the uterus following subcutaneous administration of 17β-oestradiol (2.5 μg), 17α-dihydroequiline (50 μg), oestrone sulphate (10 μg), equiline sulphate (10 μg), 17α-dihydroequiline sulphate (10 μg) or premarin (10 μg) to young female rats. The complexes formed after administration of these compounds were all detectable for periods much longer than 6 h (with the exception of those formed after administration of dihydroequiline and its sulphate) and the long-term increase in nuclear receptor content generated by those oestrogens correlated with increases in uterine growth. It was demonstrated that a single injection of 17β-oestradiol (10 μg/kg) in the mouse resulted in two increases in nuclear receptor content, 1–2 and 7–8h postinjection respectively. The second increase which is needed for full uterine growth was not observed following a single dose of oestriol (33 μg/kg)[42].

Studies in human breast cancer cells also show the relatively low stability of the oestriol–receptor complex in the nucleus. Strobl *et al.*[43] calculated the disappearance of receptor complexes from perfused cultures of human breast cancer cells and found that oestriol–receptor complexes disappeared 4 times faster than those of 17β-oestradiol. We have estimated directly the stability of the complexes between oestrogen receptor and oestriol of 17β-oestradiol in intact human MCF-7 mammary cancer cells. MCF-7 cells were incubated at 37°C with either ^{3}H-oestriol or 17β-^{3}H-oestradiol and after the oestrogen receptor sites were fully occupied (45 min) an excess of non-radioactive 17β-oestradiol was added. The results in Figure 1 show that at 37°C the half-life of the 17β-oestradiol–receptor complex was about 2–3 h, whereas a shorter half-life of 30 min was found for the oestriol–receptor complex. It can be concluded that the nuclear oestriol–receptor complex in human cells is less stable than that of 17β-oestradiol. This accounts for a shorter duration of oestriol activity since a shorter half-life of the complex reflects a shorter nuclear retention.

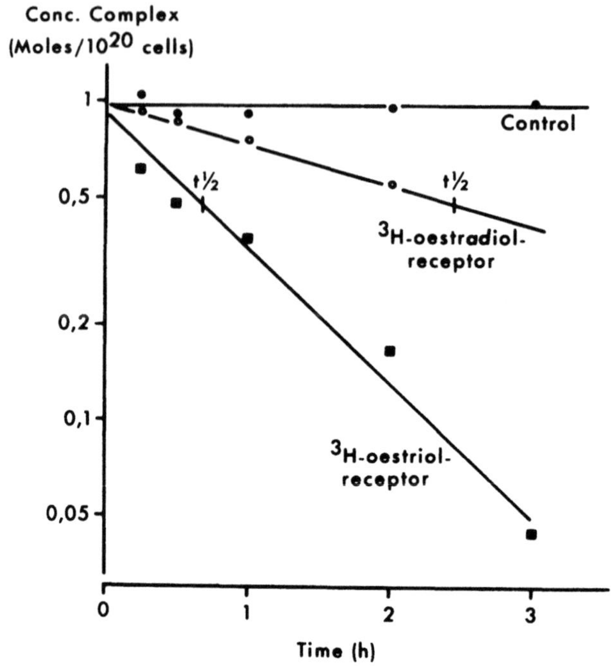

Figure 1 Dissociation of 17β-^{3}H-oestradiol and ^{3}H-oestriol from the oestrogen–receptor in the presence of excess unlabelled 17β-oestradiol in intact human MCF-7 cells at 37°C. Control is the average of the two tritiated ligands in the absence of unlabelled 17β-oestradiol. The method has been described in detail elsewhere[55]

Oestrogen receptors are not only found in the uterus but also in other target tissues. The question is whether the data obtained in uterine tissue and mammary cancer cells can be extrapolated to other target tissues. In order to answer this question we analysed the specificity of oestrogen receptors in different target tissues.

Specificity of oestrogen receptors in different target tissues

Oestrogen receptors have been found in the various target tissues known to be affected by oestrogen replacement therapy: human myometrium and endometrium[24], human breast cancer tissue[44], human liver[45], vaginal epithelium and urethra[46], human gingiva[47] and the trigone area of the human bladder[48]. The specificity of the receptors present in human myometrium, endometrium and breast cancer tissue was found to be similar[49]. The specificity of the oestrogen receptor in human myometrium was also similar to that of the oestrogen receptor found in rat uterus[44].

Oestrogen target tissues may also contain high affinity binding proteins with specificities different from that of the oestrogen receptor. Recently we have found in the human vagina a binding protein with high affinity for the natural oestrogens 17β-oestradiol, 17α-oestradiol and oestriol and low affinity for diethylstilboestrol[44,49]. The function of this protein is unknown; its presence in the human vagina could explain the preferential vaginotrophic effects of oestriol.

It may be concluded that binding studies with plasma proteins and receptor binding studies explain why oestriol, when administered in single or wide-spaced doses (interval more than 12 h), should be regarded as a short-acting oestrogen rather than a weak-acting oestrogen. A similar conclusion was obtained in pharmacological studies[16] which showed that late oestrogenic effects such as stimulation of uterine growth depend on the route of administration and the dosing regimen, and are not observed after single administration of a short-acting oestrogen.

References

1. Weinstein, M. C. (1980). Estrogen use in postmenopausal women – costs, risks, and benefits. *N. Engl. J. Med.*, **303**, 308
2. Follingstad, A. H. (1978). Estriol, the forgotten estrogen? *J. Am. Med. Assoc.*, **239**, 29
3. Meier, P. and Landau, R. L. (1980). Estrogen replacement therapy. *J. Am. Med. Assoc.*, **243**, 1658
4. Geola, F. L., Frumar, A. M., Tataryn, I. V., Lu, K. H., Hershman, J. M., Eggena, P., Sambhi, M.P. and Judd, H. L. (1980). Biological effects of various doses of conjugated equine estrogens in postmenopausal women. *J. Clin. Endocrinol. Metab.*, **51**, 620
5. Bergink, E. W., Crona, N., Dahlgren, E. and Samsioe, G. (1981). Effect of oestriol, oestradiol valerate and ethinyloestradiol on serum proteins in oestrogen-deficient women. *Maturitas*, **3**, 241
6. Maschak, C. A., Lobo, R. A., Dozono-Takano, R., Eggena, P., Nakamura, R. M., Brenner, P. F. and Mishell, D. R. (1982). Comparison of pharmacodynamic properties of various estrogen formulations. *Am. J. Obstet. Gynecol.*, **144**, 511
7. Helgason, S. (1982). Estrogen replacement therapy after the menopause. *Acta Obstet. Gynecol. Scand. (Suppl.)* **107**
8. Schwartz, U., Volger, H., Schneller, E., Moltz, L. and Hammerstein, J. (1983). Effects of various replacement oestrogens on hepatic transcortin synthesis in climacteric women. *Acta Endocrinol.*, **102**, 103
9. Lauritzen, C. (1973). The management of the premenopausal and the postmenopausal patient. In van Keep, P. A. and Lauritzen, C. (eds) *Frontiers of Hormone Res.*, Vol. 2, *Ageing and Estrogens*, pp. 2–21. (Basel: Karger)

10. Heuser, H. P. and Staemmler, H. -J. (1973). Histological investigations into the effect of oestriol succinate on the corpus uteri in postmenopausal women. *Arzneim. Forsch. (Drug Res.)*, **23**, 558
11. Myhre, E. (1978). Endometrial response to different estrogens. In van Keep, P. A. and Lauritzen, C. (eds) *Frontiers of Hormone Res.*, Vol. 5, *Estrogen Therapy*, pp. 126–144. (Basel: Karger)
12. Tzingounis, V. A., Aksu, F. and Greenblatt, R. B. (1978). Estriol in the management of the menopause. *J. Am. Med. Assoc.*, **239**, 1638
13. Campagnoli, C., Prelato Tousijn, L. P., Belforte, P., Ferruzzi, L., Dolfin, A. M. and Morra, G. (1981). Effects of conjugated equine oestrogens and oestriol on blood clotting, plasma lipids and endometrial proliferation in postmenopausal women. *Maturitas*, **3**, 135
14. Punnonen, R. and Söderström, K. -O. (1983). The effect of estriol succinate therapy on the endometrial morphology in postmenopausal women: the significance of fractionation of the dose. *Eur. J. Obstet. Gynec. Reprod. Biol.*, **14**, 217
15. Englund, D. E. and Johansson, E. D. B. (1980). Endometrial effect of oral estriol treatment in postmenopausal women. *Acta Obstet. Gynecol. Scand.*, **59**, 449
16. van der Vies, J. (1982). The pharmacology of oestriol. *Maturitas*, **4**, 291
17. Römmler, A. and Hammerstein, J. (1981). Wirkungsvergleich verschiedener Östrogene an der hypergonadotropen Hypophyse. *Arch. Gynecol.*, **232**, 648
18. Wotiz, H. H. and Müller, R. E. Estriol as an anticarcinogenic agent: experimental studies on DMBA induced breast cancer. *J. Steriod Biochem.* (In press)
19. Bergink, E. W. (1980). Oestriol receptor interactions : their biological importance and therapeutic implications. *Acta Endocrinol. (Suppl.)* **233**, 9
20. Bucala, R., Fishman, J. and Cerami, A. (1982). Formation of covalent adducts between cortisol and 16α-hydroxyestrone and protein: Possible role in the pathogenesis of cortisol toxicity and systemic lupus erythematosus. *Proc. Natl. Acad. Sci. USA*, **79**, 3320
21. Fishman, J. and Martucci, C. (1980). Biological properties of 16α-hydroxyestrone: implications in estrogen physiology and pathophysiology. *J. Clin. Endocrinol. Metab.*, **51**, 611
22. Yen, S. S. C., Martin, P. L., Burnier, M., Czekala, N. M., Greaney, M. O. and Callantine, M. R. (1975). Circulating estradiol, estrone and gonadotropin levels following the administration of orally active 17β-estradiol in postmenopausal women. *J. Clin. Endocrinol. Metab.*, **40**, 518
23. Sasson, S. and Notides, A. C. (1983). Estriol and estrone interaction with the estrogen receptor. *J. Biol. Chem.*, **258**, 8113, 8118
24. Wiegerinck, M. H. A. M., Poortman, J., Donker, T. H. and Thijssen, J. H. H. (1983). *In vivo* uptake and subcellular distribution of tritium-labeled estrogens in human endometrium, myometrium, and vagina. *J. Clin. Endrocrinol. Metab.*, **56**, 76
25. Dunn, J. F., Nisula, B. C. and Rodbard, D. (1981). Transport of steroid hormones: binding of endogenous steroids to both testosterone-binding globulin and corticosteroid-binding globulin in human plasma. *J. Clin. Endocrinol. Metab.*, **53**, 58
26. Pugeat, M. M., Dunn, J. F. and Nisula, B. C. (1981). Transport of steroid hormones: Interaction of 70 drugs with testosterone-binding globulin and corticosteroid-binding globulin in human plasma. *J. Clin. Endocrinol. Metab.*, **53**, 69
27. Laufer, L. R., Gambone, J. C., Chaudhuri, G., Pardridge, W. M. and Judd, H. L. (1983). The effect of membrane permeability and binding by human

serum proteins on sex steroid influx into the uterus. *J. Clin. Endocrinol. Metab.*, **56**, 1282

28. Vermeulen, A. and Ando, S. (1978). Metabolic clearance rate and interconversion of androgens and the influence of the free androgen fraction. *J. Clin. Endocrinol. Metab.*, **48**, 320
29. Back, D. J., Bolt, H. M., Breckenridge, A. M., Crawford, F. E., L'E Orme, M., Rowe, P. H. and Schindler, A. E. (1980). The pharmacokinetics of a large (3 mg) oral dose of ethinylestradiol in women. *Contraception*, **21**, 145
30. Whittaker, P. G., Morgan, M. R. A., Dean, P. D. G., Cameron, E. H. D. and Lind, T. (1980). Serum equilin, oestrone and oestradiol levels in postmenopausal women receiving conjugated equine oestrogens. *Lancet*, **1**, 14
31. Akpoviroro, J. and Fotherby, K. (1980). Assay of ethinyloestradiol in human serum and its binding to plasma proteins. *J. Steroid Biochem.*, **13**, 773
32. Clark, J. H., Paszko, Z. and Peck, E. J. (1977). Nuclear binding and retention of the receptor estrogen complex: Relation to the agonistic and antagonistic properties of estriol. *Endocrinology*, **100**, 91
33. Englund, D. E., Elamsson, K. B. and Johansson, E. D. B. (1982). Bioavailability of oestriol. *Acta Endocrinol.*, **99**, 136
34. Chan, L. and O'Malley, B. W. (1976). Mechanism of action of the sex steroid hormones. *N. Engl. J. Med.*, **294**, 1322, 1372, 1430
35. Weichman, B. M. and Notides, A. C. (1980). Estrogen receptor activation and the dissociation kinetics of estradiol, estriol and estrone. *Endocrinology*, **106**, 434
36. Webster, R. A. and Hamilton, T. H. (1976). Comparative effects of estradiol-17 and estriol on uterine RNA polymerases I, II, and III *in vivo*. *Biochem. Biophys. Res. Commun.*, **69**, 737
37. Müller, R. E. and Wotiz, H. H. (1979). Kinetics of estradiol entry into uterine cells. *Endocrinology*, **105**, 1107
38. Bouton, M. M. and Raynaud, J. P. (1978). The relevance of kinetic parameters in the determination of specific binding to the estrogen receptor. *J. Steroid Biochem.*, **9**, 9
39. Clark, J. H., Peck, E. J., Hardin, J. W. and Erikson, H. (1978). The biology and pharmacology of estrogen receptor binding: Relation to uterine growth. In O'Malley, B. W. and Birnbaumer, L. (eds) *Receptors and Hormone Action*, Vol. II, pp. 1–15. (New York: Academic Press)
40. Stormshak, F., Leake, R., Wertz, N. and Gorski, J. (1976). Stimulatory and inhibitory effects of estrogen on uterine DNA synthesis. *Endocrinology*, **99**, 1501
41. Stern, M. D. and Givner, M. L. (1978). Studies on the mechanism of action of conjugated equine oestrogens. In Brush, M. G., King, R. J. B. and Taylor, R. W. (eds) *Endometrial Cancer*, pp. 309–322. (London: Baillière Tyndall)
42. Korach, K., Fox-Davies, C. and Baker, V. (1980). Differential response to estriol and estradiol in the mouse uterus: Correlation to an additional nuclear event. *Endocrinology*, **106**, 1900
43. Strobl, J. S., Monaco, M. E. and Lippman, M. E. (1980). The rôle of intracellular equilibria and the effect of antiestrogens on estrogen–receptor dissociation kinetics from perfused cultures of human breast cancer cells. *Endocrinology*, **107**, 450
44. Bergink, E. W., Kloosterboer, H. J., van der Velden, W. H. M., van der Vies, J. and de Winter, M. S. (1983). Specificity of oestrogen receptors in different tissues in comparison to that of an oestrogen binding protein in human vagina. In Jasonni, V. M., Nenci, I. and Flamigni, C. (eds) *Steroids and Endometrial Cancer*, pp. 77–84. (New York: Raven Press)

45. Eisenfeld, A. J., Aten, R. F. and Weinberger, M. J. (1978). Oral contraceptives – possible mediation of side effects via an estrogen receptor in liver. *Biochem. Pharmacol.*, **27**, 2571
46. Ingelman-Sundberg, A., Rosén, J., Gustafsson, S. A. and Carlström, K. (1981). Cytosol estrogen receptors in the urogenital tissues in stress-incontinent women. *Acta Obstet. Gynecol. Scand.*, **60**, 585
47. Vittek, J., Hernandez., M. R., Wenk, E. J., Rappaport, S. C. and Southren, A. L. (1982). Specific estrogen receptors in human gingiva. *J. Clin. Endocrinol. Metab.*, **54**, 608
48. Saez, S. and Martin, P. M. (1981). Evidence of estrogen receptors in the trigone area of human urinary bladder. *J. Steroid Biochem.*, **15**, 317
49. Bergink, E. W., Kloosterboer, H. J. and van der Vies, J. (1983). Oestrogen binding protein in the female genital tract. *J. Steroid Biochem.* (In press)
50. Bhavnani, B. R., Sarda, I. R. and Woolever, C. A. (1981). Radioimmunoassay of plasma equilin and estrone in postmenopausal women following administration of Premarin. *J. Clin. Endocrinol. Metab.*, **52**, 741
51. Englund, D. E. and Johansson, E. D. B. (1978). Plasma levels of oestrone, oestradiol and gonadotrophins in postmenopausal women after oral and vaginal administration of conjugated equine oestrogens. *Br. J. Obstet. Gynaecol.*, **85**, 957
52. Englund, D. E. and Johansson, E. D. B. (1977). Pharmacokinetic and pharmacodynamic studies on oestradiol valerianate administered orally to postmenopausal women. *Acta Obstet. Gynecol. Scand. (Suppl.).* **65**, 27
53. Bergink, E. W., Holma, P. and Pyörälä, T. (1981). Effects of oral contraceptive combinations containing levonorgestrel or desogestrel on serum proteins and androgen binding. *Scand. J. Clin. Lab. Invest.*, **41**, 663
54. Bergink, E. W., van Meel, F., Turpijn, E.W. and van der Vies, J. (1983). Binding of progestagens to receptor proteins in MCF-7 cells. *J. Steroid Biochem.*, **19**, 1563.

Chapter 8

Sex steroids and lipoproteins*

U. Larsson-Cohn and L. Wallentin

INTRODUCTION

The most important factors for development of cardiovascular disease are increasing age, male gender, lipoprotein disturbances, arterial hypertension and smoking. Premenopausal women have a more advantageous pattern of serum lipoproteins than males and there is a considerably lower frequency of cardiovascular disease in females than in males of comparable ages. The variation in lipoprotein distribution between genders is mainly due to their different production of sex steroids.

Exogenously administered sex steroids influence the lipoprotein metabolism. In order to avoid increased risk of cardiovascular disease it is important that the lipoprotein alterations that may occur are taken into consideration when such treatment is considered.

PHYSIOLOGICAL BACKGROUND

In blood the lipids are transported as parts of so-called lipoprotein complexes. The lipoproteins are commonly fractionated to their hydrogenated density. The least dense particles are the triglyceride-rich chylomicrons and very low density lipoproteins (VLDL) which

* This review is based on the paper (in Swedish) 'Sexualsteroider och lipoproteiner' by Lars Wallentin, that was read at the symposium 'Klimakteriet och dess behandling' in Linköping, Sweden, on September 9, 1982

transport fat from the gastrointestinal tract and the liver respectively. After the VLDL particle has delivered triglycerides for metabolism in the musculature or for storage there remains a more dense and cholesterol-rich complex, the low density lipoprotein (LDL) particle. The LDL complexes are slowly metabolized and partly settled in various tissues including the arterial walls. Raised plasma concentrations of VLDL and LDL may thus enhance the deposition of cholesterol in the vessel walls. The high density lipoproteins (HDL), which are rich in protein and phospholipids, constitute the most dense lipoprotein fraction. HDL particles seem to take part in the transport of cholesterol to the liver from peripheral tissues and from catabolizing lipoproteins of lower density.

There is convincing epidemiological evidence that raised plasma levels of LDL and VLDL increase the risk for the development of cardiovascular disease while a high concentration of HDL reduces this risk[1].

Age and sex have a profound influence on the concentration and composition of the serum lipoproteins. Prepubertal boys and girls have similar lipoprotein patterns but after puberty males develop lower HDL levels than females. In the fertile age men have higher concentrations of LDL and VLDL than females of similar age. After the menopause the cholesterol is increased in women due to the fact that the LDL levels reach concentrations that are higher than in men of similar age. These differences between the sexes are probably mainly due to the production of sex steroids.

EFFECTS OF EXOGENOUS SEX STEROIDS ON THE LIPOPROTEIN PATTERN

Table 1 summarizes the main effects of the different sex steroids on the lipoprotein pattern. Table 2 points out other factors that are of importance for the consequences of sex steroid treatment on the plasma

Table 1 Effects of sex steroids on lipoproteins

	HDL	LDL	VLDL
Oestrogen	↑	↓	↑*
Progestogen	↓	↑*	↓
Androgen	↓	↑*	↓

* Only in high dose

Table 2 Additional factors of importance for effects of sex steroids on lipoproteins

Quantity – dose and potency of the drug
Quality – chemical structure of the drug
Route of aministration
Basic hormonal and metabolic state of the recipient

lipoproteins. These points will be further discussed below. The present discussion will mainly be based on studies from our own group[2-8] although comparable results have been obtained in some other laboratories.

DOSE AND POTENCY OF THE OESTROGEN

In the mid-seventies we[2] showed that 50 μg of ethinyloestradiol had a more pronounced influence on the lipoprotein pattern than 2 mg of oestradiol valerate. The former drug raised the HDL 20–40% and reduced the atherogenic cholesterol, e.g. the cholesterol within the two lighter lipoprotein fractions, by 25%. Oestradiol valerate gave only a 10% increase of the HDL-cholesterol and had no influence on the LDL and VLDL levels. As 50 μg of ethinyloestradiol has a much higher oestrogen potency than 2 mg of oestradiol valerate the different influences on the lipoproteins seemed quantitative rather than qualitative. Further support for a dose–response relation of postmenopausal oestrogen treatment was gained in a recent study[3] in which a raised dose of 17β-oestradiol increased the levels of triglycerides and HDL_3-cholesterol.

We conclude that the partly inconsistent results concerning the effects of oestrogens on plasma lipoproteins can mainly be explained by differences in doses and potency of the oestrogens that have been employed.

ROUTE OF ADMINISTRATION

Oral 17β-oestradiol is rapidly absorbed from the gut giving high initial oestrogen concentration in the liver. The oestradiol is in part immediately metabolized to oestrone so that the plasma levels of oestrone are considerably higher than those of oestradiol. As the half-lives of the two oestrogens are fairly short the concentrations in plasma are low 24 hours after intake of a tablet.

Percutaneously given 17β-oestradiol is absorbed much more slowly and there is less conversion into oestrone. This route of administration is also associated with a certain depot effect due to retention of oestrogen in the cutis and subcutis. Thus percutaneous treatment gives lower but more stable and lasting levels of oestrone and oestradiol. The plasma concentrations of the two oestrogens are about equal.

In order to investigate if the two routes of administration had any metabolic consequences we studied the plasma lipoproteins of postmenopausal women treated with 17β-oestradiol either orally (daily dose 2–4 mg) or percutaneously (daily dose 3 mg)[3]. Both treatments had beneficial effects on the postmenopausal symptoms and gave comparable reductions of the plasma gonadotrophin levels. The women on oral medication showed a 15% increase of the HDL-cholesterol and a similar reduction of the LDL-cholesterol while the percutaneous treatment had no significant influence on the plasma lipoproteins.

We conclude that percutaneous oestrogens have less effect on the lipoprotein metabolism than oral treatment. The difference is probably related to lower oestradiol levels and to the fact that the first liver passage is avoided during percutaneous treatment.

QUALITY OF THE PROGESTOGEN

Metabolic effects of progestogens may vary due to the chemical structure of the hormones. Hirvonen *et al.*[9] reported that the testosterone-derived progestogens norethisterone and levonorgestrel reduced the plasma HDL levels of postmenopausal women. The progesterone-derived medroxyprogesterone acetate had no such effects. We[4] have obtained similar results in postmenopausal women following percutaneous treatment with oestradiol, as 120 μg of levonorgestrel reduced the HDL_2 levels by about 30% whereas 300 mg of oral progesterone had no influence on the HDL_2 level. Levonorgestrel also reduced the VLDL triglycerides but progesterone did not.

The effects of progestogens on the lipoprotein metabolism are dose-dependent[5]. In women receiving danazol in the very high but common anti-endometriosis dose of 600 mg daily, the HDL-cholesterol levels were reduced by 60% and the HDL_2-cholesterol by as much as 80–90%.

Thus it might be concluded that testosterone-derived progestogens reduce the HDL and VLDL levels while progestogens of the progesterone-type have less influence on the lipoprotein metabolism. The alterations are dose-dependent.

BASAL HORMONAL AND METABOLIC SITUATION

Oestrogens given to women with hereditary lipid-metabolic disturbances might dramatically influence the lipoprotein metabolism. Subjects with hypertriglyceridaemia type IV can respond with a severe rise of the triglyceride levels and even with abdominal pains and with pancreatitis. Similar reactions have been reported in pregnant women with hereditary hypertriglyceridaemia types IV or V. On the other hand females with hyperlipidaemia type III and postmenopausal women with hypercholesterolaemia type II may show an amelioration of the hyperlipoproteinaemia following oestrogen administration. Such medication has therefore been suggested for treatment of hyperlipidaemia in postmenopausal women[10]. There are also data that suggest that sex steroids may influence the lipoprotein pattern differently in pre- and postmenopausal subjects[11].

COMBINED ORAL CONTRACEPTIVE TREATMENT

The influence on the lipid metabolism of combined oral contraceptives depends on the absolute and relative doses of the two components. In a randomized prospective study[6] the effects of four different combinations of levonorgestrel and ethinyloestradiol were compared. Combinations with a high dose of levonorgestrel and a high weight-per-weight ratio between the progestogen and the oestrogen reduced the HDL-cholesterol significantly. However, it was shown that it was possible to balance the doses of the progestogen and the oestrogen in such a way that the combination had no effect on the HDL-cholesterol level.

EFFECTS OF THE ENDOGENOUS SEX STEROID PRODUCTION

Both the male puberty and exogenously given steroids with androgenic properties reduce the HDL levels. It could therefore be expected that the endogenous testosterone production should diminish HDL. However, this has so far not been proven. On the contrary, several investigators have found a positive correlation between the plasma levels of HDL and testosterone[12]. In one study concerning males with carcinoma of the prostate, orchidectomy strongly reduced the plasma testosterone but had no significant effects on the plasma lipoprotein levels[7].

The physiological reduction of oestrogen production in the postmenopause could be expected to increase the LDL and reduce the HDL levels. In the postmenopause the LDL levels are increased while the HDL concentration is unchanged. It might be asked if the simultaneous loss of progesterone production would explain the unaltered HDL level in the postmenopause.

Pregnancy offers an opportunity to study the effects of changes in production of endogenous hormones. In a truly prospective investigation, in which all participants were enrolled in the study before they conceived, 20 women were followed throughout their pregnancy and also during lactation[8]. From early in pregnancy until term, triglyceride levels were raised in all the lipoprotein fractions. There was also increased cholesterol in the HDL fraction. During the latter part of the gestational period there was a marked elevation of the LDL level. The rises of triglycerides and HDL are probably consequences of the raised oestrogen production. The cause of the high LDL level in pregnancy is at present less clear.

We conclude that there are situations when probable effects of endogenous sex steroid production on the lipoprotein metabolism are not quite in concord with those observed during treatment with exogenous steroids. This may be explained by the effects of other centrally or peripherally produced substances that interfere with the lipid transport and lipoprotein metabolism.

References

1. Levy, R. I. (1981). Cholesterol, lipoproteins, apoproteins and heart disease: Present status and future prospects. *Clin. Chem.*, **27**, 653
2. Wallentin, L. and Larsson-Cohn, U. (1977). Metabolic and hormonal effects of postmenopausal estrogen replacement treatment. II. Plasma lipids. *Acta Endocrinol.*, **86**, 597
3. Fåhraeus, L., Larsson-Cohn, U. and Wallentin, L. (1982). Lipoproteins during oral and cutaneous administration of oestradiol-17β to menopausal women. *Acta Endocrinol.*, **101**, 597

4. Fåhraeus, L., Laesson-Cohn, U. and Wallentin, L. L-Norgestrel and progesterone have different influences on plasma lipoproteins. *Eur. J. Clin. Invest* (In press)
5. Fåhraeus, L., Larsson-Cohn, U. and Wallentin, L. (1984). Rapid and reversible alterations of LDL, HDL, HDL2 and HDL3 during and after danazol treatment. *Fertil. Steril.* (In press)
6. Larsson-Cohn, U., Fåhraeus, L., Wallentin, L. and Zador, G. (1981). Lipoprotein changes may be minimized by proper composition of a combined oral contraceptive. *Fertil. Steril.*, **35**, 172
7. Wallentin, L. and Varenhorst, E. (1981). Plasma lipoproteins during antiandrogen treatment by estrogens or orchidectomy in men with protastic carcinoma. *Horm. Metab. Res.*, **13**, 293
8. Fåhraeus, L., Larsson-Cohn, U. and Wallentin, L. Pronounced elevations of HDL2, LDL and VLDL in human pregnancy – results from the first truly prospective study. (Submitted for publication)
9. Hirvonen, E., Mälkönen, M. and Manninen, V. (1981). Effects of different progestogens on lipoproteins during postmenopausal replacement therapy. *N. Engl. J. Med.*, **304**, 560
10. Tikkanen, M. J., Nikkilä, E.A. and Vartiainen, E. (1978). Natural oestrogen as an effective treatment for type-II hyperlipoproteinaemia in postmenopausal women. *Lancet*, **2**, 490
11. Heiss, G., Tamir, I., Davis, C. E., Tyroler, H. A., Rifkind, B. M., Schonfeld, G., Jacobs, D. and Frantz, I. D. (1980). Lipoprotein-cholesterol distributions in selected North-American populations: The lipid research clinics program prevalence study. *Circulation*, **61**, 302
12. Mendoza, S.G., Osuna, A., Zerpa, A., Gartside, P. S. and Glueck, C. J. (1981). Hypertriglyceridemia and hypoalphalipoproteinemia in azoospermic and oligospermic young men: Relationships of endogenous testosterone to triglyceride and high density lipoprotein cholesterol metabolism. *Metabolism*, **30**, 481

Chapter 9

Oestrone sulphatase activity in normal and pathological endometria

G. Agnani, O. Prost, A. Petitjean and G. L. Adessi

INTRODUCTION

Recent studies suggest that oestrone sulphate plays the role of prehormone in different human or animal tissues. The first stage of its intracellular activation is its hydrolysis by membrane-bound oestrone sulphatase. In view of the role played by oestrogens in the development of endometrial hyperplasia, the oestrone sulphatase activity was measured in normal and pathological endometria: endometrial hyperplasia and neoplasia.

MATERIAL

The reference group used consisted of 23 biopsies of morphologically normal endometria. The tissues were collected during laparoscopy or from cases of vaginal prolapse. The 23 patients presented no sign of uterine bleeding or infection. No distinction was made in cyclic women between the follicular and luteal phases.

In pathological biopsies, oestrone sulphatase activity was measured in 19 cases of endometrial hyperplasia and three cases of endometrial neoplasia.

The hyperplasia were classified according to Sommers into four subgroups:[1]

- simple hyperplasia : 11 cases
- cystic hyperplasia : 1 case
- polyps : 4 cases
- adenomatous hyperplasia : 3 cases

In three cases of polyps the biopsy was taken from normal tissue. In the fourth case, two biopsies were performed: one biopsy on the normal area and the other on a mild hyperplastic area. As hyperplasia can benefit from progestogen treatment the sulphatase activity was measured in patients treated with lynestrenol, demegestone or chlormadinone acetate from the 15th to the 25th day of the menstrual cycle.

METHOD

The oestrone sulphatase assay has been previously described[3]. For each biopsy, part of the fresh tissue was fixed in Bouin's solution for routine histological examination.

RESULTS

Sulphatase activity was significantly increased in simple and cystic hyperplasia (Table 1). In normal endometrial biopsies associated with polyps, oestrone sulphatase activity was in the same range as in the

Table 1 Oestrone sulphatase activity measured according to the standard assay in normal and pathological endometrial biopsies

Type of endometria	*n*	*Age* (years)[a]		*Oestrone sulphatase activity*[b] (pmol E_1/min/mg protein)
Normal endometrium	23	33.0	$p < 0.01$	23.13 ± 8.44 (4.9–43)
Simple hyperplasia	11	45.2		64.20 ± 22.47 (42.1–110)
Cystic hyperplasia	1	60		47.20
Normal endometrium associated with polyps	4	45.5		19.10 ± 5.33 (13.2–25.3)
Adenomatous hyperplasia	3	42.0		25.30 ± 11.4 (14.3–37.2)
Endometrial neoplasia	3	60.6		30.30 ± 9.57 (19.8–38.6)

Endometrial biopsies were classified according to Sommers[1]

[a] Mean

[b] Mean ± SD (extreme values)

Table 2 Oestrone sulphatase activity measured in endometrial biopsies (simple hyperplasia) of progestogen-treated patients

Progestogen	*n*	*Age* (years)[a]	*Oestrone sulphatase activity*[b] (pmol E_1/min/mg protein)
Lynestrenol	2	39.5	86.2 ± 46.9
Demegestone	1	44	46.4
Chlormadinone acetate	4	43.7	24.8 ± 9.57

[a] Mean
[b] Mean ± SD

reference group. In one patient, two endometrial biopsies were simultaneously performed. One specimen was slightly hyperplastic and the other was judged as normal. Higher oestrone sulphatase activity was found in the first specimen. No increase was found in the adenomatous hyperplasia, nor in the three cases of endometrial neoplasia. After progestogen treatment (Table 2) oestrone sulphatase activities were normal whenever the hyperplasia disappeared; in the other cases the activities remained at an increased level.

COMMENT

The pathogenesis of endometrial hyperplasia is not entirely understood. However, from a histological point of view the simple hyperplasia corresponds to an accentuation of the modifications which are observed at the end of the proliferative phase. Therefore, current research concerns:

- circulating oestrogen levels
- oestrogen receptors
- enzymes which control the metabolism of oestrogens

The first two items have not provided a conclusive explanation. Among the enzymes, two are progesterone induced and vary according to the menstrual cycle: 17β-oestradiol-dehydrogenase and oestrone sulphotransferase. 17β-E_2-dehydrogenase is probably not implicated in the genesis of hyperplasia[2]. The third enzyme, oestrone sulphatase, converts oestrone sulphate into oestrone. Its potential effects should be taken into account, since oestrone sulphate is quantitatively the major circulating oestrogen. Oestrone sulphatase is a membrane-bound enzyme. Moreover clinical observation[3] has confirmed that the sulphatase activity does not vary in relation to the menstrual cycle, that the activity increases in patients with an irregular cycle and that, rather strangely, the activity also increases in patients with chronic salpingitis.

Using *in vitro* incubation techniques, it has also been possible to show that the sulphatase activity is inhibited by high concentrations (50 μmol/l) of the major unconjugated steroids; the most potent inhibitor being oestradiol. Oestrone sulphatase activity was also strongly inhibited by copper acetate. Our results show that oestrone sulphatase activity is consistently increased by hyperplastic endometrium. Such an increase is not found in adenomatous hyperplasia nor in neoplasia.

Only the use of the electronic microscopy can, as Ferenczy has demonstrated[4], distinguish between adenomatous hyperplasia and *in situ* carcinoma. In the latter case there is a large decrease of the organelle membranes, i.e. microvilli, endoplasmic reticulum, Golgi and mitochondria complexes. This decrease is more obvious in adenocarcinoma. Thus the transformations accompanying adenocarcinoma do not correspond to the histological changes found in hyperplasia that appear to be directly linked to hyperoestrogenic states. In our cases the use of the optic microscopy was unable to distinguish between the adenomatous hyperplasia and *in situ* carcinoma.

Our results also suggest that synthetic progestogens have different influences on the activity rate. In peri- and postmenopausal women, the hydrolysis of plasma oestrone sulphate, the major circulating oestrogen, by oestrone sulphatase, provides a continuous supply of unconjugated oestrone particularly when oestrone sulphatase activity is increased. Due to the low progesterone levels an unopposed oestrogenic stimulation may be responsible for a continuous endometrial proliferation and a simple hyperplasia.

References

1. Sommers, S. C. (1982). Defining the pathology of endometrial hyperplasia, dysplasia and carcinoma. *Pathol. Res. Pract.*, **174**, 175
2. Gurpide, E., Gusberg, S. B. and Tseng, L. (1976). Estradiol binding and metabolism in human endometrial hyperplasia and adenocarcinoma. *J. Steroid Biochem.*, **7**, 891
3. Prost, O. and Adessi, G. L. (1983). Estrone and dehydroepiandrosterone sulfatase activities in normal and pathological human endometrium biopsies. *J. Clin. Endocrinol. Metab.*, **56**, 653
4. Ferenczy, A. (1977). Ultrastructural pathology of the uterus. In Wynn, R. M. (ed.) *Biology of the Uterus*, pp. 545–585. (New York: Plenum Press)

Chapter 10

Considerations on the output of pituitary gonadotrophins in the perimenopause

D. Vandekerckhove, M. Dhont and R. Serreyn

Unlike the menarchal age, the timing of the onset of the climacteric in our studied population displayed no variation over a considerable period of time. For a given population a statistically predictable mean can easily be determined. The onset occurs invariably at the very end of the fourth decade of life.

In an era of contraceptive behaviour, however, it does not actually tell the individual patient what she wants to know if the end of reproductive life has come, or is in sight. Although fertility drops sharply with increasing age the possibility of ovulatory cycles being present remains high[1] and is related to cycle length[2].

In the well-established postmenopausal state the clinical features and biochemical findings offer no difficulties regarding correct diagnosis of the condition. Apart from the clinical data which are so different from the data relating to cyclic events in younger age, the lasting hypergonadotrophic and hypo-oestrogenic values are highly characteristic.

In some cases a sudden onset of the postmenopausal condition can occur, in a way not so different from the events resulting from surgical castration. Most often, however, the very last menstruation is preceded by a period, variable in length, marked by aberrant menstrual patterns[3] mostly due to luteal insufficiency, changes in the follicular phase and anovulation[4].

The hormonal events of the menstrual cycle are well known and the steady state of high gonadotrophins and low oestrogens in the postmenopausal condition well established, but much less is known about the period at the end of reproductive life which sometimes precedes the onset at the menopause.

Recently some authors have drawn attention to the hormonal condition in the perimenopausal period[2,5-8]. For obvious reasons the number of patients in the reproductive studies have been small. Cycles of women in the transitional period sometimes varied widely in length, sometimes not, and they displayed several types of hormonal patterns. In some, no clear hormonal changes were present whereas in others monotrophic elevations of FSH or LH or of both gonadotrophins could be found.

Although the average cycle length did not differ significantly mean serum levels increased with age in all phases of the cycles[9]. A striking phenomenon was the not uncommon association of high gonadotrophin levels (FSH) with elevated oestrogens.

To explain this finding several hypotheses have been put forward, including increasing age, related disturbed feedback mechanism, the lowering of follicular inhibin, etc. Even an endometrial factor in determining the final absence of menstruation has been considered.

The finding of postmenopausal values of biochemical parameters offers no guarantee of the postmenopausal state and at a given time its diagnosis can be missed. In the transitional period from a practical point of view, and based on clinical data alone, the probability that the menopause is present, is related to the duration of the amenorrhoea, and for a given interval with age[10].

In the past too much attention has been paid, in our institution as well as in others, to isolated elevations of gonadotrophin levels in amenorrhoeic women in the transitional period. Far from being in the well-established menopausal condition some of them continued to menstruate with changing levels of gonadotrophins and oestrogens.

The foregoing data from the literature and our own experience incited us to explore the hormonal condition of women in the transitional perimenopausal period by determining serum levels of gonadotrophins and of oestradiol.

MATERIAL

Out of more than 1000 perimenopausal patients, only those women

Table 1 Perimenopausal women in the study and hormonal treatment

	n
Continuous progestogen treatment	43
Intermittent progestogen and combined hormonal treatment	28
No treatment	79
Total	150

who could be followed during the transitional period up to one year after the established menopause were selected for study. During the interval at least one clinical and hormonal examination was performed annually. Finally 150 patients were chosen for our study, of which 79 did not take hormonal preparations during the perimenopausal period (Table 1).

DURATION OF THE PERIMENOPAUSAL PERIOD

In women presenting with amenorrhoea following progestogen treatment the real onset of the menopause could not be determined. The length of the perimenopausal period could be calculated only in the 79 untreated patients as well as in 28 others after a limited period of progestational or combined contraceptive treatment. The onset of the perimenopausal period was objectively fixed at the moment FSH levels exceeded the postmenopausal value of 40 mIU/ml. At that moment changes in the menstrual pattern had occurred in some. The mean age when postmenopausal values were obtained was 49.3 years, i.e. some months earlier than the menopausal age of the group. The interval between the time where postmenopausal values of FSH were obtained and the onset of the menopause is given in Figure 1.

As can be seen, in nearly 50% of the patients postmenopausal values of FSH preceded the onset of the menopause by 0 to 1 year. In decreasing numbers the interval was spread over 1 to 5 years. In 32 patients no postmenopausal values of FSH were found during the year preceding the menopause. However, in this group the mean FSH level was far higher than the postmenopausal values in younger individuals (28 mIU as against 15 mIU/ml).

Although it is highly probable that in some women high levels of gonadotrophins were not detected due to the large intervals of hormonal evaluation, it is clear from Table 2 that the length of the

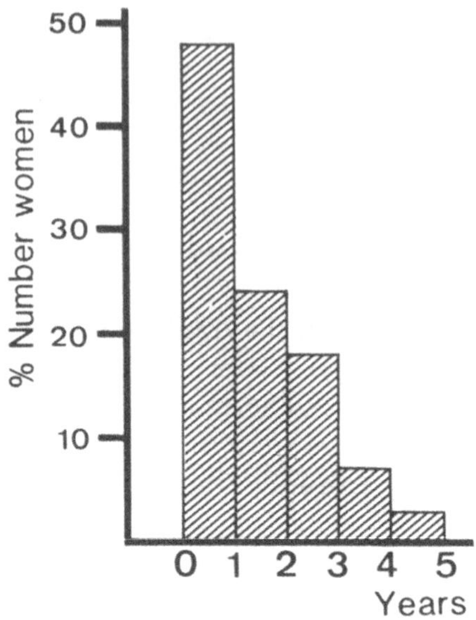

Figure 1 Histogram of the interval in years between first rise of FSH and onset of menopause

Table 2 Interval in months between first rise of FSH and onset of menopause related to age

Age of first rise of FSH	40–42	43–45	46–48	49–51	52–54	55–57
Number of women	4	12	30	33	21	7
Interval menopause in months	25.7	23.3	19.2	12.1	9.5	14.3
Standard error	7.6	4.2	3.3	2.1	2.3	7.4
% of patients with interval < 1 year	25	21.4	43.3	48.6	64.5	57.1

perimenopausal period was inversely correlated with the age of the patient.

THE HORMONAL PROFILE IN THE PERIMENOPAUSE

The concentration of serum FSH, LH and of oestradiol in untreated women ranged over yearly intervals starting at one year before the perimenopause and going up to one year after the onset of the menopause are shown in Figures 2 and 3. As can be seen there is a

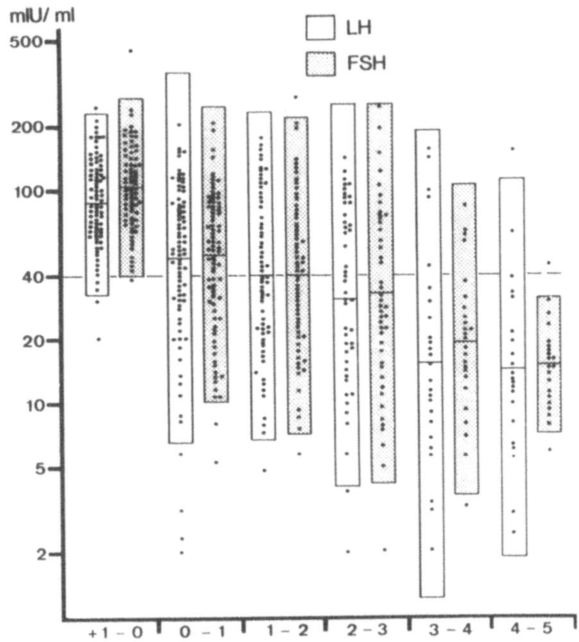

Figure 2 Individual values (mean ± SD) of LH and FSH concentrations in 79 untreated patients ranged according to yearly intervals until onset menopause

gradual rise of the gonadotrophic values during the years of the transitional period to reach finally the postmenopausal values of 90 mIU/ml LH, 108 mIU/ml FSH within the first year of the menopause.

The mean values indicate that the gradual increase of gonadotrophic hormones is accompanied by a sudden decrease of oestradiol at the very moment of the menopause. The general trend, however, takes no account of possible time-linked variations in the individual patients. In 30 women where gonadotrophic and oestrogen levels were frequently available, different periods of high and low values of both gonadotrophins and oestradiol were demonstrated (Figure 4). Although the fluctuations are dependent mainly on the frequency of hormonal evaluation, the variability of the perimenopausal gonadotrophic secretion is well illustrated. Generally a good correlation was found between LH and FSH levels ($r = 0.71$).

Oestradiol levels seem to be higher at the moment of low gonadotrophin values although a considerable overlapping of high values occurs in the presence of high postmenopausal values. Only a

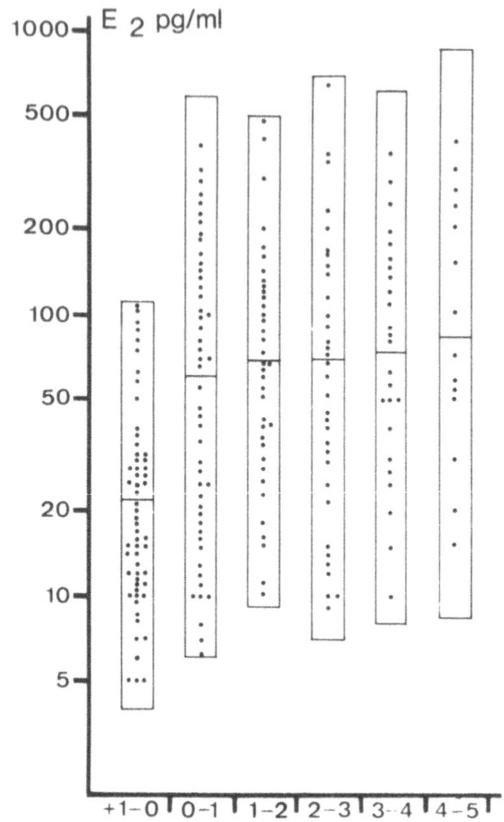

Figure 3 Oestradiol concentrations in plasma in the patients of Figure 2

weak negative correlation was found between FSH and oestradiol levels in the perimenopausal transition ($r = -0.37$; $p < 0.05$).

Frequently high oestradiol levels were found in the presence of high concentrations of gonadotrophins as can be seen in the highly fluctuating individual patterns (Figures 5, 6 and 7) and in the daily values over a two-week period (Figure 8) where FSH gradually rose in the presence of non-menopausal oestradiol concentrations.

THE INFLUENCE OF PROGESTOGENS ON HORMONE LEVELS OF THE PERIMENOPAUSAL TRANSITIONAL PERIOD

In our series 71 women were treated over periods of months or years by means of progestogens for different reasons (contraception,

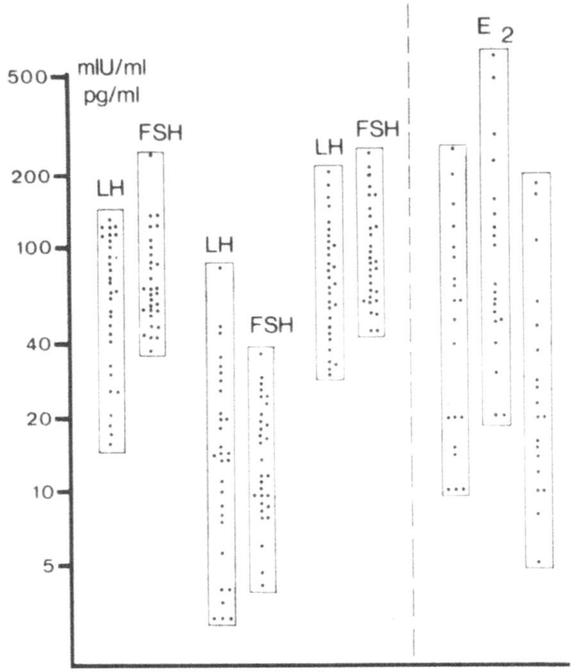

Figure 4 LH, FSH and E2 levels in 30 perimenopausal women during three periods where postmenopausal, premenopausal and postmenopausal values were observed successively

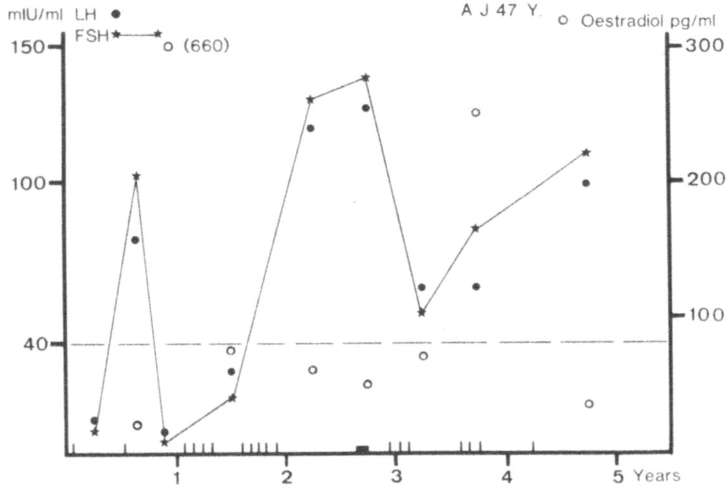

Figure 5 Highly changing levels of FSH and E2 during an observation period of 4 years in an individual of 47 years, together with the altered menstrual cycle. The highest FSH levels are observed in the amenorrhoeic periods

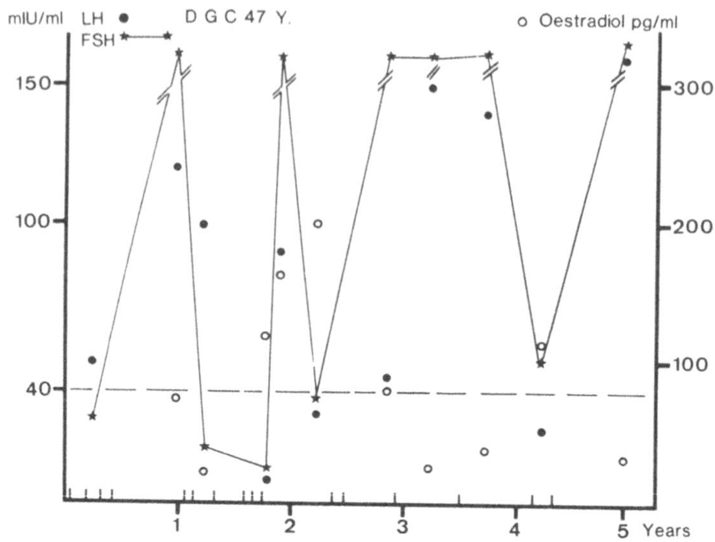

Figure 6 In this patient the interval between the first cycle disturbance and the menopause was about 4 years. At some periods there was no parallelism between LH and FSH levels. A high level of E_2 occurs in the presence of high FSH levels

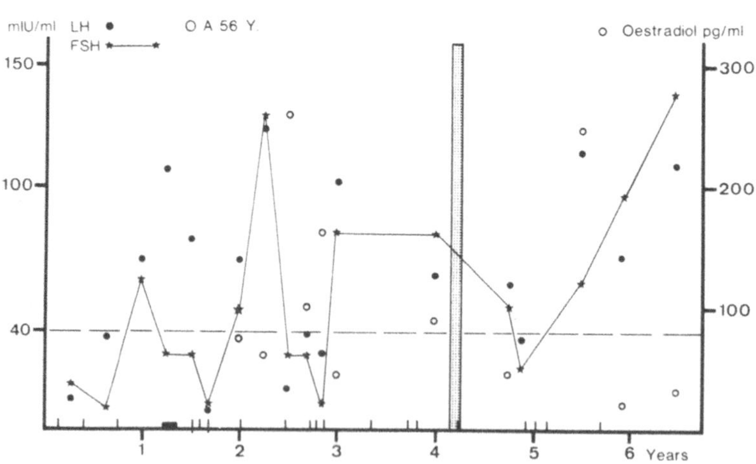

Figure 7 Highly fluctuating FSH and LH levels over a considerable period of time in a case where the menopause occurred at age 61, together with changing levels of E_2 and the altered cycle pattern. A period of 2 weeks is studied in detail in Figure 8

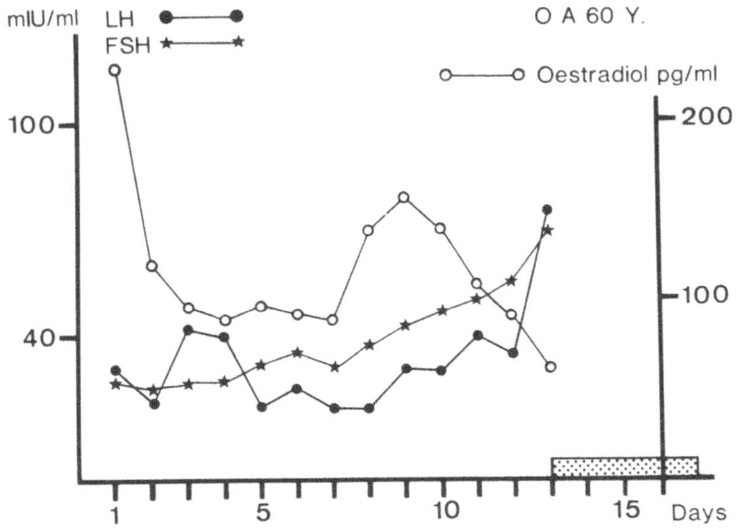

Figure 8 Daily concentrations of LH, FSH and E_2 in a 60-year-old patient, over a 2 week observation period

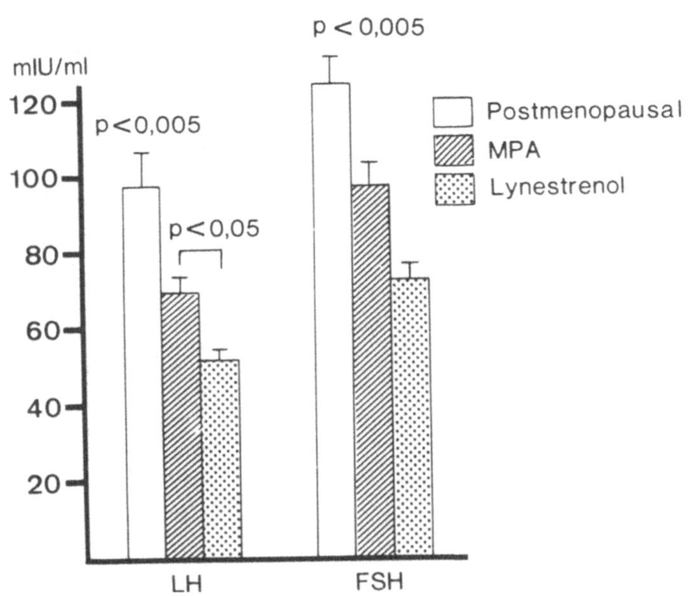

Figure 9 Comparison between LH and FSH levels in untreated postmenopausal women and progestogen-treated ones (lynestrenol 5 mg/day and MPA 150 mg/3 months)

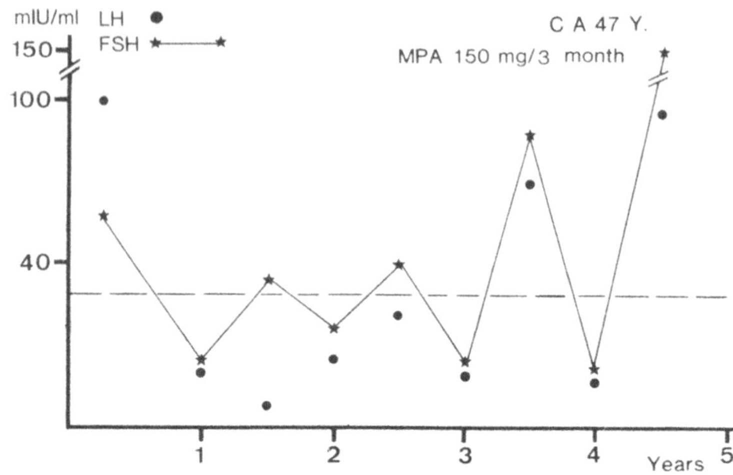

Figure 10 Gonadotrophic levels in a perimenopausal woman treated by MPA during 5 years. Gonadotrophic fluctuations persist under treatment

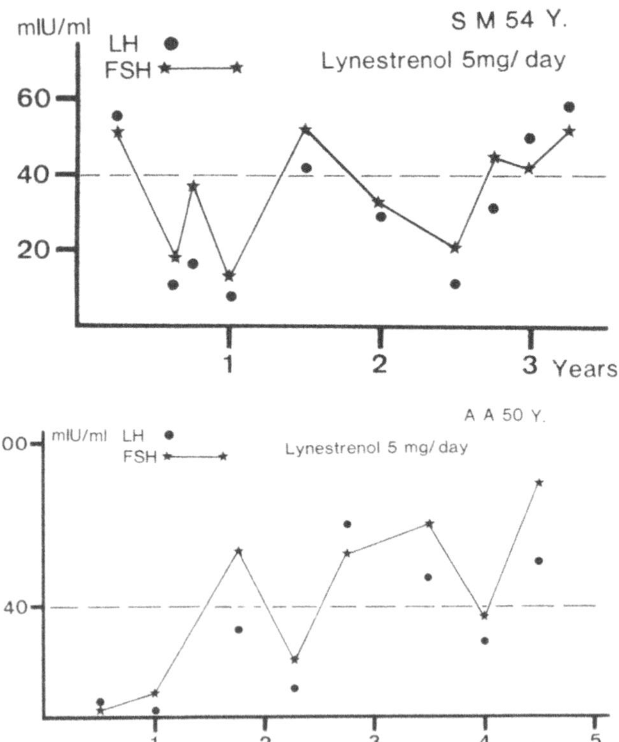

Figure 11 Two examples of patients treated orally by lynestrenol. No suppression of LH and FSH fluctuations under treatment

fibrocystic mastopathy, dysfunctional bleeding, endometriosis). A large number of them (43) were under treatment (lynestrenol 5mg/day, or MPA 150 mg/3 months) until after the menopause as is evidenced by the lasting subsequent hypergonadotrophic amenorrhoea. When comparing the postmenopausal gonadotrophin levels of progestogen-treated patients with non-treated individuals, it can be seen (Figure 9) that a progestogen treatment in no way prevents postmenopausal levels to be reached, although the values are significantly lower for both gonadotrophins and more marked for lynestrenol than for MPA. Furthermore during both types of progestogen treatment in perimenopausal women gonadotrophin fluctuations are not suppressed (Figures 10 and 11).

COMMENT

The results of our longitudinal and retrospective study on gonadotrophic and oestrogen levels in the transitional perimenopausal condition indicate a gradual increase of gonadotrophic values, more marked, however, for FSH levels during the years preceding the menopause. They are consistent with data in the literature showing elevations of both gonadotrophins or a monotrophic increase of FSH during most stages of the menstrual cycle, starting early in late reproductive life[5,7-9].

In untreated patients, the extreme variability of the gonadotrophic condition could well be illustrated and may give an explanation of the unpredictable variation of the menstrual cycle noted in some individuals. In a majority of patients high gonadotrophin levels are found at some time. Nevertheless ovulation subsequently occurred in these patients. In the transitional period the association of high levels of oestradiol and high FSH can be seen in some cases possibly indicating altered feedback mechanism.

After the onset of the menopause, however, the sudden decrease in oestradiol was invariably associated with high gonadotrophin levels. In patients under continuous progestogen treatment, considerable variations in the gonadotrophic levels, especially of FSH, were present just as they were in untreated patients, although the levels were significantly lower in the treated patients. The attainment of postmenopausal values was not prevented.

Although fertility is markedly impaired in advanced age, corpora lutea were frequently found (reference 11 and own observations). Conception, however, occurred only exceptionally even after hypergonadotrophic periods[12] or marked follicular depletion[13].

In addition to the major role of quantitative changes due to follicular depletion in the ageing ovary[14,14] qualitative aspects may be equally important. Furthermore, as a matter of speculation, alterations to the concentration of follicular inhibin[16] which impairs the production of FSH *in vitro*[17] may be considered. In Booroola Merino Sheep, lowered ovarian inhibin content was associated with a high ovulation rate[18]. In this respect are to be noted a higher incidence of dizygote twins[19] with advancing age and the occurrence of functional cysts in the premenopausal ovary[20]. Undoubtedly age itself and its resultant alterations in the genital tractus must also play an important role[21].

In view of the changes during the perimenopausal period, and from a clinical and biochemical point of view, predicting the onset of the menopause is extremely difficult. Not less difficult is the decision to withhold contraception. In this respect the use of progestogens may be of use.

However, by combining clinical data (age, duration of amenorrhoea, etc.) and the biochemical findings, a better estimation of the onset of the menopause is possible.

References

1. Aertsens, W. and Vandekerckhove, D. (1980). Unpublished data
2. Metcalf, M. G. and Donald, R. A. (1979). Fluctuating ovarian function in a perimenopausal woman. *N. Z. Med. J.*, **89**, 45
3. Treloar, A. E., Boynton, R. E., Behn, B. G. and Brown, B. W. (1967). Variation of the human menstrual cycle through reproductive life. *Int. J. Fertil.*, **12**, 77
4. Döring, G. K. (1969). The incidence of anovular cycles in women. *J. Reprod. Fertil. (Suppl.)*, **6**, 77
5. Sherman, B. W., West, J. K. and Korenman, S. G. (1976). The menopausal transition: Analysis of LH, FSH, estradiol and progesterone concentrations during menstrual cycles of older women. *J. Clin. Endocrinol. Metab.*, **42**, 629
6. Adamopoulos, D. A., Loraine, J. A. and Dove, G. A. (1971). Endocrinological studies of women approaching the menopause. *J. Obstet. Gynaecol. Br. Commonw.*, **78**, 62
7. Van Look, P. F. A., Lothian, H., Hunter, W. M., Michie, E. A. and Baird, D. T. (1977). Hypothalamic–pituitary–ovarian function in perimenopausal women. *Clin. Endocrinol.*, **7**, 13
8. Metcalf, M. G., Donald, R. A. and Livesey, J. H. (1982). Pituitary–ovarian function before, during and after the menopause: a longitudinal study. *Clin. Endocrinol.*, **17**, 489
9. Reyes, F. I., Winter, J. S. D. and Faiman, Ch. (1977). Pituitary–ovarian relationships preceding the menopause. I. A cross-sectional study of serum follicle-

stimulating hormone, luteinizing hormone, prolactin, estradiol, and progesterone levels. *Am. J. Obstet. Gynecol.*, **129**, 557

10. Wallace, R. B., Sherman, B. M., Bean, J. A., Treolar, A. E. and Schlabaugh, L. (1979). Probability of menopause with increasing duration of amenorrhea in middle-aged women. *Am. J. Obstet. Gynecol.*, **135**, 1021
11. Novak, E. R. (1970). Ovulation after fifty. *Obstet. Gynecol.*, **36**, 903
12. O'Herlihy, C., Pepperell, R. J. and Evans, J. H. (1980). The significance of FSH elevation in young women with disorders of ovulation. *Br. Med. J.*, **281**, 1447
13. Block, E. (1952). Quantitative morphological investigations of the follicular system in women. Variations at different ages. *Acta Anat.*, **14**, 108
14. Thomas, P. R., Winstanley, D., Peckham, M. J., Austin, D. E., Murray, M. A. and Jacobs, H. S. (1976). Reproductive and endocrine function in patients with Hodgkin's disease: effects of oophoropexy and irradiation. *Br. J. Cancer*, **33**, 226
15. Nielsen, J., Sillesen, I. and Hansen, K. B. (1979). Fertility in women with Turner's syndrome. Case report and review of literature. *Br. J. Obstet. Gynecol.*, **86**, 833
16. de Jong, F. H. and Sharpe, R. M. (1976). Evidence for inhibin-like activity in bovine follicular fluid. *Nature (Lond.)*, **263**, 71
17. Lagacé, L., Labrie, F., Schwartz, N. B., Lorenzen, J. and Dorrington, J. H. (1978). Similar selective inhibitory effect of ovarian fluid and Sertoli cell culture medium on FSH secretion *in vitro*. *Endocrinology*, **102** (Suppl.), Abstr. 727
18. Cummins, L. J., O'Shea, T., Bindon, B. M., Lee, V. W. and Findlay, J. K. (1983). Ovarian inhibin content and sensitivity to inhibin in Booroola and control strain Merino ewes. *J. Reprod. Fertil.*, **67**, 1
19. Parkes, A. S. (1969). Multiple births in men. *J. Reprod. Fertil. (Suppl.)*, **6**, 105
20. Schröder, R. (1954). Endometrial hyperplasia in relation to genital function. *Am. J. Obstet. Gynecol*, **68**, 294
21. Henderson, S. A. and Edwards, R. G. (1968). Chiasma frequency and maternal age in mammals. *Nature*, **218**, 22

Chapter 11

Problems of the untreated menopause

W. H. Utian

INTRODUCTION

If the human life cycle were simple, then certain things would be obvious and predictable. All individuals, however, are affected during their life cycles by a wide range of variables. Apart from being prisoners of their genes and the 'internal milieu', humans are exposed during their lives to potent variables ranging from climate to radiation, from drugs to diet, poverty to riches, a sedentary life of ease to a life of physical hard work and drudgery, and always there is the threat of coincidental infection, disease, trauma and metabolic derangement. Moreover, changing social habits such as 'jogging', smoking, diet and obesity, continually change the status quo and make follow-up of natural history even more difficult to elucidate.

Menopause is merely one milestone in this highly complex life cycle in women. Because it occurs at a time of life when there is a rising incidence of degenerative disease, it is not surprising that a causal relationship between some of these degenerative disorders and climacteric endocrine changes should have been postulated. Proof of direct relationship is generally lacking between climacteric-related hormone changes and the development of any particular metabolic derangement or degenerative process. In some instances, only indirect evidence is available. Moreover, despite an intense interest generated in recent years over the metabolic effects of perimenopausal ovarian failure, little is yet known for certain about the true natural history of the untreated menopause.

The purpose of this presentation is to review and place in perspective the little that is known[1].

Numerous endocrine changes are associated with menopause[1]. The actual mechanism by which the hormonal steroids influence the gene activity is largely unknown, but information in this respect is developing at an exciting pace.

Target tissues are defined as being tissues characterized by the presence of highly specific protein receptor molecules within the cells that are able to bind firmly to the specific circulating steroid. As a result of the presence of these specific receptors, target tissues can be triggered into action by the hormones which circulate in very low concentrations. The absence of a specific hormone receptor in a tissue would result, theoretically at least, in that tissue being immune to the relevant hormone effect. It is possible, however, that such a tissue may be indirectly affected by changes in the endocrinological profile. For example, until now no oestrogen receptors have been demonstrated to be present in the osseous tissue, although ovarian function appears to have a definite effect on bone resorption. In this instance, oestrogens may indirectly affect osseous tissue by alternate mechanisms.

Receptors have been identified in many tissues, including ovary, endometrium, vaginal epithelium, and hypothalamus. These tissues will thus respond to the presence or absence of steroid hormones by definitive alterations in structure or function. It is these peripheral target tissue responses that are of interest in evaluating the natural history of menopause and the problems that may result therefrom.

DISCUSSION

For the purposes of discussion, the specific pelvic and extrapelvic target tissues will now be considered individually in terms of their response to ovarian function and its ultimate failure at the climacteric. These sites with potential problems in the long term are listed in Table 1.

PELVIC ORGANS

Vulva

Sexual intercourse, pregnancy, and childbirth produce a number of changes in the vulva. Stretching or tearing of the perineum usually

Table 1 Potential problems of the untreated menopause

Organ/structure affected	*Potential problem*
Vulva	?Dystrophy, pruritus
Vagina	Atrophy, vaginitis, dyspareunia
Bladder and urethra	Cysto-urethritis Ectropion ?Stress incontinence
Pelvic floor	Utero-vaginal prolapse
Neuro-endocrine	Hot flushes
Skin	Atrophy, dryness, wrinkles
Mucous membranes	Dry mouth
Vocal chords	Reduction in upper register
Skeleton	Osteoporosis related backache and fracture
Breasts	Atrophy
Psychological equilibrium	Unknown

results in it becoming shorter, making the vaginal orifice appear wider and more exposed. After the menopause the vulval structures gradually undergo atrophy. Pubic hair loss is progressive, and the skin becomes thinner, often in old age having a glazed or shiny appearance. The subcutaneous tissues all but disappear so that the labia majora become very small and the labia minora almost non-existent. Dystrophy and pruritis of the vulva are much more frequent in postmenopausal women but there are no good data to confirm a direct relationship[1].

Vagina

The presence of oestrogens stimulates the maturation of the vaginal epithelium from the basal layers through to the superficial layer. The absence of oestrogen stimulation results in lack of epithelial growth, confirmed by the presence of parabasal cells on the vaginal smear[2].

During the reproductive age, the vaginal epithelium demonstrates a cyclic response parallel to the changing endocrine profile. Glycogen-rich cells are produced which are acted upon by Döderleins bacilli with the production of lactic acid and a resultant vaginal pH of 4.0 to 5.5.

Regular intercourse results in some stretching of the vaginal walls, which is also aggravated by pregnancy and childbirth. The latter tends to reduce the number of vaginal rugae, particularly if there is uterovaginal prolapse.

The vagina shows several specific responses to the climacteric.

Vaginal epithelial maturation decreases. There is a failure of production of the glycogen-containing superficial cells and ultimately an increase in vaginal pH to ranges between 6.0 and 8.0. The resistance of the vagina to pyogenic organisms becomes reduced, and atrophic vaginitis may result. Even in the absence of this, the vagina will tend to become shorter and narrower with obliteration of the vaginal fornices and an eventual loss of vaginal rugae. The ultimate problems include susceptibility to infection and dyspareunia.

It should be emphasized that some of the above changes may be prevented or slowed by a continuance of regular intercourse. This may be due to purely mechanical reasons, or could be a result of absorption of steroids from the ejaculate itself.

Uterus–endometrium

Following the climacteric the uterus becomes smaller and the walls thinner. The weight reduces from about 120 g to 50–60 g, and can be as little as 25–30 g in advanced years. The endometrium, however, maintains the ability to respond to oestrogenic stimulation. Normally it becomes cuboidal and thin, with short glands and fibrotic stroma, but it will proliferate following endogenous or exogenous oestrogen stimulation. The relationship between endometrial hyperplasia, carcinoma and persistently raised blood oestrogen concentrations is an important one.

Fallopian tube

The fallopian tube is functionally quiet after menopause. In essence the muscular and endosalpingeal changes in structure and function are similar to those of the uterus, and need not be discussed further.

Ovary

The ageing of the ovary is the prime cause of the menopause. The morphological and functional changes have been previously reviewed[1].

Bladder and urethra

The bladder's transitional epithelium demonstrates a similar response to ovarian hormones as does the vaginal epithelium. With ageing the bladder and urethra can be affected by atrophic cysto-urethritis, urethral caruncle, ectropion, and early stress-incontinence. Surprisingly, there is little valid documentation for an increase in stress incontinence while there is at least one good study which shows little change in micturition patterns with advancing age[3].

The distal urethra does appear to be sensitive to changing hormone profiles during the climacteric. This could result in atrophic distal urethritis and stricture formation resulting in obstructive cystopathy with an increase in residual urine[4]. This can result in ascending infection. Detrusor dysynergia is also a possible problem in such patients, although urethral pressure studies in postmenopausal patients taking oestrogens would suggest that more is involved than just the periurethral tissues[5].

Much more information is needed on the effects of the climacteric on bladder and urethral function before any meaningful statements can be made about changed urodynamics after the menopause.

The pelvic floor

The pelvic floor can become stretched or damaged following pregnancy and vaginal delivery, and the muscular tissue appears to lose tone with the decline of oestrogen production. The increased incidence of postmenopausal vaginal prolapse is probably related to tissue ageing as much as to the alterations in hormone function and production.

The ultimate effect of this combination of ageing tissues and loss of hormonal stimulus is an increase in the incidence of cystocoele, rectocoele, enterocoele, uterine prolapse, and combinations thereof.

EXTRAPELVIC EFFECTS

The hormonal changes after the menopause or after castration also appear to be associated with widespread effects on general target tissues or organs. Reports into direct aetiological relationships and mechanisms are still lacking in some specific areas, but information is beginning to accumulate about some organ system changes.

Vasomotor symptoms

Numerous reviews, studies, and descriptions of 'hot flushes' have failed to reveal the natural history of this troublesome symptom[1]. While anything between 15 and 80% of the women interviewed in various studies have reported hot flushes, it is not clear why some women are more susceptible than others to the problem, nor why the symptom persists for years in some women and for only a few months in others.

Skin

Of all major body organs, skin best illustrates the difficulties in differentiating the general ageing and environmental processes from the specific hormonal target tissue responses. Thus skin, on the one hand, is a major hormone target tissue; on the other hand, it is one of the most abused body organs in terms of exposure to environmental hazards, particularly the sun. Both factors become cumulative from the menopause onward.

(1) Oestrogen receptors. Oestrogen receptors do exist on skin, although there is a distinct need for precise identification[6,7]. Oestrogens appear to have actions on all skin components and have been demonstrated to be actively bound and metabolized[7,8].

(2) Evaluation of skin. Specific changes in the appearance of skin are difficult to document scientifically over a period of time. The fact that a man's skin differs from a woman's, or that a baby's differs from an adult's, is readily apparent. But how does one compare the skin of one 45-year-old woman to that of another aged 50? Or even to that of the same woman two or three years later? Therein lies the research difficulty, and the explanation for the dearth of literature in this respect. The following are some factors that are considered experimentally:

(a) Skin thickness
(b) Number of mitoses
(c) Degree of hyperaemia or perfusion, measured by taking skin temperature or measuring perfusion by xenon clearance
(d) Degree of water retention
(e) Alteration of carbohydrate metabolism

Despite the difficulties in evaluation, there is information worthy of consideration.

(3) Skin changes with age. The epidermis becomes progressively thinner after menopause. On microscopic section the epidermal

ridges and dermal papillae become less prominent. Parallel with this change is a progressive decrease in the density of scalp and body hair follicles[9]. Sebaceous gland function appears to decline as well after loss of ovarian function[10]. Sweat glands also undergo a reduction in function and become less responsive to triggering stimuli[11].

Diminution in sweat and sebaceous gland activity associated with epidermal thinning results in a dry, easily traumatized skin. This dryness will be aggravated in conditions of low humidity. A usual complaint in this situation will be itching.

The dermis, too, becomes thinner, and several changes in collagen metabolism have been demonstrated. In particular, there are reduced amounts of soluble collagen with slower rates of collagen synthesis and turnover. There is, therefore, a reduced excretion of urinary hydroxyproline with age. Inevitably, there is loss in the resilience and pliability of the skin[12].

The mucous membranes also appear to be sensitive to ovarian function. Dry mouth, for example, has been described as a menopausal disorder[13]. Van Keep and Haspels feel that the voice alters with a reduction in the upper register and a loss of timbre – hardly a problem to the average woman, but of potentially serious consequence for professional singers[14].

In summary, therefore, it would appear from the limited information available that oestrogens are actively bound and metabolized in all components of skin. Alteration in the function after the menopause may contribute to the ageing of skin by an effect additional to the concomitant ageing process.

Cardiovascular system

Castration and normal climacteric appear to be related to change in blood-lipid profile, the development of atheromatisis, increase in hypertension, and the incidence of clinical coronary heart disease. There is no uniform agreement. This entire topic is still open to further research, and dogmatic conclusions are not justified.

The skeleton

Strong evidence exists to relate ovarian function to bone metabolism. Castration or normal climacteric leads to a negative calcium balance, increased bone resorption, osteoporosis, and an increased incidence of bone fractures.

Miscellaneous

(a) *Breasts.* One physical characteristic demonstrating a significant relationship to menopause and oophorectomy is that of breast configuration[15]. The mature breast undergoes cyclic changes during the normal reproductive cycle. Oestrogen, growth hormone, and deoxycortone probably determine duct development, while glandular formation is under the influence of progesterone, prolactin, and glucocorticoids. Thus, in the luteal phase of the cycle there is increased epithelial activity which regresses during menstruation. Breast volume increases by as much as 100 ml in the second half of the menstrual cycle by a combination of glandular proliferation and water retention[16]. These cyclic changes explain the symptom production normally described during the reproductive cycle, e.g. fullness or tenderness.

Following the menopause the glandular tissue of the breast becomes atrophic. Breasts of thin women will thus tend to reduce in size and becoming flat, whereas those in obese woman can remain large and pendulous. The breasts will also become atrophic following surgical castration. This change would seem to occur fairly rapidly. Indeed, atrophy of the breasts becomes obvious in as short a span as six months after removal of functional ovaries from premenopausal women[15].

The loss of elasticity in the Cooper's ligament aggravates the tendency of the breast to droop. The nipples become smaller and flatter, and lose their erectile properties.

(b) *Thyroid function.* Changes may occur with age in thyroid function, but they are not sex related. However, no definitive evidence seems to exist linking any change in thyroid function with menopausal status. This is an unexpected finding in view of the profound effects that increased circulating oestrogen levels, whether of exogenous or endogenous origin, have on thyroid function tests. Protein-bound iodine (PBI) increases with pregnancy or with exogenous oestrogen administration, an effect due to an oestrogen-induced increase in the binding proteins. However, thyroxine (T4) values tend to lie within relatively narrow limits during the normal reproductive cycle[17]. A re-evaluation of thyroid status and menopausal status is probably worthwile, although present indications are that failing ovarian function is unlikely to be associated with any dramatic change in thyroid function.

(c) *Mood and psychological status.* The relationship between ovarian function, menopause, oophorectomy and mental (psychic) status has proved extraordinarily difficult to evaluate[1].

Sexuality should also be mentioned in this context. While sexual responsiveness appears to decrease as a function of age, the true significance of sexual dysfunction in the menopause is difficult to assess. There would seem to be no evidence to support hormonal deprivation as a primary cause for this reduced sexual activity.

CONCLUSION

A considerable amount of research is still necessary to define all the specific sites where sex steroid hormone receptors may be present, and to clarify the response of these tissues to the altered endocrine state of climacteric. Nonetheless, more than enough evidence does exist to define the climacteric as an endocrinopathy in which changes in hormonal profile are associated with extensive pelvic and extrapelvic target tissue effects.

The longer these effects are allowed to continue without corrective therapy, the more likely there is to be expression of a pathological process and clinical symptom. The exact profile of these problems remains to be completely elucidated.

References

1. Utian, W. H. (1980). *Menopause in Modern Perspective.* (New York: Appleton–Century–Crofts)
2. Utian, W. H. (1970). Use of vaginal smear in assessment of oestrogenic status of oophorectomized females. *S. Afr. Med. J.*, **44**,69
3. Osborne, J. L. (1976). Post-menopausal changes in micturition habits and in urine flow and urethral pressure studies. In Campbell, S. (ed.) *Management of the Menopause and Post-menopausal Years*, pp. 285–289. (Lancaster: MTP Press)
4. Smith, P. J. B. (1976). The effect of estrogens on bladder function in the female. In Campbell, S. (ed.) *Management of the Menopause and Post-menopausal Years*, pp. 291–298. (Lancaster: MTP Press)
5. Harrison, R. F. (1976). Urethral profile studies on menopausal women and the effects of estrogen treatment. In Campbell, S. (ed.) *Management of the Menopause and post-menopausal Years*, pp. 299–305, (Lancaster: MTP Press)
6. Frost, P., Weinstein, E. D. and Hsia, S. L. (1966). Metabolism of oestradiol and oestrone in human skin. *J. Invest. Dermatol.*, **46**, 584

7. Stumph, W. E., Madhabananda, S. and Joshi, S. G. (1974). Oestrogen target cells in the skin. *Experientia*, **30**, 196
8. Punnonen, R. (1972). Effect of castration and peroral estrogen therapy on the skin. *Acta Obstet. Gynecol. Scand. (Suppl.)*, **21**
9. Ferriman, D. (1971). *Human Hair Growth in Health and Disease*. (Springfield, Ill.: Thomas)
10. Hamilton, J. B. and Mestler, G. E. (1963). Low values for sebum in eunuchs and oophorectomized women. *Proc. Soc. Exp. Biol. Med.*, **112**, 374
11. Silver, A. F., Montagna, W. and Karacan, I. (1965). The effect of age on human eccrine sweating. In Montagna, W. (ed.) *Advances in Biology of Skin*. pp. 129–150. (Oxford: Pergamon)
12. Kirk, J. E. and Chieffi, M. (1962). Variation with age in elasticity of skin and subcutaneous tissue in human individuals. *J. Gerontol.*, **17**, 373
13. Hertz, D. G., Steiner, J. E., Zuckerman, S. and Pizanti, S. (1971). Psychological and physical symptom formation in menopause. *Psychoter. Psychosom.*, **19**, 47
14. van Keep, P. A. and Haspels, A. A. (1977). *Oestrogen Therapy During the Climacteric and Afterwards*, p. 21. (Amsterdam: Excerpta Medica)
15. Utian, W. H. (1970). Clinical and metabolic effects of the menopause and the role of replacement oestrogen therapy. *Unpublished Ph.D. Thesis*, University of Capetown.
16. Milligan, D., Drife, J. O. and Short, R. V. (1975). Changes in breast volume during normal menstrual cycle and after oral contraceptives. *Br. Med. J.*, **4**, 494
17. Chan, V., Besser, G. M. and Landon, J. (1972). Effects of oestrogen on urinary thyroxine secretion. *Br. Med. J.*, **4**, 699

Chapter 12

The perimenopausal woman: guidance and treatment

P. Nijs

INTRODUCTION

Physicians are easily led to reduce problems of the menopause to an endocrinological dysfunction. But, even if hormonal change is the causal factor, the menopause itself remains the experience of the individual woman. The physician may be able to understand this very personal reaction of the woman if he is able to relate her reactions to her social environment and her personal perspective. Hormonal treatment may be the first and essential step, but it is not the only one. Women also need a doctor who will guide them through the perimenopausal years.

Ageing can be seen as a conflict, or as Buyse[1] said: 'A difficult season for the human being who looks ahead'. Until that phase of life this woman has known the challenge of growth, development and fulfilment. At this time a different future gradually comes into view: involution, decrease of abilities and opportunities, illness or incapacitation, inevitably leading towards death. Naturally women will experience an emotional reaction towards these physical changes because today's society values more highly the qualities of youth, physical beauty, sexual attractiveness and performance. On the other hand the same society has little time for the elderly with their experience and wisdom, qualities that are highly valued in some other cultures. Women's self-confidence is therefore put to the test in our society. Menstruation signifies to the majority of women (and men) youth, femininity and fertility. As long as she menstruates a woman feels young and attractive. The cessation of the monthly period causes her to reflect on her life, asking herself such questions as 'What has life brought me?' 'What is still in store for me – only illness and incapacitation?' This leads to increased concern for her own body, to unspoken inferiority feelings and also to loss of libido and a decline in sexual reaction. She thinks of herself as too old for sex and judges her sexual longings to be inappropriate, a view strongly influenced by the prejudice that sex has meaning only when procreating is still possible[2].

The role of emotional attitudes in human sexual behaviour is as important as that of hormonal factors. Moreover, every human being, whether young or old, has a need for tenderness and intimate body contact.

Postmenopausal women will often feel unsure about their sexuality, largely because they are unprepared and often uninformed. In the 19th century the myth of the sexless child was widespread. To-day we are confronted with the myth of the sexless elderly; both myths rise from the strong link between sex and procreation.

The ageing female cannot be dismissed with statements such as 'There is a time for arrival and a time for departure'; or 'What do you expect at your age?' It is the comprehensive life situation – including the partner, the children – that determines the well-being of the ageing person and not sexuality alone. At this time of life the children will often have left home one after another and the woman's own parents may have died. Retiring from professional life offers security in the form of a pension on the one hand but brings along the risk of a general decrease in social and sexual activity on the other.

REDISCOVERY

Throughout the climacteric a woman experiences, step by step, a lessening of biological, emotional and sexual activities as well as of her social involvement[3]. A primary effort for the postmenopausal woman should be put into helping her rediscover her own individuality and re-establishing her own place in the social environment. All this can be done if new opportunities for social contact, recreation and activity present themselves or are identified. It should also be remembered that the changes of postmenopausal life can revive previous inferiority feelings or complexes that seemed to have been overcome.

To cope with the climacteric in a positive way the woman should acknowledge the need to change her way of life and accept that certain things are now impossible, whilst remaining committed to and involved in life. Jung has pointed out the increase of introspection at the time of middle age as male and female begin to weigh up the balance of life, with its achievements and failures. Many women are able to develop their lives in new directions after they have been relieved of the burden of procreation and bringing up the children.

One can sometimes also observe that women begin to develop their own potential after their husbands have died and inhibitions and limitations previously imposed by the partner come to an end. There is evidence that those women who have proved to be flexible enough to adapt to previous changes in life will have less difficulty in determining a new course for the postmenopausal life.

The postmenopausal woman who has a problem in adapting will of course be more likely to consult a physician, her general practitioner, or gynaecologist, or perhaps even an internist, the orthopaedic surgeon or the urologist. Some women who have climacteric problems escape into a state of hyperactivity or 'mental turgor' (H. Deutsch) and behave strangely and erratically perhaps by joining a militant political movement or a religious sect. She may plunge vehemently into business adventures and, particularly in the case of the unmarried perimenopausal woman, may engage in uncontrolled sexual activity due to the so-called 'Torschluss-Panik' caused by previous sexual frustration.

This last phenomenon also occurs in married women who have been badly disappointed in their marriage, and the 'late' child is not always born because of failing contraception in the perimenopausal years.

It should be borne in mind that hypersexuality often remains associated with embarrassment and guilt feelings in the same way that overeating, leading to obesity and caused by emotional disillusionment, is often related to feelings of guilt.

Due to the perceived decrease in vitality a woman may also become completely apathetic, disinterested in life generally and display inability to think any more, to take positive action of any kind, to sleep or to enjoy sex any more. Such a disillusioned woman may appear to those around her as ill-humoured, easily irritated and petty by complaining constantly about matters of little consequence – her ill-fitting dentures for instance. She often appears also to be very spiteful and jealous towards younger women, including her own daughters. The woman who fears to recognize the reality of the climacteric and the menopause, and may deny even to herself that it is happening, will easily find support from her own partner, relatives or even doctors, who will gladly promise her extended youth.

Out of fear of being lonely the ageing woman may stubbornly hang on to children and grandchildren by making herself, often to the dismay of the children, indispensible. This unhappy behaviour can lead to stronger rejection.

Feelings of desperation can also come to a woman even if she does accept the existence of the climacteric and the menopause, if she comes to the conclusion that she has not been able to achieve self-realization in her life so far. This troublesome period that has come in her life has entirely different characteristics which cannot be dealt with as she has previously handled her life, by using the perspective of the future because that perspective is not there any more. From living a life of happy anticipation of what the future might bring this woman seeks the instant relief of eating, alcohol or drug abuse.

The climacteric woman is often met with a lack of attention when she explains these problems to health care professionals, because they are not of a somatic nature. Hot flushes, excessive transpiration and palpitation can be directly linked to hormonal changes and their vasomotor syndrome must of course be treated with hormone substitution. Emotional hypersensitivity, irritability, sudden changes of mood, inability to concentrate, amnesia and sudden headaches accompany the vegetative syndrome and are also probably directly caused by the abrupt hormonal changes. Nevertheless they require a different approach.

The plaintive (or ever-accusing) way in which she presents her symptoms is often taken to be indicative of a hypochondriacal reaction, reflecting an anxious or even a paranoid attitude. Of course all of this cannot be explained by the known hormonal changes because it represents the individual reaction of an individual woman who feels threatened and betrayed by her own body[3].

Depression in climacteric women is well known to the physician and even a psychosis with depressive and paranoid elements is not a rare phenomenon. In this case knowledge of the family history should be enough to warn the doctor in good time to administer neuroleptic as well as antidepressant medication. The vast majority of depressions in this particular phase of life are, however, of the reactive type and caused by the overburdening of the mind with seemingly important problems and questions of life occurring at a time when biological changes lessen her resistance. As was mentioned before, hypochondriacal or paranoid symptoms are often present and these should hopefully be recognized in good time and treated bearing in mind that the risk of successful suicide is enhanced by the tendency of older women to use more radical methods (drowning, hanging, cutting their wrists) rather than taking overdoses of tranquillizers or mild sleeping drugs on the one hand, and by the social isolation that may prevent help coming in time on the other.

Finally, the 'masked depression' is something also to be looked out for[4]. In this type of depression the word itself remains hidden behind a series of somatic and 'functional' complaints and is truthfully not recognized by the patient, although the family often reports a gradual change for the worse. Slight changes in appetite, insomnia and obstipation often occur. A depression of this type can also be hidden by overcompensation in some form or another – mainly overeating, alcohol abuse, excessive and chronic use of the telephone or hypersexuality.

GUIDANCE

Since the climacteric is a phase of life marked by changes, the doctor's treatment should take the form of continuous guidance, including biological, psychological and social solutions. As a well functioning body is a necessary condition for a sound mind and a good social life, the smallest physical ailment should be properly treated.

Thorough physical examination by the doctor is needed to track down and eliminate possible disease of the gall-bladder, the liver, the cardiovascular system, metabolic malfunctions and diabetes. The patient needs to feel that her own complaints are being taken seriously.

Hormone therapy, however, is almost always insufficient where a depressive component is present. Early diagnosis of masked depression can avoid chronic misuse of tranquillizers, sleeping pills or even neuroleptics. Although antidepressants must be the chosen therapy in treating these patients, every aspect must be taken into account and every type of symptom must be treated in its own way[4].

This is why we value guidance over treatment. Guidance can be described as a series of short counselling sessions to be scheduled in advance so that the patient will not just come at any time when she feels unwell. This method confirms in the patient's mind that she will receive the right amount of attention and will not be dismissed with only a prescription.

Guidance requires the proper attitude from the doctor, because although he will not necessarily be aware of it himself he will be inclined to keep at a distance those patients complaining of ageing and loss of vitality. This gloomy type of patient tends to be silenced with medication. However, letting her speak is a form of treatment in itself because given the opportunity to express her feelings she will stop complaining. In using the brief consultation method the doctor is recommended to try to limit the number of complaints discussed and the speed of progress, rather than make available extra consultation time.

In doing this the doctor will help the patient to gain an insight into her various problems and she will thus more easily learn to adapt to her new life and obtain a new perspective to hold on to. A new perspective is of prime importance, especially if the patient is virtually immobilized by depression. Ideally a new lifestyle should be found and the physician can help to guide her there. She has to learn, for example, to let the children go their own way whether or not this fits in with her own plans. She should be encouraged to find new vocational or even professional activities. In doing so the woman will need a lot of support, especially from her husband.

In general it is good policy to invite the husband along to the consultations if only to minimize the impact of the seemingly unimportant complaints of his wife.

The average perimenopausal woman is perfectly capable of speaking for herself. As a well-informed patient she also will want to have a say when it comes to choosing between therapies. Medical treatment should be explained in the broad sense, including information that is perhaps not specifically requested, e.g. the fact that a hysterectomy operation does not change sexual response. The necessity for detailed information is even greater when a mastectomy is indicated. Together with her husband the patient should receive information about the various steps which constitute the treatment and should be offered support in dealing with the emotional as well as the physical aspects of the therapy.

From a preventive point of view the general practitioner or the gynaecologist, who may often meet with the woman for contraceptive counselling until around the age of 40, should start at the appropriate time to orientate his patient on the likely future lifestyle.

It is a known fact that women who perform only the mother role have more difficulty in coping with the climacteric than those who are happily engaged in social and professional life. A similar difference is seen between women who have less satisfying jobs in the lower categories and those who have a higher category, professional and more satisfying job.

The menopausal woman may be unsure about her own sexuality. Masters and Johnson have stated that 'there is no age limit for female sexuality' even if they find changes in physical response, such as a decrease in the intensity of the reactions and the rapidity and duration of the biological changes. Regular sexual activity is important to maintain the sexual function. For instance Masters and Johnson also found that regular intercourse in women over 60 remained agreeable by good lubrication even if the decrease in production of female sex hormones cause thinning of the vaginal mucosa[5].

This should be kept in mind when abstinence is necessary and the period of abstinence should be as brief as possible. As already mentioned, hysterectomy does not put an end to sexual desire and activity. A follow-up study has proved that in general more than 60% of women interviewed in a study who had had a hysterectomy showed no change in libido after the operation; 20% showed an increased libido and the remaining 20% a decline. The last group, however, also showed a predominance of marital problems.

When sexual desire declines after a hysterectomy underlying emotional factors are the cause. When the ovaries are also removed general symptoms of hormone shortage *may* occur and influence the libido incidentally. In this case hormone substitution is indicated. This again calls for thorough counselling with the patient and her husband. It should be re-emphasized that the sudden change in hormone production at the time of the menopause does not induce a decrease in the libido. The sexual functions will gradually slow down with age. The lessening of the physical intensity can, however, be amply compensated by a deepening of the emotional intensity borne out of a lifetime together as husband and wife.

References

1. Buyse, G. (1977). Een moeilijk seizoen voor de verwachtende mens. In Nijs, P.

and Christiaens, M. (eds) *Man en vrouw in de tweeds leeftijd, Leuvense Cahiers voor Seksuologie*, nr. 1, pp. 43–53. (Leuven: Acco)

2. Nijs, P. (1977). Wie is te oud voor seksualiteit? In Nijs, P. and Christiaens, M. (eds) *Man en vrouw in de tweede leeftijd*, Leuvense Cahiers voor Seksuologie, nr. 1, pp. 31–42. (Leuven: Acco)
3. Hertz, D. G., and Molinski, H (1980). *Psychosomatik der Frau*, p. 159. (Berlin, Heidelberg, New York: Springer Verlag)
4. Nijs, P. and Steppe, A. (1980). De huisarts en de gemaskeerde depressie. *T. Geneesk.*, **36**, 223
5. Masters, W. and Johnson, V. (1966). *Human Sexual Response.* (Boston: Little, Brown & Co.)

Chapter 13

Oral oestrogen treatment of the climacteric and the postmenopausal period

C. Campagnoli, A. Sandri and P. Belforte

In Europe, the most widely used oral oestrogens in the treatment of the climacteric and postmenopausal period are: oestradiol valerate (EV), conjugated equine oestrogens (CEE) and oestriol (E_3), or oestriol succinate. Nowadays, synthetic oestrogens such as ethinyloestradiol and diethylstilboestrol are rarely used because of their side-effects[1], at least at the dosages normally used until recently. Other preparations such as micronized oestradiol and piperazine oestrone sulphate are used in some countries.

The effect of natural oestrogens (EV, CEE, E_3) regarding vasomotor and psychic disturbances in the climacteric period is well documented[1-3]. These natural oestrogens are also effective in the treatment of vaginal atrophy, and, as far as CEE and EV are concerned, in the prevention of osteoporosis[2,3].

Oestriol has gained much in popularity in recent years due to its weak endometriotrophic action[3]. Figure 1 shows the response to the progestogen challenge test (medroxyprogesterone acetate 10 mg for 10 days) after different oral treatments in three groups of selected postmenopausal women[4]. In all cases, a negative pretreatment test indicated absence of a basal endometrial proliferation. The progestogen, given in the second phase of the fifth cycle to the women treated with CEE (0.625 mg/day for cycles of 21 days) produced a withdrawal

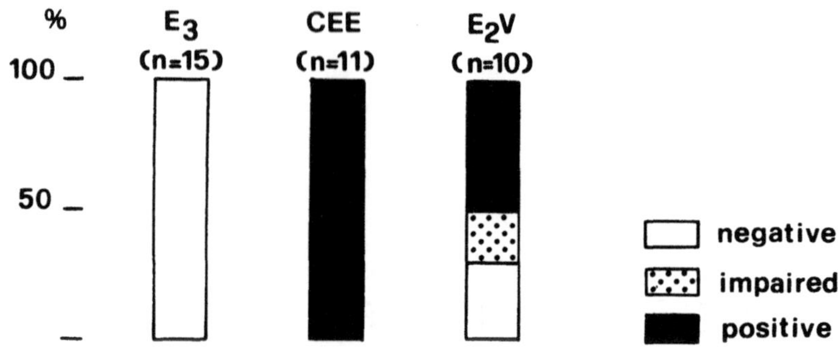

Figure 1 Response to medroxyprogesterone acetate (MPA) challenge test after different oral oestrogen treatment in postmenopausal women with negative pre-treatment test. Type of treatment: E_3: oestriol: 2 mg/day, continuously, MPA: 10 mg/day from 124 to 133rd day of treatment; CEE: conjugated equine oestrogens: 0.625 mg/day, for cycles of 21 days and 7 days off, MPA: from 12 to 21st day of the fifth cycle of therapy; EV: oestradiol valerate: 2 mg every other day, for cycles of 20 days and 8 days off, MPA: from 11 to 20th day of the fifth cycle of treatment. The results are classified according to Hull *et al.*[28]

bleeding in all cases, showing that the treatment induced endometrial proliferation. As far as EV is concerned (2 mg every second day for cycles of 20 days) the findings suggest an endometriotrophic action, although this was not present in every case, and an altogether lesser effect than that of CEE at a dosage of 0.625 mg/day. Conversely, none of the patients treated with E_3 (2 mg in single daily dose, administered continuously for the same period of time) had a withdrawal bleeding after progestogen administration, suggesting an absence of endometrial proliferation. In fact, oral E_3 – even if showing a certain proliferative effect on the endometrium when administered in repetitive daily doses – does not induce such proliferation when administered in a single daily dose, even with dosages of 8 mg/day[5].

Oral treatment has the following *advantages*:

- the dosage can be easily adjusted to the needs of the patient;
- treatment can be rapidly stopped;
- the dosage can be slowly and progressively reduced until complete discontinuation, minimizing the probability of the recurrence of complaints.

Oral treatment can, on the other hand, present certain *disadvantages* for some women:

- psychological disturbance caused by daily tablet ingestion and by the need to follow closely the eventual cyclic schedule (should such be prescribed);

- concern at the use of a hormonal 'pill', partly stimulated by reports of an increased incidence of cardiovascular accidents in women taking oral contraceptives, especially when over the age of 40[6-8]. This is despite the fact that the evidence is that the natural oestrogen used to alleviate climacteric complaints does not appear to carry such a risk[9,10].

Among the main effects of oestrogens (Table 1), hepato-mediated effects are of particular importance when oestrogen is administered orally. In effect, oral therapy results in a 'bolus' of oestrogen being delivered directly to the liver via the portal circulation[11]. Another consequence of this 'first liver passage' is faster metabolism, viz., conjugation[11]. However, this rapid conjunction does not seem to be a problem in itself, because the dose is flexible. A third possible clinical consequence, although this is debatable, could be a certain increase in gall-bladder disease[9,10].

Of the principal *hepato-cellular effects* of oestrogens (Table 2), the increase of binding globulins for cortisol and for sex hormones seems to have little clinical importance. Other effects, such as the influence on the synthesis of renin substrate, of antithrombin III, and lipoproteins, have important clinical implications because of a potential influence on cardiovascular risk[11]. The intensity of the effects of oestrogens varies greatly depending on the type of preparation and the dosage[11]. Additionally, at least with regard to lipoproteins, the action can differ completely with different preparations and/or dosages[12].

Table 1 Main actions of oestrogens

- Direct action on target tissues (hypothalamic–hypophyseal system; breast; uterus; vagina; etc.)
- Hepato-mediated actions
- Actions mediated by other organs (regulation of bone metabolism)

Table 2 Principal hepato-cellular effects of oestrogens

Influence on the synthesis of:
- Cortisol binding globulin (CBG)
- Sex hormone binding globulin (SHBG, TeBG)
- Renin substrate
- Antithrombin III
- Lipoproteins

The synthetic oestrogens, diethylstilboestrol and ethinyloestradiol, have an effect on the liver which is decisively greater than that of natural oestrogens, i.e. between four- and eighteen-fold in excess of that estimated from their suppression of FSH[13]. In effect, probably by virtue of their structure, the synthetic oestrogens are more resistant than their natural counterparts to the process of intracellular metabolism and degradation, and thus their activity may be prolonged[11]. Among 'natural' oestrogens, the CEE are those which have a greater effect on the liver[13]. This is probably a consequence of the presence, in the CEE, of the equilin and 17α-dihydroequilin, which are not 'natural' oestrogens in women[11].

CEE, even at a dosage of 0.3 mg/day, cause a significant increase of the *renin substrate*[14]. It bears mentioning, however, that this biochemical change does not necessarily result in clinical complications, such as an increase in arterial pressure. Such a complication has been noted in only a minority of cases[3,9].

Another hepato-cellular effect caused by oestrogens is the influence on the production of *antithrombin III*. Unlike the effects of percutaneous administration of oestradiol, orally administered CEE, in a dosage of 1.25 mg/day, significantly reduces the levels of antithrombin III[15]. In our study of selected groups[4], using the more common dosage of 0.625 mg/day, we did not find this reduction of antithrombin III levels.

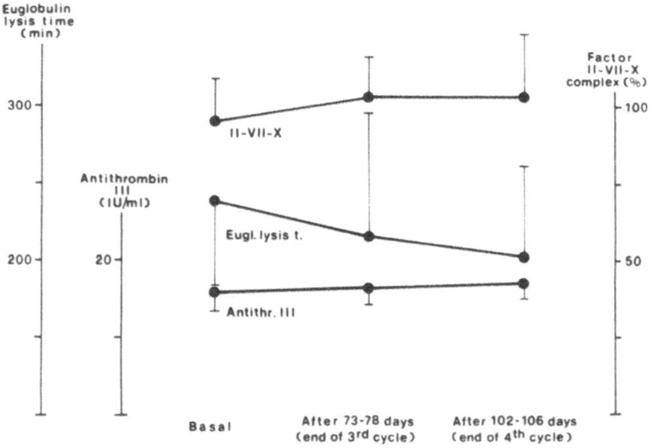

Figure 2 Activity of the factor II-VII-X complex, euglobulin lysis time and antithrombin III levels, before and during treatment with conjugated equine oestrogens (0.625 mg/day, for cycles of 21 days on and 7 off), in a selected group of postmenopausal women (n = 12). (Adapted from Campagnoli *et al.*[4])

At the end of the third and fourth cycles of treatment we found only an insignificant increase of activity of the factor II-VII-X complex, counterbalanced by an insignificant decrease of the euglobulin lysis time (Figure 2). In addition, no such changes were noted with the use of E_3 (2 mg in single daily dose) administered continuously for the same period of time (Figure 3). Equally no changes in blood-clotting factors or in antithrombin III during long-term therapy with CEE[16] or with E_3 succinate[17] have been observed. Moreover, overall clinical evidence indicates no increased risk of thromboembolic diseases from oestrogen replacement therapy[10].

The effects of oral oestrogens on *hepatic synthesis of lipoproteins* are of great clinical importance. As is well known, the risk of cardiovascular disease is increased with low HDL (high density lipoprotein)-cholesterol levels and/or high LDL (low density lipoprotein)-cholesterol levels[12]. A study by Silfverstolpe *et al.*[18] shows that, unlike ethinyloestradiol, 20 μg/day, which causes an increase of all lipoprotein fractions, EV, at 2 mg/day, produces a significant increase of the high density lipoproteins, with a significant reduction of the other fractions. These findings are consistent with data from both long- and short-term studies[12,19].

In summary, the hepato-mediated effect of oral oestrogens on lipids

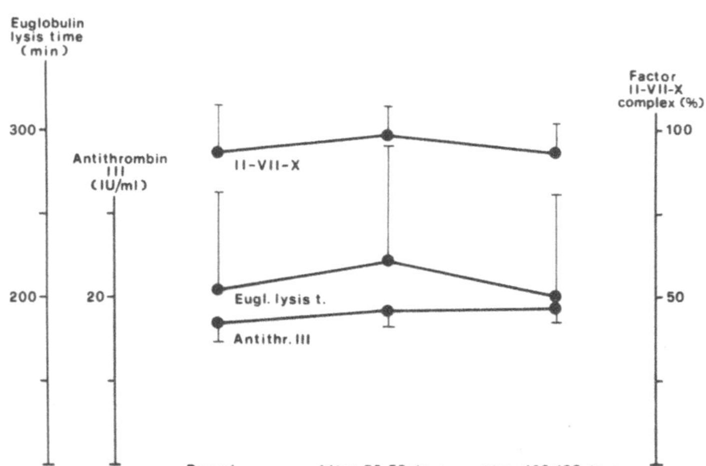

Figure 3 Activity of the factor II-VII-X complex, euglobulin lysis time and antithrombin III levels, before and during treatment with oestriol (2 mg/day, continuously), in a selected group of postmenopausal women (n = 10). (Adapted from Campagnoli *et al.*[4])

(at doses currently used in the treatment of climacteric symptoms) is beneficial with regard to cardiovascular risk[12]. Such an effect seems to override the other potentially adverse effects, even if the overall epidemiological evidence is still not conclusive[9,10]. For instance in a recent study performed in an American retirement community women using oestrogens showed a risk-ratio of death from ischaemic heart disease of 0.43 when compared with control groups[20]. In another American study, all-cause mortality rates were consistently reduced in women using oestrogens in the postmenopause; some of the lower risks could be accounted for by increased levels of HDL-cholesterol in oestrogen users[21].

It must be noted, however, that the results of a large part of the two studies we have cited refer to women using CEE without the use of a progestogen. As is well known, since 1975 – when epidemiological data began to suggest an increased incidence of endometrial cancer in postmenopausal women treated with unopposed oestrogens over a long period of time[22,23] – the use of highly endometriotrophic oestrogens, such as CEE, is currently combined with cyclic administration of a progestogen[10,24]. This could cause an interference with the beneficial effects of oestrogens on the cardiovascular system as a consequence of a negative effect of progestogens on lipoproteins, particularly a decrease of HDL-cholesterol, as first evidenced by Hirvonen *et al.*[25]. The effect on HDL-cholesterol is greatest when the androgenic progestogens of the 19-nortestosterone series are used, whereas it is less important with medroxyprogesterone acetate or with natural progesterone[12,25]. Obviously, such an effect may create few clinical problems when a very weakly endometriotrophic oestrogen, like E_3 in single daily dose, is used. In this case, there is no need for cyclic progestogen treatment (or, at most, this need is limited to a brief period, until the residual endogenous oestrogen production stops). It is probable that the above-mentioned benefits will outweigh the problems, even for women who take a progestogen cyclically for many years, due to the use of highly endometriotrophic oestrogens. Nevertheless, the clinical consequences of prolonged administration of progestogens (especially those of the 19-nortestosterone series at the dosage currently used), particularly the possible interference with the beneficial effects of oral oestrogens on the cardiovascular system, await clarification[26].

An analogous clarification is necessary for those oestrogens parenterally administered. In fact, non-oral oestrogens, while practically lacking a beneficial effect regarding lipids, as a consequence of their weaker influence on the liver[12], necessitate the use of cyclic progestogens, to compensate for their endometriotrophic effect[11,27]. An adverse action on the levels of high density lipoproteins, at least with the use of a 19-nortestosterone derivative, has been noted[12], and a potential increase of cardiovascular risk could follow.

References

1. Lauritzen, C. (1973). The management of the premenopausal and the postmenopausal patient. In van Keep, P. A. and Lauritzen, C. (eds.) *Frontiers of Hormone Reasearch*, Vol. 2, *Ageing and Estrogens*, pp. 2–21. (Basel: Karger)
2. Kopera, H. (1979). Effects, side-effects, and dosage schemes of various sex hormones in the peri- and postmenopause. In van Keep, P. A., Serr, D. M. and Greenblatt, R. B. (eds) *Female and Male Climacteric*. pp. 43–68. (Lancaster: MTP Press)
3. Utian, W. H. (1980). *Menopause in Modern Perspective. A Guide to Clinical Practice.* (New York: Appleton – Century – Crofts)
4. Campagnoli, C., Prelato-Tousijn, L., Belforte, P., Ferruzzi, L., Dolfin, A. M. and Morra, G. (1981). Effects of conjugated equine oestrogens and oestriol on blood clotting, plasma lipids and endometrial proliferation in postmenopausal women. *Maturitas*, **3**, 135
5. Punnonen, R. and Söderström, K. O. (1983). The effect of oral estriol succinate therapy on the endometrial morphology in postmenopausal women: The significance of fractionation of the dose. *Eur. J. Obstet. Gynecol. Reprod. Biol.*, **14**, 217
6. Vessey, M. P. and Doll, R. (1968). Investigation of relation between use of oral contraceptives and thromboembolic disease. *Br. Med. J.*, **2**, 199
7. Masi, A. T. (1978). Myocardial infarction in young women: review of United States data on possible contributory factors including use of oral contraceptive drugs. In Sciarra, J. J., Zatuchni, G. I. and Speidel, J. J. (eds) *Risks, Benefits, and Controversies in Fertility Control*, pp. 138–155. (Hagerstown: Harper and Row)
8. Mann, J. I. (1978). Oral contraception and myocardial infarcation in younger women: data from countries other than the United States. In Sciarra, J. J., Zatuchni, G.I. and Speidel, J. J. (eds) *Risks, Benefits, and Controversies in Fertility Control*, pp. 129–137. (Hagerstown: Harper and Row)
9. Hammond, C. B. and Maxson, W. S. (1982). Current status of estrogen therapy for the menopause. *Fertil. Steril.*, **37**, 5
10. Gambrell, R. D., Jr. (1982). The menopause: benefits and risks of estrogen-progestogen replacement therapy. *Fertil. Steril.*, **37**, 457
11. Campbell, S. and Whitehead, M. I. (1982). Potency and hepato-cellular effects of oestrogens after oral, percutaneous, and subcutaneous administration. In van Keep, P. A., Utian, W. H. and Vermeulen, A. (eds) *The Controversial Climacteric*, pp. 103–126. (Lancaster: MTP Press)
12. Larsson-Cohn, U. (1982). Some biochemical consequences of postmenopausal hormone replacement treatment. In van Keep, P. A., Utian, W. H. and Vermeulen, A. (eds) *The Controversial Climacteric*, pp. 29–38. (Lancaster: MTP Press)
13. Mashchak, C. A., Lobo, R. A., Dozono-Takano, R., Eggena, P., Nakamura, R. M., Brenner, P. F. and Mishell, D R., Jr. (1982). Comparison of pharmaco-

dynamic properties of various estrogen formulations. *Am. J. Obstet. Gynecol.*, **144**, 511

14. Geola, F. L., Frumar, A. M., Tataryn, I. V., Lu, K. H., Hershman, J. M., Eggena, P., Sambhi, M. P. and Judd, H. L. (1980). Biological effects of various doses of conjugated equine estrogens in postmenopausal women. *J. Clin. Endocrinol. Metab.*, **51**, 620
15. Elkik, F., Gompel, A., Mercier-Bodard, C., Kuttenn, F., Guyenne, P. N., Corvol, P. and Mauvais-Jarvis, P. (1982). Effects of percutaneous estradiol and conjugated estrogens on the level of plasma proteins and triglycerides in postmenopausal women. *Am. J. Obstet. Gynecol.*, **143**, 888
16. Notelovitz, M. (1977). Coagulation, oestrogen and the menopause. *Clin. Obstet. Gynecol.*, **4**, 107
17. Toy, J. L., Davies, J. A. and McNicol, G. P. (1978). The effects of long-term therapy with oestriol succinate on the haemostatic mechanism in postmenopausal women. *Br. J. Obstet. Gynaecol.*, **85**, 363.
18. Silfverstolpe, G., Gustafson, A., Samsioe, G. and Svanborg, A. (1980). Lipid metabolic studies in oophorectomized women: effects induced by two different estrogens on serum lipids and lipoproteins. *Gynecol. Obstet. Invest.*, **11**, 161
19. Barrett-Connor, E., Brown, W. V., Turner, J., Austin, M. and Cruqui, M. H. (1979). Heart disease risk factors and hormone use in postmenopausal women. *J. Am. Med. Assoc.*, **241**, 2167
20. Ross, R. K., Paganini-Hill, A., Mack, T. M., Arthur, M. and Henderson, B. E. (1981). Menopausal oestrogen therapy and protection from death from ischaemic heart disease. *Lancet*, **1**, 858
21. Bush, T. L., Cowan, L. D., Barrett-Connor, E., Criqui, M. H., Karon, J. M., Wallace, R. B., Al Tyroler, H. and Rifkind, B. M. (1983). Estrogen use and all-cause mortality. Preliminary results from the lipid research clinics program follow-up study. *J. Am. Med. Assoc.*, **249**, 903
22. Smith, D. C., Prentice, R., Thompson, D. J. and Herrmann, W. L. (1975). Association of exogenous estrogen and endometrial carcinoma. *N. Engl. J. Med.*, **293**, 1164
23. Ziel, H. K. and Finkle, W. D. (1975). Increased risk of endometrial carcinoma among users of conjugated estrogens. *N. Engl. J. Med.*, **293**, 1167
24. Gambrell, R. D., Jr. (1978). The prevention of endometrial cancer in postmenopausal women with progestogens. *Mauritas*, **1**, 107
25. Hirvonen, E., Mälkönen, M. and Manninen, V. (1981). Effects of different progestogens on lipoproteins during postmenopausal replacement therapy. *N. Engl. J. Med.*, **304**, 560
26. Notelovitz, M. (1982). Progestins in the perimenopause. In van Keep, P. A., Utian, W. H. and Vermeulen, A. (eds) *The Controversial Climacteric,* pp. 127–136. (Lancaster: MTP Press)
27. Whitehead, M. I., Townsend, P. T., Pryse-Davies, J., Ryder, T. A. and King, R. J. B. (1981). Effects of estrogens and progestins on the biochemistry and morphology of the post-menopausal endometrium. *N. Engl. J. Med.*, **305**, 1599
28. Hull, M. G. R., Knuth, U. A., Murray, M. A. F. and Jacobs, H. S. (1979). The practical value of the progestogen challenge test, serum oestradiol estimation or clinical examination in assessment of the oestrogen state and response to clomiphene in amenorrhoea. *Br. J. Obstet. Gynaecol.*, **86**, 799

Chapter 14

Percutaneous oestrogen therapy

R. Sitruk-Ware, A. Basdevant, B. de Lignières and P. Mauvais-Jarvis

INTRODUCTION

Oestrogen therapy includes several groups of compounds that differ substantially in their chemical structure and general properties but display one common biological activity : the ability to stimulate and maintain the female sex characteristics.

The potential benefits of oestrogen replacement therapy (ERT) for postmenopausal women are recognized and no member of the international scientific community involved in the menopause research field will refute the gratifying results of this hormone therapy. However, the debate weighing risks against benefits continues in 1983.

Knowledge of side-effects and their mechanisms improves day by day, with evaluation of the theoretical aspects of innocuity of substitution oestrogen therapy and substantial improvement of therapeutic regimens. Most of the harmful side-effects of ERT have been related (1) to the absence of progestational balance; and (2) to the fact that most of the oestrogens available for clinical use are synthetic and administered orally, resulting in intensive metabolism in the liver, leading to metabolic disturbances[1].

During the last five years therapeutic improvements have included the addition of a sequential progestogen and the use of natural oestrogens, such as oestradiol, together with the search for a means of administration other than the oral route, thus avoiding the effect of the hepatic passage.

WHY SYNTHETIC OESTROGENS SHOULD BE AVOIDED: THE CASE FOR NATURAL VERSUS SYNTHETIC OESTROGENS

Two different types of oestrogens, classified as natural and synthetic oestrogens are used in the treatment of climacteric symptoms. However, the classification into natural and synthetic is somewhat false as 'natural' oestrogens have to be synthesized in order to be produced in tablet form. Therefore the term 'artificial' oestrogens (i.e. not physiologically produced by any known mammals) would be more appropriate than 'synthetic'.

The pharmacological modification of the oestradiol molecule resulted in the synthesis of 17α-ethinyl-17β-oestradiol (EE) which represents the most potent oestrogen in oral therapy and one of the most widely used. The attachment of the ethinyl group on C-17 enables the molecule to resist hepatic inactivation and after one oral single dose the steroid can be active for up to 24 hours or even for as long as 48 hours[2]. But these favourable pharmocokinetics, mainly due to a decrease in hepatic inactivation, lead to accumulation in the liver of active metabolites and an overstimulation of hepatic oestrogen dependent enzymatic activities[1]. It should be kept in mind that the liver partially under oestrogenic control, regulates the metabolism of renin substrate (RS), high density lipoproteins (HDL), low density lipoproteins (LDL), several plasma coagulation factors and antithrombin III (AT III). Deregulation by oestrogens may therefore enhance the risk of hypertension, hyperlipidaemia and hypercoagulability.

Even low doses of EE have been demonstrated to have supraphysiological effects on the synthesis of plasma renin substrate[3], very low density lipoproteins (VLDL)[4] and also to decrease AT III activity[5,6]. These adverse metabolic effects have been proposed as a possible basis for the occurrence of hypertension[7], cardiovascular disease[8] and increased incidence of thrombosis[9]. Moreover, a direct deleterious effect of synthetic oestrogens on the vascular wall has been reported[10]. Thus recommendations have been made on the avoidance of these artificial oestrogens in women over 40 and, therefore, similarly in postmenopausal women. Consequently, natural oestrogens are preferred for the oestrogen substitute therapy in postmenopausal women who run a higher risk of contracting metabolic and cardiovascular disease.

WHY SHOULD ORAL THERAPY BE AVOIDED?

Natural oestrogens include 17β-oestradiol (E_2), oestrone (E_1), oestriol (E_3) and the conjugated oestrogens obtained from the urine of pregnant mares, the main components of which are E_1 and also equiline and equilinine. These 'equine oestrogens' have been the most popular form of ERT in past years in the USA. However, conjugated oestrogens are 'natural' only in the horse and the same metabolic side-effects as produced by artificial oestrogens have been described after oral administration to women. They have been shown to increase plasma triglycerides and VLDL[11,4], impair several coagulation factors[12], decrease AT III[13] and presumably enhance vascular morbidity in non-selected populations[14].

Also, E_1 binds preferentially to the liver receptor sites[15] and appears to be twice as active as E_2 on the liver side-effects[16]. Unfortunately, all the other natural oestrogens available are, when administered orally, rapidly metabolized in the liver, leading to high circulating levels of E_1 and to an inversion of the E_2/E_1 ratio[17]. The administration of micronized E_2 does not solve the problem. After oral administration of micronized E_2, the plasma levels of E_1 are tremendously increased[18,19]; the same effect is observed after oral administration of oestradiol valerate[18,17]. Thus, after oral therapy the bolus of oestrogens reaching the portal vein and the conversion of E_2 and E_1 in the gut transforms the liver cell into a preferential target.

Hence, it has been proposed that these hepato-cellular effects were related not only to the type of oestrogen, but also to the route of administration. Oral therapy actually results in a large, unphysiological bolus of oestrogens being delivered into the portal circulation, while in a physiological state oestrogens are secreted into the circulation and delivered to the target organs before they reach the liver. Therefore, routes of administration other than the oral route have been sought to bypass the liver and avoid the excessive stimulation of liver metabolism.

WHY PERCUTANEOUS THERAPY?

Parenteral administration of oestrogens

Parenteral routes of administration such as subcutaneous implants, percutaneous or vaginal application of oestrogens, deliver the steroids into the systemic circulation and therefore may cause less marked changes in liver enzymatic activities, as the portal system is bypassed. The available methods studied were intramuscular injections, subcutaneous implantation[20], vaginal rings[21], vaginal creams[22,23], transdermal application units[24,25] and percutaneous administration of oestradiol[26,27].

Intramuscular injections are no longer used not only because they are uncomfortable for the patient but also because the oestrogen plasma levels obtained are not stable, with initial peaks followed by very low levels of oestrogens[28].

Subcutaneous implantation of oestradiol leads to a rise in plasma E_2 values and the E_2/E_1 ratio is close to physiological values. According to some authors the plasma levels increase to the proliferative phase range and remain stable[20]. However, an irregular resorption of the steroid may occur in some patients and once inserted they are difficult to remove in the case of over-dosage or intolerance.

Vaginal epithelium rapidly resorbs oestrone and oestradiol and the use of vaginal rings[21] or vaginal creams[22,23] lead to high plasma steroid values with physiological E_2/E_1 ratios. However, the oestradiol plasma levels are quite unstable throughout the course of the day or from one day to another, probably because of coincidental striking changes in vaginal secretion and vascularization. Furthermore prolonged topical application of oestrogens in high dosage directly to a target organ, such as the uterine cervix, should not be recommended without further knowledge of long-term tolerance.

Percutaneous absorption of oestradiol

The ability of the skin to absorb steroids has been recognized since the beginning of this century and has been extensively studied[29,30]. The use of appropriate vehicles allows the penetration through the stratum corneum which has the principal 'barrier function'of the epidermis[29]. Different processes occur in sequence. First, absorption of the molecules within the stratum corneum; second, retention in the stratum corneum (reservoir effect); and third, diffusion through the epidermis and papillary dermis until they reach the capillary plexus and are transferred to the circulating blood. Each step of these different events is essential and individual variations at any stage can influence the rate of absorption[29].

Steroids penetrate the stratum corneum quite easily from an appropriate polar vehicle which can affect permeation[29]. The reservoir function of human skin for steroids is localized in the stratum corneum, as demonstrated by Vickers[31]. This role of a reservoir of the stratum corneum induces a sustained release of the steroid percutaneously applied extended to more than 24 hours.

Oestradiol, when applied to human skin in an alcoholic solution, rapidly penetrates the stratum corneum (within ten minutes of application). Then diffusion of the steroid through the epidermis and dermis according to the pathway described above occurs with a delay of several hours[26,32]. The rate of absorption depends upon the dose topically applied, and about 10% of the total dose passes through the cutaneous barrier, is transferred to the vascular system, and eliminated in the urine over the following 72 hours[33].

In women, application of a single dose of 3 mg of 17β-oestradiol in a hydroalcoholic solvent leads to a plasma E_2 increase within 12 hours of administration. The plasma levels obtained vary considerably from one individual to another[26]. However, after three daily repeated applications, the mean plasma concentrations of E_2 become stable and reach levels of 110 + 24 pg/ml, that is within the follicular phase range[27]. No peak increments are observed and this is mainly due to the 'reservoir effect' of the skin, which allows a progressive and constant diffusion of the steroid.

The E_2/E_1 ratio observed after percutaneous application of oestradiol gel remains around 1, close to the physiological values observed during the follicular phase of a normal cycle[13,18,27]. In addition, the levels of E_2 around 100 pg/ml, are able to relieve climacteric complaints and to prevent hypo-oestrogenic consequences[26,27]. The plasma levels of FSH and LH, exhibit a significant decrease[13,27], even if, as with other oestrogenic therapy, the gonadotrophins do not decrease to premenopausal levels. However, it is known that a decrease in plasma gonadotrophins is not necessary to obtain the relief of climacteric complaints[34].

Efficacy of percutaneous oestradiol at the target level

The obtained stable plasma oestradiol values, in the proliferative range correct predictably the oestrogen deficiency, and ensure the efficacy of the treatment at the target level. The relief of hot flushes and night sweats comes rapidly, within the first few days of treatment, and vaginal dryness is reversed[26,27]. Psychological symptoms, and particularly the depressive mood, can be reversed provided the levels of plasma E_2 remain between 50 and 150 pg/ml[35].

As far as the endometrium is concerned, it has been shown by Whitehead *et al.*[36] that percutaneous E_2 induced an increase in nuclear oestradiol receptors (REN) and in soluble progesterone receptors (RPC) within the proliferative phase range, demonstrating the efficacy of this therapy on the target organ. Thus progestogen therapy should be added on a sequential basis, to avoid endometrial hyperplasia, as with any other (active) oestrogenic therapy.

Finally, the activity of percutaneous oestradiol on the breast has not been assessed by *in vitro* studies. However, the appearance of breast tenderness and mastodynia which have been correlated with high oestradiol levels in premenopausal women[37] have been observed in some postmenopausal women treated with percutaneous oestradiol. In these cases E_2 plasma levels reached high values, over 150 pg/ml[38]. Whilst the percutaneous administration of oestradiol is efficient on most of the target organs its efficacy in preventing osteoporosis remains to be demonstrated: this is at the moment under investigation. Preliminary results are encouraging.

Hepato-cellular effects of oestradiol: oral versus percutaneous

In a previous study done by our group it was observed that percutaneous administration of oestradiol was not associated with an increase in serum triglycerides[39], as had been demonstrated by others with vaginal rings[21] or implants[20]. This observation was related to the liver bypass. Other studies have been carried out which confirm the importance of the route of administration of oestradiol to avoid metabolic effects.

Elkik *et al.*[13] studied 18 postmenopausal subjects who received either oral conjugated equine oestrogens (1.25 mg/day) or percutaneous oestradiol cream (5 g of gel/day, i.e. 3 mg oestradiol/day). Conjugated equine oestrogens significantly elevated plasma renin substrate (PRS), sex hormone binding globulin (SHBG), and reduced significantly plasma AT III levels, while no changes were observed after percutaneous oestradiol except a slight increase in SHBG, the most sensitive marker for oestrogenic effect.

Previously, Geola *et al.*[40] reported that even low doses of conjugated equine oestrogens exhibited supraphysiological effects on renin substrate synthesis. Thus the differences in the effects of oral conjugated oestrogens and percutaneous oestradiol cannot be explained solely by a greater hepato-cellular potency of conjugated oestrogens. Oestrone sulphate or 17β-estradiol, the natural molecule, when given orally in effective dosages exhibit a supraphysiological hepato-cellular effect according to the excessive increase in PRS and SHBG plasma levels[30].

Fåhraeus *et al.*[41] studied 38 postmenopausal women receiving either oestradiol cream, 5 g/day (i.e. 3 mg E_2) or micronized oestradiol (2 mg then 4 mg/day). They demonstrated that oral treatment increased the HDL and decreased the LDL levels, thus raising the HDL/LDL ratio, and increased the triglycerides (TG) concentration, while the cutaneous treatment did not induce any significant change in the lipoprotein pattern. Furthermore, they showed in a subsequent study that oral therapy increased preferentially the HDL_2 fraction[42]. Therefore, they concluded that oral therapy was more beneficial, as high HDL/LDL ratios were reported as offering protection against cardiovascular disease in the general population[43]. However, it must be pointed out that:

(1) A decrease in HDL level is not observed after menopause nor implicated in the common risk factors of cardiovascular diseases in postmenopausal women[14]. Evidently the mechanisms and consequences of the increase of HDL subfraction to supraphysiological levels are not clear and not necessarily favourable. In the 1960s, the dramatic increase of α-lipoproteins (HDL-like) induced by oral oestrogen therapy in men coincided with a dramatic increase in the incidence of cardiovascular accidents. Moreover, the oral administration of large doses of ethinyloestradiol increases HDL-cholesteral to very high levels but also increases the morbidity of the thromboembolism.

(2) Other potentially adverse effects of oral therapy could neutralize the supposedly 'benefical' increase of HDL/LDL ratio, namely TG increase, hypertension and thrombogenic effect.

Indeed, Basdevant *et al.*[18] recently demonstrated that oral administration of micronized oestradiol or oestradiol valerate leads to an increase in VLDL-TG while it increased HDL/LDL ratios as observed by Fåhraeus *et al.*[41]. Conversely, percutaneous oestradiol induced a significant decrease in TG and VLDL-TG and no change in cholesterol levels. Furthermore, these authors[44] were able to demonstrate that oral oestradiol induced a dramatic decrease in serum AT III activity while percutaneous oestradiol had no effect as previously observed by Elkik *et al.*[13]

Finally, Whitehead[45] also measured peripheral oestrone 3-glucuronide concentrations. As glucuronidation of oestrogens occurs almost exclusively in hepatic tissues, any change in these values would prove a hepatic interaction. Whitehead compared percutaneous oestradiol to oestradiol implant therapy or to oral therapy with oestradiol valerate and observed a surge in oestrone 3-glucuronide levels the morning following the oral treatment while no changes occurred after parenteral treatment.

In the light of these data, it appears clear that the route of administration of oestradiol is of the greatest importance in oestrogen replacement therapy. Very low levels of ethinyloestradiol (10 μg) of conjugated oestrogens or even of micronized 17β-oestradiol show almost the same adverse metabolic effects if they are administered orally[30,46,47]. The considerable oestrone production observed after oral administration of these steroids corresponds to unphysiologically high concentrations of oestrogens at the hepatic receptor level and may account for the exaggerated hepato-cellular effects of orally administered natural oestrogens. The increase in HDL/LDL ratios should be interpreted with caution in the particular case of oestrogen therapy and obviously the other adverse metabolic disturbances which occur could not be regarded as favourable. The aim of treating a climacteric woman should be to maintain the metabolic conditions at the same level as in the physiological premenopausal state. Any metabolic modification induced by treatment, above or below physiological values, cannot be, *a priori*, considered as desirable.

Mode of administration and compliance to percutaneous therapy

17β-Oestradiol used in topical treatment is dissolved in a hydro-alcoholic solvent and presented in a gel form (60 mg of oestradiol for 100 g of gel). Each tube contains 80 g of gel. Calibration of the tube indicates quantities of 5 g of gel containing 3 mg of E_2. The gel is applied to the skin of the abdomen, arms or shoulders on a surface greater than 70 cm^2. The patient must let the gel dry for five minutes after application and is informed of the symptoms of overdosing, i.e. mastodynia, or underdosing, i.e. persistence of night sweats. She herself is then able to modify the dosage of oestrogens but the finest control is maintained by a plasma determination. The woman informed about the side-effects of oral therapy accepts a new form of drug administration fairly well. Patients are usually less surprised by the mode of administration than the prescribing doctor, and the rate of compliance is very high even on a long-term basis.

The transdermal therapeutic system (TTS)

A new system of delivery of E_2 through the skin has been developed recently. This system consists of two membranes approximately 3 cm in diameter enclosing a reservoir of oestradiol. The lower membrane is covered by adhesive tape and is permeable to the steroid, being applied to the skin for periods of between 24 and 72 hours. The upper membrane is occlusive and impermeable. Two systems have been developed, one to deliver 15 – 30 μg of oestradiol/day and the other of 30 – 60 μg/day. A significant increase in plasma E_2 is observed indicating that E_2 is absorbed but the levels are quite low and decrease immediately to baseline levels after removal of the TTS[24,25]. The difference between this system and percutaneous application of E_2 can be explained by the fact that the use of an occlusive membrane to cover the area of skin where the steroid is applied greatly increases the diffusion through the stratum corneum, which looses its 'reservoir effect'. Also, the surface of application of the total dose of E_2 is important to consider. Nevertheless, the TTS leads to a physiological E_2/E_1 ratio and represents a novel approach in oestrogen administration that warrants further evaluation, with the use of greater surface areas. However, the economic and psychological acceptance of the larger TTS, staying day and night on the skin, remains doubtful for most of the postmenopausal patients.

CONCLUSION

It is widely recognized that the oral administration of oestrogens is responsible for unfavourable metabolic side-effects and many scientists have focused their interest on parenteral routes of administration of oestradiol, mostly for women over 50. The percutaneous therapy appears to be a simple, safe method of delivering oestrogens, since a natural molecule can be used, the plasma E_2 levels can be checked easily, and the therapy easily adjusted. The E_2/E_1 ratios obtained are physiological and ultimately no hepatic or metabolic toxicity has been observed. This therapy represents a novel approach to the treatment of the climacteric woman and to all other forms of substitutive oestrogen therapy.

Acknowledgements

We warmly thank Mrs. Charlotte Vial for her help in preparing the manuscript and Miss Yolaine Desjardins for excellent technical assistance.

References

1. Adlercreutz, H., Martin, F., Pulkkinen, M., Dencker, H., Rimer, U., Sjöberg, N. and Tikkanen, M. (1976). Intestinal metabolism of estrogens. *J. Clin. Endocrinol. Metab.*, **43**, 497
2. Cortés Gallegos, V., Carranco, A., Sojo, I., Navarrete, M., Cervantes, C. and Parra, A. (1979). Accumulation of ethinylestradiol in blood and endometrium of women taking oral contraceptives: the sequential therapy. *Fertil. Steril.*, **32**, 524.
3. Menard, J. and Catt, K. J. (1973). Effects of estrogen treatment on plasma renin parameters in the rat. *Endocrinology*, **92**, 1382
4. Glueck, C. J., Fallat, R. W. and Scheel, D. (1975). Effects of estrogenic compounds on triglyceride kinetics. *Metabolism*, **24**, 537
5. Sagar, S., Stamatakis, J. D., Thomas, D. P. and Kakkar, V. V. (1976). Oral contraceptives, antithrombin-III activity, and postoperative deep-vein thrombosis. *Lancet*, **1**, 509
6. Wessler, S. (1983). *Contraceptive steroids and thrombosis.* Workshop on steroidal contraception, April 1983, Bethesda
7. Laragh, J. H. (1976). Oral contraceptive-induced hypertension. Nine years later. *Am. J. Obstet. Gynecol.*, **126**, 141
8. Stern, W. P., Brown, B. W., Haskell, W. L., Farquhar, T. W., Wehrle, C. L. and Wood, P. D. S. (1976). Cardiovascular risk and use of estrogens or estrogen/progestagen combination. *J. Am. Med. Assoc.*, **235**, 811
9. Von Kaulla, E. and Von Kaulla, K. N. (1970). Oral contraceptives and low antithrombin-III activity. *Lancet*, **1**, 36
10. Gammal, E. B. (1976). Intimal thickening in arteries of rats treated with synthetic sex hormones. *Br. J. Exp. Pathol.*, **57**, 248
11. Furman, R. H., Alaupovic, P. and Howard, R. P. (1967). Effect of androgens and estrogens on serum lipids and the composition and concentration of serum

lipoproteins in normolipemic and hyperlipidemic states. *Prog. Biochem. Pharmacol.*, **2**, 215

12. Poller, L., Thompson, J. M. and Coope, J. (1977). Conjugated equine estrogens and blood clotting: A follow-up report. *Br. Med. J.*, **1**, 935
13. Elkik, F., Gompel, A., Mercier-Bodard, C., Kuttenn, F., Guyenne, P. N., Corvol, P. and Mauvais-Jarvis, P. (1982). Effects of percutaneous estradiol and conjugated estrogens on the level of plasma proteins and triglycerides in post-menopausal women. *Am. J. Obstet. Gynecol.*, **143**, 888
14. Gordon, T., Kannel, W. B., Hjortland, M. C. and McNamara, P. M. (1978). Menopause and coronary heart disease. The Framingham Study. *Am. Intern. Med.*, **89**, 157
15. Stone, G. M., Baggett, B. and Donnelly, R. B. (1963). The uptake of tritiated estrogens by various organs of the ovariectomized mouse following intravenous administration. *J. Endocrinol.*, **27**, 271
16. Gallagher, T. F., Mueller, M. N. and Kappas, A. (1966). Studies on the structural basis for estrogen-induced impairment of liver function. *Medicine*, **45**, 471
17. Whitehead, M. T., McQueen, J., Minardi, J. and Campbell, S. (1978). Clinical considerations in the management of the menopause: the endometrium. *Postgrad. Med. J.*, **54**, 69
18. Basdevant, A., de Lignières, B. and Guy-Grand, B. (1983). Differential lipemic and hormonal responses to oral and parenteral 17β-estradiol in post-menopausal women. *Am. J. Obstet. Gynecol.*, **147**, 77.
19. Yen, S. S. C., Martin, P. L., Burnier, A. M., Czekala, N. M., Greaney, M. O., Jr. and Callantine, M. R. (1975). Circulating estradiol, estrone and gonadotrophin levels following the administration of orally active 17β-estradiol in postmenopausal women. *J. Clin. Endocrinol. Metab.*, **40**, 518
20. Greenblatt, R. B. and Bryner, J. R. (1977). Estradiol pellet implantation in the management of menopause. *J. Reprod. Med.*, **18**, 307
21. Mishell, D. R., Jr., Moore, D. E., Roy, S., Brenner, P. F. and Page, M. A. (1978). Clinical performance and endocrine profiles with contraceptive vaginal rings containing a combination of estradiol and d-norgestrel. *Am. J. Obstet. Gynecol.*, **130**, 55
22. Rigg, L. A., Hermann, H. and Yen, S. S. C. (1978). Absorption of estrogens from vaginal creams. *N. Engl. J. Med.*, **298**, 195
23. Whitehead, M. I., Minardi, J., Kitchin, Y. and Sharples, M. J. (1978). Systemic absorption of estrogen from Premarin vaginal cream. In Cooke, I. (ed.) *The Role of Estrogen/Progestogen in the Management of the Menopause*, pp. 63–71. (Lancaster: MTP Press)
24. Laufer, L., De Fazio, J., Lu, J., Meldrum, D., Eggena, P., Sambhi, M., Hershman, J. M. and Judd, H. L. (1983). Estrogen Replacement Therapy (ERT) by transdermal estradiol administration. *Am. J. Obstet. Gynecol.*, **146**, 533
25. Schenkel, L. (1981). A new method of controlled, percutaneous oestradiol administration. In van Keep, P. A., Utian, W. H. and Vermeulen, A. (eds) *The Controversial Climacteric*, p. 111. (Lancaster: MTP Press)
26. Basdevant, A. and de Lignières, B. (1980). Treatment of menopause by topical administration of estradiol. In Mauvais-Jarvis, P., Vickers, C. F. H. and Wepierre, J. (eds) *Percutaneous Absorption of Steroids*, pp. 249–258. (London: Academic Press)
27. Sitruk-Ware, R., de Lignières, B., Basdevant, A. and Mauvais-Jarvis, P. (1980). Absorption of percutaneous oestradiol in post-menopausal women. *Maturitas*, **2**, 207

28. Somerville, B. W. (1975). Estrogen-withdrawal migraine. Duration of exposure required and attempted prophylaxis by premenstrual estrogen administration. *Neurology*, **25**, 239
29. Scheuplein, R. J. (1980). Percutaneous absorption: Theoretical aspects. In Mauvais-Jarvis, P., Vickers, C. F. H. and Wepierre, J. (eds) *Percutaneous Absorption of Steroids*, pp. 1–17. (London: Academic Press)
30. Mashchak, C. A., Lobo, R. A., Dozono-Takano, R., Eggena, P., Nakamura, R. M., Brenner, E. F. and Mishell, D. R., Jr. (1982). Comparison of pharmacodynamic properties of various estrogen formulations. *Am. J. Obstet. Gynecol.*, **144**, 511
31. Vickers, C. F. H. (1980). Reservoir effect of human skin: pharmacological speculation. In Mauvais-Jarvis, P., Vickers, C. F. H. and Wepierre, J. (eds) *Percutaneous Absorption of Steroids*, pp. 19–29. (London: Academic Press)
32. Wendker, H., Schaefer, H. and Zesch, A. (1976). Penetrations kinetics and distribution of topically applied estrogens. *Arch. Dermatol. Res.*, **256**, 67
33. Feldmann, R. J. and Maibach, H. I. (1969). Percutaneous penetration of steroids in man. *J. Invest. Dermatol.*, **52**, 89
34. Utian, W. H., Katz, M., Davey, D. A. and Carr, P. J. (1978). Effect of premenopausal castration and incremental dosages of conjugated equine estrogens on plasma follicle-stimulating hormone, luteinizing hormone and estradiol. *Am. J. Obstet. Gynecol.*, **132**, 297
35. de Lignières, B. and Vincens, M. (1982). Differential effects of exogenous estradiol and progesterone on mood in post-menopausal women: individual dose/effect relationship. *Maturitas*, **4**, 67
36. Whitehead, M. I., Townsend, P. T., Pryse-Davies, J., Ryder, T. A. and King, R. J. B. (1981). Effects of estrogens and progestins on the biochemistry and morphology of the postmenopausal endometrium. *N. Engl. J. Med.*, **305**, 1599
37. Sitruk-Ware, R., Sterkers, N. and Mauvais-Jarvis, P. (1979). Benign breast diseases. I. Hormonal investigation. *Obstet. Gynecol.*, **53**, 457
38. de Lignières, B. and Mauvais-Jarvis, P. (1981). Hormonal dependence of benign breast disease, gynecomastia and breast cancer. In Hollman, K. H., de Brux, J. and Verley, J. M. (eds) *New Frontiers in Mammary Pathology*, pp. 287–308. (New York: Plenum Press)
39. Loeper, J., Loeper, J., Ohlgiesser, C., de Lignières, B. and Mauvais-Jarvis, P. (1977). Influence de l'estrogénothérapie sur les triglycérides. *Nouv. Presse Méd.*, **6**, 2747
40. Geola, F. J., Frumar, A. M., Tataryn, I. V., Lu, K. H., Hershman, J., Eggena, P., Sambhi, M. P. and Judd, H. L. (1980). Biological effects of various doses of conjugated equine estrogens in post-menopausal women. *J. Clin. Endocrinol. Metab.*, **51**, 620
41. Fåhraeus, L., Larsson-Cohn, U. and Wallentin, L. (1982). Lipoproteins during oral and cutaneous administration of oestradiol-17β to menopausal women. *Acta Endocrinol.*, **101**, 597
42. Fåhraeus, L. and Wallentin, L. (1983). High density lipoprotein subfractions during oral and cutaneous administration of 17β-estradiol to menopausal women. *J. Clin. Endocrinol. Metab.*, **56**, 797
43. Gordon, T., Castelli, W. P., Hjortland, M. C., Kannel, W. B. and Dawber, T. R. (1977). High density lipoprotein as a protective factor against coronary heart disease. *Am. J. Med.*, **62**, 707
44. Conard, J., Samama, M., Basdevant, A., Guy-Grand, B. and de Lignières, B. (1983). Differential AT III-response to oral and parenteral administration of 17β-estradiol. *Thromb. Haemostas.*, **49**, 252

45. Whitehead, M. I. (1982). Comparative studies of oral, vaginal, subcutaneous and percutaneous oestrogen administration on plasma oestrogen levels, SHBG and endometrial receptors. In van Keep, P.A., Utian, W. H. and Vermeulen, A. (eds) *The Controversial Climacteric*, pp. 110–116. (Lancaster: MTP Press)
46. Campbell, S. (1982). Potency and hepato-cellular effects of oestrogens after oral, percutaneous and subcutaneous administration. In van Keep, P. A., Utian, W. H. and Vermeulen, A. (eds) *The Controversial Climacteric*, pp. 103–125. (Lancaster: MTP Press)
47. Mandel, F., Geola, F., Lu, J., Eggena, P., Sambhi, M., Hershman, J. and Judd, H. (1982). Biologic effects of various doses of ethinylestradiol in postmenopausal women. *Obstet. Gynecol.*, **59**, 673

Chapter 15

Clinical effects of vaginally applied oestrogens

S. Wesel

The problems related to vulvo-vaginal atrophy in the perimenopause are often disregarded or even disdained for reasons that are mostly determined culturally. Women brought up on a sexually restrictive climate of embarrassment often hesitate to mention such problems even to their gynaecologist. The gynaecologist, usually male, in turn tends to consider the decrease of sexual activity caused by these problems as simply to be expected.

The vaginal application of oestrogens is a rewarding therapy for the problems and complaints caused by atrophy of the uro-genital organs. This treatment is well accepted by patients and is easy to administer.

Oestrogens, also oestriol, have proven their effectiveness when administered orally[1,2]. However, relatively high doses are required to obtain a locally satisfactory effect and the sometimes just irksome but sometimes truly serious side-effects of high doses of oestrogens are well known.

For vaginal problems it is therefore logical to prefer locally applied oestrogen therapy in smaller doses, from which one can expect a satisfactory result without side-effects, either general or local. The local application of ointment or of vaginal suppositories containing synthetic or natural conjugated equine oestrogens has produced very good results, but resorption through the vaginal mucosa has been seen to be sufficiently high as to produce a significant rise in the blood concentration of oestrogens and to cause an inhibition of FSH and LH[3-7].

Luisi has shown, in 1980 at the International Symposium on the Menopause held in Viareggio, Italy, a considerable rise of E_1, E_2 and sex hormone binding globulin (SHBG) during treatment with locally applied conjugated equine oestrogens, while oestriol did not produce any change in these three parameters[7]. Both preparations produced a slight rise of the E_3 level and an inhibition of FSH and LH but this inhibition was significantly higher with conjugated equine oestrogens (Figures 1 and 2). When treated with oestriol the patients' endometrium remained atrophic, while a slight proliferation occurred during treatment with conjugated equine oestrogens. These results were confirmed

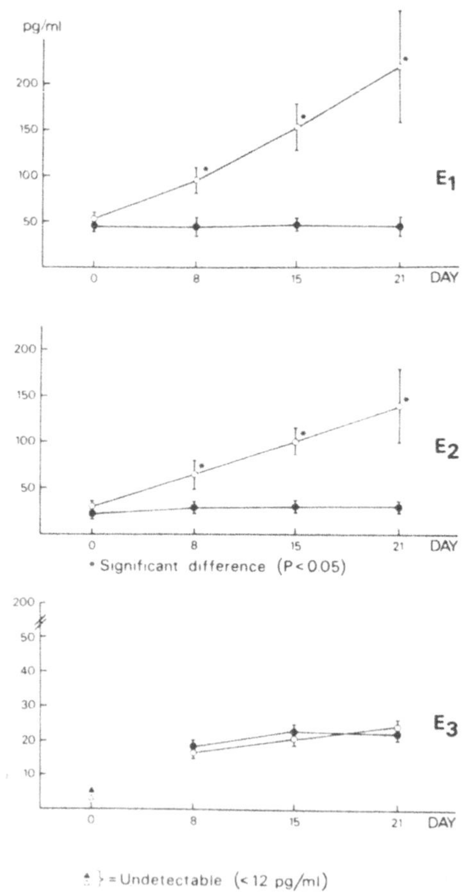

Figure 1 Mean plasma levels (±SD) of E_1, E_2 and E_3. E_1 = oestrone; E_2 = oestradiol; E_3 = oestriol. o—o, Conjugated equine oestrogen, •—•, oestriol. (Adapted from Luisi *et al.*[7])

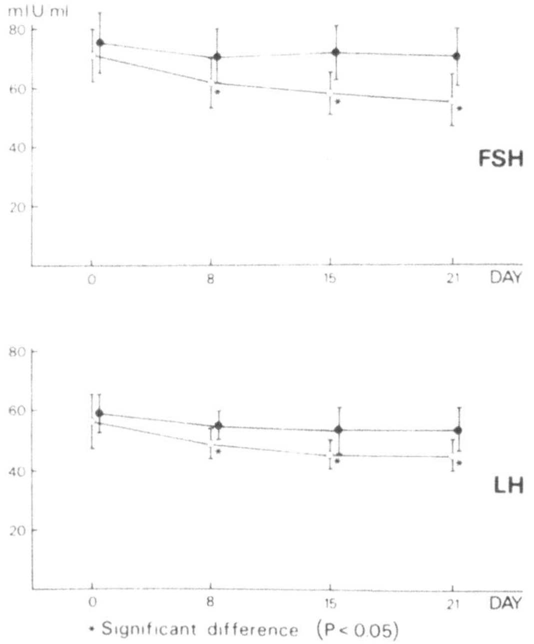

Figure 2 Mean plasma levels (±SD) of FSH and LH. o—o, Conjugated equine oestrogen, •—•, oestriol. (Adapted from Luisi *et al.*[7])

by Kicovic *et al.*[8]. In an earlier study[4] the author had to perform curettages on two patients suffering from metrorrhagia after treatment with locally applied conjugated equine oestrogens. It seems therefore that preparations for local use based on oestriol combine the required conditions for treatment of relatively minor problems. Only a therapy that brings ease and comfort and adds to the quality of life, whilst on the other hand not producing any irksome or even dangerous side-effects, is acceptable.

Clearly the effects of locally applied oestriol remain to be established.

Michalas *et al.*[9] treated 20 patients suffering from vaginal atrophy with vaginal suppositories containing 0.5 mg of oestriol for a period of 13 weeks with a dose of one suppository per day during the first week and one suppository every second day during the remaining 12 weeks. Table 1 shows the clinical results of the treatment. Marked improvement was observed in most patients.

The maturation index showed a significant shift towards the intermediate and superficial cell types (Table 2).

Feldman[10] reported in 1980 on a study carried out on 62 patients

Table 1 The objective complaints and therapeutic effects after 1, 4 and 12 weeks

Patient number	*Diagnosis*	*After 1 week*	*After 4 weeks*	*After 12 weeks*
1	Atrophy	†	††	†††
2	Atrophy	†	††	†††
3	Atrophy	○	††	††
4	Dyspareunia	†	††	†††
5	Colpitis senilis	††	†	††
6	Colpitis senilis	†	††	††
7	Atrophy	†	††	†††
8	Atrophy			
9	Atrophic genitals	○	○	†
10	Atrophic genitals	††	††	†††
11	Dyspareunia	○	††	†††
12	Early atrophy	†	†	††
13	Atrophy of vulva and vagina	†	†	†
14	Atrophy	††	††	†††
15	Atrophy	○	†	††
16	Early atrophy	†	††	†††
17	Dry vagina	○	†	††
18	Atrophy of vulva and vagina			
19	Atrophy	†	††	†††
20	Colpitis senilis	††	†††	†††

††† Cured
†† Marked improvement
† Slight improvement
○ No improvement
(Adapted from Michalas *et al.*[9])

treated once daily with ointment or vaginal suppositories for a period of two weeks. The clinical results were as follows: cured 52, improved 10. The cytological results indicated a better maturation index (Table 3).

Anger[11] treated 25 patients over two weeks with one ointment application per day. His results were even more impressive: three patients with dyspareunia were cured and so were 17 with senile colpitis and five with vaginal descensus. The cytological tests showed a normalization in all cases (Table 4)

Our own study[12] included 47 patients treated with one vaginal suppository daily for three weeks and one suppository every second day for the following month. Table 5 shows the evolution of the subjective complaints and symptoms.

Table 6 shows the development of the maturation index. These results confirm conclusively the effectiveness of locally applied oestriol in patients with vulvo-vaginal disease in the postmenopause.

Table 2

	Findings prior to therapy: Maturation index (MI)			*Findings after 12 weeks of therapy: Maturation index (MI)*		
Patient number	*Parabasal cells*	*Intermediate cells*	*Superficial cells*	*Parabasal cells*	*Intermediate cells*	*Superficial cells*
1	100	0	0	0	70	30
2	100	0	0	0	70	30
3	80	20	0	0	80	20
4	100	0	0	0	70	30
5	80	20	0	0	85	15
6	80	20	0	0	90	10
7	60	40	0			
8	80	20	0	0	90	10
9	100	0	0	60	40	0
10	80	20	0	0	85	15
11	100	0	0	0	90	10
12	100	0	0	0	90	10
13	100	0	0	0	90	10
14	80	20	0	0	70	30
15	100	0	0	0	90	10
16	100	0	0	0	70	30
17	100	0	0	0	90	10
18	80	20	0			
19	80	20	0	0	85	15
20	70	30	0	0	80	20

(Adapted from Michalas *et al.*[9])

Table 3

Administration form	cream/pessaries	
Number of patients:	62	
Length of study:	2 weeks	
Therapeutic scheme		
Cream: 1 application/day	2 weeks	
Results		
Clinical:	recovery	52
	improving	10
Cytological:	restoring of an eutrophic maturation index	

(Adapted from Feldman[10])

We prescribed oestriol in the form of one vaginal suppository per week by way of continuous treatment; we have never observed side-effects due to this treatment. Some women do have an occasional irritation but in all probability this is due to the excipient.

Table 4

Administration form	cream	
Number of patients:	25	
Length of study:	2 weeks	
Therapeutic scheme		
1 application/day	2 weeks	
Results		
Clinical:	dyspareunia	3/3
	senile colpitis	17/17
	descensus vaginalis	5/5
Cytological:	smear normalization	

(Adapted from Anger[11])

Table 5 Evolution of the subjective symptoms of atrophic vaginitis in 47 patients

Week			*Improvement*			*No. of*
(dosage)	*Aggravation*	*Status quo*	*Slight*	*Pronounced*	*Cure*	*patients*
1 (0.5/day)	—	8	21	16	2	47
3 (2 × 0.5/wk)	—	1	4	19	22	46 *
5 (2 × 0.5/wk)	—	0	2	16	28	46 *
7 (2 × 0.5/wk)	—	0	1	9	34	44 **

* One patient discontinued treatment because of intercurrent bleeding
** Two patients did not return for the last control
(Adapted from Wesel[12])

Table 6 Evolution of the maturation index (as a percentage)

	Type of cells (data in %)		
Test	*Superficial*	*Intermediary*	*Basal/parabasal*
Before treatment	2.8	35.2	56.5
Week 1	29.3	66.0	4.2
Week 3	38.1	61.2	0.7
Week 5	20.1	79.1	0.1
Week 7	18.2	79.2	2.3

(Adapted from Wesel[12])

CONCLUSION

We would emphasize the importance of using local oestrogen therapy on women with problems of vulvo-vaginal atrophy in the peri- and postmenopause. This method of treatment is reliable, effective, harmless and contributes considerably to the comfort and well-being of women whose role in society is still growing. Among locally applied drugs oestriol, prepared in several different forms, would appear to be the first choice.

References

1. Tzingounis, V. V., Aksu, M. F. and Greenblatt, R. B. (1978). Estriol in the management of the menopause. *J. Am. Med. Assoc.*, **239**, 1638
2. Perovic, D., Kopajtic, B. and Stankovic, T. (1975). Treatment of climacteric complaints with estriol. *Arzneim.-Forsch.*, **25**, 962
3. Falk, H. C. and Hassid, R. (1963) Atrophic or senile vaginitis: treatment with dienestrol cream. *J. Am. Geriatr. Soc.*, **11**, 1152
4. Widholm, O. and Vartiainen, E. (1947). The absorption of conjugated oestrogen and sodium oestrone sulphate from the vagina. *Ann. Chir. Gynaecol. Fenn.*, **63**, 186
5. Englund, D. E. and Johansson, E. D. B. (1978). Plasma levels of oestrone, oestradiol and gonadotrophins in postmenopausal women after oral and vaginal administration of conjugated equine oestrogens (Premarin). *Br. J. Obstet. Gynaecol.*, **85**, 957
6. Rigg, L. A., Hermann, H. and Yen, S. S. C. (1978). Absorption of estrogens from vaginal creams. *N. Engl. J. Med.*, **298**, 195
7. Luisi, M., Franchi, F. and Kicovic, P. M. (1980). A group-comparative study of effects of Ovestin cream versus Premarin cream in post-menopausal women with vaginal atrophy. *Maturitas*, **2**, 311
8. Kicovic, P. M., Cortes-Prieto, J., Milojevic, S., Haspels, A. A. and Aljinovic, A. (1980). The treatment of postmenopausal vaginal atrophy with Ovestin vaginal cream or suppositories: clinical, endocrinological and safety aspects. *Maturitas*, **2**, 275
9. Michalas, S., Papandrikos, A., Koutselini, E. and Tzingounis, V. (1980). Local therapy of atrophic vaginal conditions with oestriol suppositories. *J. Int. Med. Res.*, **8**, 358
10. Feldman, H. U. (1980). Häufig reicht die alleinige topische Applikation von Östriol aus. *Gynecologie 10*. (Essen: HUF Verlag)
11. Anger, H. (1980). Atrophie des Vaginalepithels. Therapeutische Erfahrungen mit Ortho-Gynest. *Gynecologie 9*. (Essen: HUF Verlag)
12. Wesel, S., Etienne, J. and Lestienne, M. C. (1981). Clinical, cytological and biological study of the intra-vaginal administration of oestriol (Ortho-Gynest) in postmenopausal patients. *Maturitas*, **3**, 271

Chapter 16

Hormone implants in women following hysterectomy and bilateral salpingo-oophorectomy

J. W. W. Studd, L. D. Cardozo, D. M. F. Gibb, S. M. Tuck, A. L. Magos, M. Brincat and D. J. Cooper

INTRODUCTION

Hormone replacement therapy is becoming an accepted form of treatment for menopausal symptoms and the prevention of osteoporosis[1,2]. There are various routes of administration available. Oral therapy will undoubtedly remain the most frequent mode of administration, but percutaneous routes using either oestrogen cream or subcutaneous hormone pellets seem to have an advantage in that they avoid the first pass liver effect. Pellets of oestradiol, with or without testosterone, are inserted under local anaesthesia as an outpatient. The technique is simple, fast and painless[3]. The blood hormone values obtained have been described[4] and it should be noted that physiological levels of plasma oestradiol and oestrone equivalent to those found in the proliferative phase are found following the use of a 50 mg oestradiol implant. This is opposite to the high and unphysiological concentration of oestrone that occurs after oral oestrone or oestradiol therapy[5].

Over the last seven years, more than 2000 women have had over 10 000 implants in our clinic. We believe that the presence of a uterus is not a contraindication to this form of hormone replacement therapy, as long as the patient has from five to ten days of progestogen each month to produce a withdrawal bleed and prevent endometrial hyperplasia[6]. Our experience of this has been reported elsewhere[7]. This paper is a study of hormone implants in women who have previously undergone a hysterectomy and bilateral salpingo-oophorectomy.

PATIENTS AND METHODS

A total of 55 women who had previously had a total abdominal hysterectomy and bilateral salpingo-oophorectomy attending Dulwich Hospital Menopause Clinic, and receiving hormone implant therapy for their climacteric symptoms were admitted to the study. Of the patients 67% had previously taken oral hormone replacement therapy which was considered unsatisfactory for a variety of reasons. None had any contraindications to hormone treatment and all had received between one and five consecutive implants of oestradiol 50 mg and testosterone 100 mg (Organon Laboratories) over a period of up to four years.

A full history was taken and a general examination, including breasts, abdomen and pelvis, was performed on entry to the study and before hormone administration. Weight and blood pressure were recorded. A proforma was completed comparing symptoms before and after implant therapy. Side-effects and other complications were noted. A 20 ml sample of venous blood was withdrawn at five to seven months after the previous implant, when most patients were complaining of a recurrence of symptoms. Plasma levels of follicle stimulating hormone (FSH), luteinizing hormone (LH), oestrone (E_1), oestradiol (E_2) and testosterone (T) were measured.

RESULTS

The mean age of the study group at the time of assessment was 48.4 years (range 28–63), and a total of 245 implants had been administered. There was significant relief of all symptoms (Student's t test on paired samples, $p < 0.05$), and hot flushes were relieved to some extent in all patients (Table 1). The duration of symptomatic relief was six months in 80% of patients (range 3–12 months). There

Table 1 The effects of oestradiol and testosterone implants on climacteric symptoms in 55 castrated women

Symptoms	*Present before implants* (%)	*Complete relief* (%)	*Incomplete relief* (%)	*No relief* (%)
Hot flushes	89.1	95.9	4.1	0.0
Headaches	72.7	67.5	25.1	7.5
Insomnia	70.9	79.5	18.8	7.7
Palpitation	45.5	76.0	20.0	4.0
Bone pains	65.5	63.9	19.4	16.7
Dyspareunia	65.5	69.4	27.7	2.8
Loss of libido	87.3	68.7	29.2	2.1
Irritability	81.8	73.4	24.4	2.2
Poor concentration	63.6	60.0	28.6	11.4
Depression	76.4	81.0	16.7	2.3
Lethargy	72.7	72.5	25.0	2.5
Urethral syndrome	25.5	50.0	21.4	28.6

were no significant changes in systolic or diastolic blood pressures during implant treatment (Tables 2 and 3). A statistically significant proportion of women showed an increase in weight following this treatment (Student's t test on paired samples, $p < 0.05$; Table 4). The commonest side-effect was breast tenderness (32.7%), but only two patients (3.6%) complained of severe discomfort. Slight hirsutism was noted by 9.1% of patients and acne by one. There were no complaints of nausea and vomiting. No patient had to discontinue treatment because of side-effects. There were no cases of venous thrombosis but two patients (3.6%) developed benign breast pathology.

Blood hormone levels after varying numbers of implants are shown

Table 2 Changes in systolic blood pressure after implant treatment

Change in systolic blood pressure (mmHg)	*Patients* (%)
+ > 40	3.7
+ 31 – 40	7.4
+ 21 – 30	11.1
+ 11 – 20	11.1
No change	42.6
– 11 – 20	7.4
– 21 – 30	13.0
– 31 – 40	3.7
– > 40	0.0

Table 3 Changes in diastolic blood pressure after implant treatment

Change in diastolic blood pressure (mmHg)	*Patients* (%)
+ > 40	3.7
+ 31 - 40	3.7
+ 21 - 30	9.3
+ 11 - 20	13.0
No change	50.0
- 11 - 20	16.5
- 21 - 30	1.9
- 31 - 40	0.0
- > 40	1.9

Table 4 Changes in weight after implant treatment

Change in body weight (kg)	*Patients* (%)
+ > 10	0.0
+ 6 - 10	16.4
+ 1 - 5	30.9
No change	23.6
- 1 - 5	23.6
- 6 - 10	5.5
- > 10	0.0

Table 5 Plasma hormone concentrations after implant treatment

	Concentration 6 months after index implant				
	Number of implants (n)				
Hormone	1 (8)	2 (4)	3 (7)	4 (10)	5 (14)
FSDH (IU/l)*	27.9	26.2	3.2	16.2	2.4
LH (IU/l)*	30.1	7.4	5.5	13.4	3.0
Oestrone (pmol/l)Δ	462	365	370	363	369
Oestradiol (pmol)/l)Δ	364	467	409	610	821
Testosterone (nmol)/1)Δ	2.5	2.6	2.5	1.9	2.2

* Arithmetic mean
Δ Geometric mean

in Table 5. Plasma FSH fell markedly after two implants, although plasma LH concentrations declined after only one. Following the first implant plasma oestrone was higher than oestradiol, but the ratio was reversed following subsequent implants, the concentration of oestradiol increasing progressively with successive implants. There were no significant changes in plasma testosterone levels.

DISCUSSION

The natural cessation of ovarian function during the climacteric occurs gradually, and many women may be asymptomatic or only have mild symptoms which do not require treatment. However, premenopausal women who have been castrated suffer severe and prolonged symptoms from acute hormone withdrawal[8]. These patients require treatment which may be life-long. The major climacteric symptoms fall into five categories: (a) vasomotor; (b) emotional; (c) psychosexual; (d) genito-urinary; and (e) musculo-skeletal[9]. The classical vasomotor symptom is the hot flush, which has been shown unequivocally to respond to oestrogen therapy[10]. Other studies have shown that conjugated equine oestrogens given orally cure hot flushes in over 90% of cases. Our data show that oestradiol implants give complete relief from hot flushes in 96% of patients.

Emotional factors are more difficult to assess as they may be due to reasons not directly associated with the menopause. In castrated women depression may occur due to the operation itself rather than hormone withdrawal, so it is difficult to assess the effects of replacement therapy. Campbell and Whitehead[10] suggested that these symptoms often respond by a 'domino effect' after the hot flushes had been cured. Nevertheless, a large proportion of patients (81%) thought that their depression was cured by oestradiol implants, which suggests that in this type of patient this symptom is hormone dependent. Similarly, insomnia was cured in 80% of patients. It is possible that some of these were able to sleep more easily because they no longer suffered from night sweats, as well as the change in their emotional state.

It is significant that 67% of our patients had implants because of unsatisfactory oral therapy. There may be good metabolic reasons why this is so, as percutaneous treatment, whether it is oestrogen cream or subcutaneous implants of oestradiol, avoids the first pass effect through the liver and the unwanted metabolic changes of clotting factors and lipoproteins which occur with oral therapy. Also, physiological plasma levels and normal ratio of oestradiol to oestrone occur with oestradiol implants rather than the excessively high concentration of oestrone which follow oral oestrone or oestradiol administration[5]. No valid comparison should be made at this time of symptomatic changes after oral and implant treatments, but the apparent preference of over half of our patients to hormone pellets suggests that a randomized trial of the different routes of oestrogen administration is long overdue.

Psychosexual problems occurring at the menopause have been shown to respond to testosterone[11]. During the natural climacteric the ovaries continue to secrete testosterone indefinitely, whereas in a castrated patient there is immediate withdrawal and severe symptoms occur. 87% of our patients complained of loss of libido. Oral methyltestosterone can cause cholestasis and liver adenomata[12], whereas disorders of liver function are not found with implants of crystalline testosterone[13]. Of our patients receiving implants of testosterone 70% reported that their psychosexual symptoms were completely cured. Dyspareunia may be improved by testosterone but is also helped by oestrogens. There is new work suggesting that testosterone is no more effective than oestradiol alone in the correction of loss of libido when studied under controlled conditions[14] and this aspect of post-menopausal hormone replacement therapy requires further study.

Loss of body calcium after the menopause is responsible for osteoporosis. Bone and joint pains are often part of the syndrome. Only 65% of our castrated patients experienced this, and of these only 64% found that hormone treatment cured the 'arthritis'. Lindsay *et al.*[15] showed that osteoporosis could be prevented in nearly all cases by oral oestrogens. Thus it may be that our patients complained of bone pains for some reason other than osteoporosis.

The incidence of all side-effects in our study was low. Although 32.7% of patients complained of breast tenderness, in the majority of cases it was mild and disappeared within four weeks. Hirsutism was rarely volunteered as a symptom, but on direct questioning occurred in 9.1%; it was no more than an increase in downy hair on the side of the face which was not troublesome, and disappeared immediately if testosterone was excluded from subsequent implants.

There can be no doubt that percutaneous implant therapy is an effective means of treating climacteric symptoms, especially in patients without a uterus where there is no risk of abnormal vaginal bleeding. The symptoms return at approximately six months when it is our practice to reinsert the hormone pellets. It is reassuring that the slight cumulative effect of repeated implants on plasma hormone levels do not reach the abnormal range.

An intriguing finding is that symptoms recur at a time when plasma oestradiol, oestrone, FSH and LH are all in the normal premenopausal range. Subsequent unpublished work by us shows that an active implant removes symptoms at this stage, while a placebo is not effective. Our conclusion is that these climacteric symptoms are not the result of absolute low levels of oestrogen, but are a product of a change of plasma concentrations, presumably from high to normal. We believe that the association of symptoms with a 'flux' of hormone concentrations is an important concept in the understanding of the aetiology of the symptoms of the climacteric.

References

1. Greenblatt, R. B. and Suran, R. R. (1949). Indications for hormone pellets in the therapy of endocrine and gynaecological disorders. *Am. J. Obstet. Gynecol.*, **57**, 294
2. Studd, J. W. W. (1976). Management of the menopause. *Practitioner*, **216**, 546
3. Thom, M. H. and Studd, J. W. W. (1980). Prodecures in practice–Hormone implantation. *Br. Med. J.*, **280**, 848
4. Thom, M. H., Collins, W. P. and Studd, J. W. W. (1981). Hormonal profiles in post-menopausal women after therapy with subcutaneous implants. *Br. J. Obstet. Gynaecol.*, **88**, 426
5. Jacobs, H. S., Hutton, J. D., Murray, M. A. F. and James, V. H. T. (1977). Plasma hormone profiles in postmenopausal women before and during oestrogen therapy. *Br. J. Obstet. Gynaecol.*, **84**, 314
6. Studd, J. W. W. and Thom, M. H. (1981). Oestrogens and endometrial cancer. In Studd, J. W. W. (ed.) *Progress in Obstetrics and Gynaecology,* Vol. 1, pp. 182–198. (Edinburgh: Churchill Livingstone)
7. Cardozo, L. D., Gibb, D. M. F., Thom, M. H. and Studd, J. W. W. (1983). Treatment of the climacteric with hormone implants of oestradiol and testosterone. *Am. J. Obstet. Gynecol.* (In press)
8. Chakravarti, S., Collins, W. P., Newton, J. R., Oram, D. H. and Studd, J. W. W. (1977). Endocrine changes and symptomatology after oophorectomy in premenopausal women. *Br. J. Obstet. Gynaecol.*, **84**, 769
9. Studd, J. W. W., Chakravarti, S. and Oram, D. H. (1977). The climacteric. In Greenblatt, R. B. and Studd, J. W. W. (eds) *Clinics in Obstetrics and Gynaecology,* Vol. 4, 1, pp. 3–29. (London: W. B. Saunders)
10. Campbell, S. and Whitehead, M. I. (1977). Oestrogen therapy and the menopausal syndrome. In Greenblatt, R. B. and Studd, J. W. W. (eds) *Clinics in Obstetrics and Gynaecology,* Vol. 4, 1, pp. 31–47. (London: W. B. Saunders)
11. Studd, J. W. W., Collins, W. P., Chakravarti, S., Newton, J. R., Oram, D. H. and Parsons, A. (1977). Oestradiol and testosterone implants in the treatment of psychosexual problems in the postmenopausal woman. *Br. J. Obstet. Gynaecol.*, **84**, 314
12. Westaby, D., Ogle, S. J., Paradinas, F. J., Randell, J. B. and Murray-Lyon, I. M. (1977). Liver damage from long-term methyltestosterone. *Lancet*, **2**, 261
13. Studd, J. W. W. (1981). The hepatic effects of crystalline pellets of testosterone. In van Keep, P. A., Utian, W. H. and Vermeulen, A. (eds) *The Controversial Climacteric,* p. 35. (Lancaster: MTP Press)
14. Dow, M. G. T., Hart, D. M. and Forrest, C. A. (1983). Hormonal treatments of sexual unresponsiveness in postmenopausal women: a comparative study. *Br. J. Obstet. Gynaecol.*, **90**, 361
15. Lindsay, R., Hart, D. M., Aitken, J. M., MacDonald, E. B., Anderson, J. B. and Clarke, A. C. (1976). Long-term prevention of postmenopausal osteoporosis by oestrogen. *Lancet*, **1**, 1038

Chapter 17

Osteoporosis and its treatment

J. Dequeker, P. Geusens and A. Verstraeten

INTRODUCTION

Osteoporosis is the most common of the diseases that affect bones. One out of four women will develop osteoporosis after the menopause. But first, what is osteoporosis? Osteoporosis is defined clinically as the loss of bone (ostopaenia) sufficient to result in fractures with minimal trauma, generally of the spine, but also of the hip and wrist.

Although men and women lose bone when they age[1,2], women are more prone to osteoporosis than are men. This may be because of hormonal factors and because women have smaller, more fragile skeletons to begin with. Even in postmenopausal women osteoporosis is a heterogenous syndrome. Osteoporosis may be the end result of different pathological mechanisms on top of physiological bone loss with ageing, e.g. oestrogen/progestogen deficiency, reduction in intestinal calcium absorption, renal calcium loss, immobilization, imbalance in vitamin D metabolites, parathyroid hormone, calcitonin, growth hormone, thyroid hormone, endogenous corticosteroids and alcohol consumption.

Heterogenesis of osteoporosis is further characterized by the apparent difference in fracture sites, trabecular (spine) or cortical (femoral neck) and the bone remodelling activity, low or high turnover at the time of bone failure[3]. Because treatment may differ depending on the cause and type of osteoporosis, cortical or trabecular failure, differential diagnosis remains important.

Given the heterogenesis in the osteoporotic syndrome, what is known in the literature to prevent, to reduce or to cure osteoporosis? Clinical studies with different treatment regimens have been numerous. Few studies have clearly defined the factors responsible for osteoporosis in the patient population studied, but then few studies have included double-blind controls. Many studies were short, too short to show clear-cut changes in bone density or structure. Furthermore, short-term studies do not take into account the concept of basic multicellular units, in which there is a definite coupling between bone resorption and formation[4]. In these studies false conclusions can thus be made. For example if one observes a reduction in resorption, this does not mean an improvement for the patient since bone formation will follow resorption in time and will also be reduced, resulting in a low bone mass.

The maximal reduction of fracture incidence was not determined in most studies and even then one has to be careful not to include final cases with most vertebrae collapsed. Almost all studies evaluate the effect of treatment on one parameter – bone mineral density at the peripheral skeleton, total body calcium or histomorphometry – while there might be different effects at different sites, trabecular or cortical.

Regardless of these criticisms, the weight of evidence in long-term studies (conducted over more than one year) supports the following points:

(1) Postmenopausal bone loss can be prevented
(2) Bone loss can be halted
(3) Trabecular bone mass can be increased

PREVENTION OF OSTEOPOROSIS

Epidemiological considerations

If, as is suggested from cross-sectional data, 25% of white women older than 60 years suffer vertebral compression fractures, and one fifth will suffer a fractured hip by the age of 90, the social, medical and economic implications of providing therapy for such a large group are enormous and must be measured against the possible side-effects of a long-term treatment. The morbidity and mortality resulting from the complications of the disease process must also be taken into account. For example the mortality rate associated with hip fractures is as high as 17%, which is about 20 times that expected for a population of this age[5].

Whether or not any individual patient requires long-term treatment must depend on the recognition of bone loss or, alternatively, of those factors which are likely to result in the patient being particularly at risk.

Identification of those who are at risk

If osteoporosis is to be prevented the first step is to identify in good time those at risk. The bone-losing effect of oestrogen deficiency is well documented[6-8]. Patients at high risk of osteoporosis are women with premature oestrogen deficiency, surgical or natural, who clearly require oestrogen substitution treatment. Knowledge of factors other than oestrogen deficiency likely to cause or aggravate age- and sex-related bone loss is of clinical value for prediction and counselling.

Clinical criteria

There seems to be general agreement that small, thin, fair, light-skinned women, especially of Northern European extraction, spinsters or mothers of only one or two children, those with strong family histories of hip and spine fracture, and possibly those who, in addition to the foregoing, are heavy smokers, appear to have significantly higher fracture risk[9].

Of clinical interest in those context is the observation that osteoporosis and generalized osteoarthrosis are rarely seen together although both are common in the older age group. Actual data suggest that real differences between the two conditions exist[10]. Significant differences in some anthropometric indices between osteoarthrosis and osteoporosis have been found. In studies women with osteoarthrosis have been shown to have an excess of body weight, skin-fold thickness and muscle girth and strength, while women with osteoporosis scored below average for these indices[11]. Are these differences of pathogenetic importance for the development of the two diseases? Is the excess of body weight and excess of fat, or a factor related to these, associated with reduced bone resorption? In previous studies [12-14], the observation by Foss and Byers[15] that osteoarthrosis cases had a higher bone mass than osteoporosis as matched for age and sex could be confirmed. A logical hypothesis for this difference could be that patients with osteoarthrosis, with their excess of fat, have an increased peripheral aromatization of androstenedione to oestrone, with a reduced bone resorption as a result[16].

Since the first clinical signs of generalized osteoarthrosis are readily observable in the hand joints – Heberden and Bouchard nodes – in the perimenopausal period, these changes can be useful in eliminating a group of women who are probably not at risk of developing symptomatic osteoporosis and thus do not need preventive treatment.

Objective criteria

Objective identification of the fracture risk group is a goal of great practical significance since treatment of a group larger than necessary would be difficult, expensive and in certain instances fraught with needless risk.

Refinements in bone mass measurements of a sort readily available in medical practice, such as radiogrammetry, single and dual photonabsorptiometry, would aid in identification of preosteoporotic women with low bone mass. (It remains to be seen whether these women are those most at risk.)

In the 1960s radiogrammetry of the second metacarpal and in the 1970s single photonabsorptiometry of the radius were developed, allowing reasonably accurate quantification of cortical bone mass in the forearm. These methods have been found very useful for epidemiological research and follow-up measurements in groups of people[17].

However, some fractures of postmenopausal osteoporosis involve areas of predominantly trabecular bone in the spine and there is now abundant evidence that forearm bone mass measurements poorly discriminate cases with vertebral crush fractures, but discriminate better femoral neck fracture cases where a predominantly cortical bone area is involved[10].

For clinical evaluation and for therapeutic trials it is a must to employ two or more measurements of bone at different sites including the more metabolically active trabecular bone in the spine and the more compact cortical bone bank at the periphery.

Two new fundamentally different techniques, dual-photonabsorptiometry and computed tomography, make it possible now to measure bone mass in areas affected by postmenopausal osteoporosis. The newer methods allow corrections for soft tissue absorption and thus allow bone density measurement in such cortical areas as the lumbar spine and proximal femur. There are major discrepancies amongst clinical studies using these techniques and it is unclear to what extent the differences result from patient selection, study design, or technical factors in the measurements, such as insufficient correction for low absorption coefficient for fat, present in the cortical area[17]. It is certain however that sensitive, accurate and clinically meaningful assays of bone mass in selected skeletal regions will soon be more widely available. The main role of such measurements will be to detect people already at high risk of fracture. At present, a person who has a bone mass measurement 20% below the average of an age–sex-matched control population can be considered to have a low bone mass and to be a candidate for preventive treatment.

Preventive treatment

Prevention refers here primarily to the slowing, or cessation, of the age-related bone loss in postmenopausal women. Prevention of fracture is of course the only goal of practical importance, but no controlled prospective studies bearing on this outcome have been carried out, and for logistic reasons may never be carried out. Rich *et al.*[18] estimated that demonstration of a 40% reduction in fracture frequency would require 1400 patients followed over a 3-year period. Hence we are left with a fairly reasonable presumption, but a presumption nonetheless, that prevention of bone loss is a necessary condition for prevention of bone fracture.

Oestrogens

There is now evidence to suggest that preventing the accelerated bone loss in postmenopausal women is practical and effective. Several double-blind, placebo-controlled studies of oestrogen prophylaxis have recently been reported[19–22]. These studies have shown significant protection against age-related bone loss, i.e. reduction in rate of loss to undetectable levels and even an increase in peripheral bone mass of 1.2%/year[22]. Treatment duration ranged from two to five years. Hutchinson *et al.*[23], using case control methods, were able to demonstrate, apparently for the first time, protection against hip and radius fractures in women given postmenopausal oestrogen therapy. Weiss *et al.*[24] calculated, based on an epidemiological study that the risk of fracture was 50% to 60% lower in women who had received oestrogen treatment for six years or longer than in women who had not received the treatment. Persistence of the protective effect after many years of oestrogen treatment had been documented[25]. Oestrogen treatment of postmenopausal bone loss is effective at doses as low as 0.625 mg of conjugated equine oestrogen, or the equivalent, daily[21,26].

Side-effects associated with prolonged oestrogen treatment are well known and need no further mention. There is new evidence that cyclic administration of oestrogens with an added progestogen may reduce the risk of breast and endometrial cancer[27-28].

A point of concern is the finding[29] that in 14 postmenopausal oophorectomized women, withdrawal of oestrogen therapy was followed by a phase of rapid bone loss (2.5%/year) which largely negated the benefit to bone of oestrogen therapy. This finding was confirmed by Horsman *et al.*[30] in a small group of 12 postmenopausal women. However, Christiansen *et al.* [31], in a controlled randomized cross-over study in 74 postmenopausal women, could not confirm the increased bone loss after withdrawal of oestrogen. The annual rate of bone loss after discontinuation of hormone therapy (oestrogen) in combination with cyclic administration of a progestogen, was almost identical with the bone loss in the placebo group, (2.3% vs 1.9% per year). These results indicate that even temporary hormone replacement therapy after the menopause will have a lasting beneficial effect on bone mass. How long preventive oestrogen therapy has to be given is still a matter of discussion and in most cases has to be governed by individual judgement. At least five years, but preferably ten to fifteen years treatment would bring the patient at risk beyond the natural fracture time.

If then, as seems possible, 10 to 15 years' treatment is required to defer the impact of osteoporosis, women at risk will need to be encouraged to take treatment until perhaps the age of 65. Treatment has proved acceptable in the short term in highly motivated younger women supported by convinced doctors, but there is little evidence for its long-term acceptability in the older woman who still has her uterus.

Is there an alternative? The case for progestogen and calcium has been made as preventive agents for postmenopausal bone loss.

Progestogens

Lindsay *et al.*[32] in a one-year study in 10 postmenopausal women, found that gestranol prevented postmenopausal bone loss in a similar way to oestrogen. In a cross-sectional and longitudinal study over a mean of 4.5 years, we found a reduced bone loss in perimenopausal women who were taking lynestrenol[33,34]. Although lynestrenol's effectiveness in inhibiting bone loss seemed to be similar to that of oestrogen, the effect is less than that observed in postmenopausal women treated with conjugated equine oestrogens (1.25 mg) or ethinyloestradiol (0.025 mg)[25]. That progestogens inhibit bone resorption is biochemically shown by Gallagher[35] who found that norethesterone effectively lowered the plasma calcium/urine calcium/creatinine ratio and hydroxyproline/creatinine ratio in normal postmenopausal women and this in the same way as observed in oestrogen-treated postmenopausal women.

The bone-protecting effect of progestogens is important enough to warrant the consideration of a progestogen as a substitute for oestrogens, especially since the side-effects of progestogens are probably less serious than those of oestrogen and since the continuous administration of a progestogen induces an atrophic endometrium and no intermittent bleeding. Further studies on the effect of progesterone on bone and its interaction with other hormones are necessary, especially in view of the recent discovery that low progesterone levels may be much more important than previously believed[36].

Mechanism of action of oestrogens and progestogens on bone

The mechanism of action of oestrogens on bone is unclear, since no investigator has been able to demonstrate the presence of oestrogen receptors in bone, despite the very obvious effect that oestrogens have in reducing bone loss to low levels. Probably therefore, oestrogen controls bone resorption indirectly. Recent studies have shown that oestrogens increase the secretion of calcitonin, a hormone which does act directly on bone to reduce resorption[37]. For a long time the main mechanism of postmenopausal bone loss has been attributed to an increase of skeletal sensitivity to parathyroid hormone in the presence of oestrogen deficiency[38]. Furthermore, this increased sensitivity to bone-resorbing hormones, PTH and probably 1,25-$(OH)_2$Vit D_3 is unopposed because the loss of ovarian function also accelerates the decline in the secretion of calcitonin which occurs with age[39].

As far as progesterone is concerned, there do appear to be receptors for progesterone in bone tissue[40]. Because progesterone competes effectively with dexamethasone for the glucocorticoid receptor in bone cells, it has been suggested that the action of progesterone is to function as a glucocorticoid antagonist as shown in other systems[41]. The decline in progesterone secretion at the menopause may therefore be very important in that it allows corticosteroids to act fully on bone. The observation by Johnston *et al.*[36] that women who lose bone mass quickly, as compared with those who show a slower rate of loss, have significantly lower levels of serum progesterone but not serum oestrogens, confirms the importance of cortisone/progesterone interaction.

Calcium

There is evidence that simple calcium supplementation may slow bone loss in postmenopausal women[21,42], but to a lesser degree than does oestrogen therapy. Longitudinal studies of patients with deliberately elevated calcium intake have shown that high intakes of about 1.5 μg of calcium per day will inhibit age-related bone loss in postmenopausal white women, when observed for two years[21]. The rationale for calcium therapy is that in Western populations there is a suboptimal dietary intake of calcium, and that calcium balance, under the same intake of calcium, is different in the pre- and postmenopausal period[43]. Calcium balance was about 25 mg more positive in the non-oestrogen deficient groups, both the premenopausal women and the oestrogen treated ones. The deterioration in the calcium balance in the oestrogen deprived group was in about half of the cases due to decreased intestinal absorption and in the other half to decreased kidney retention. Interestingly, calcium intake had the same influence on balance in both groups; on average, for each gram increase in calcium intake, calcium balance was 54 mg positive in either group. These data suggest that calcium balance is influenced by calcium intake even in the hormone deficient state and that increase in calcium intake may be able to compensate for the disturbance of the calcium economy occurring at the menopause.

Further, in Yugoslavia it has been shown that inhabitants of a community with lifelong high calcium intake (1.087 mg/day) have a lower incidence of fractures and a higher bone mass than those of a similar community with a lower calcium intake [44].

Calcium 'deficiency' should be considered as one of the factors contributing to the development of osteoporosis and in some individuals it may be the principal one. However, it is not the most powerful factor. Black women in the United States have a considerably lower calcium intake than white women, yet have a larger bone mass and rarely suffer from postmenopausal osteoporosis[45].

It should be noted that calcium supplements alone have not been shown to increase bone mass, and in the studies that directly compared the effect of calcium supplements with that of oestrogens, the oestrogens came out slightly better[21,42]. In contrast to oestrogen a rebound effect after withdrawal of calcium was not seen[30]. Since calcium in the form of dietary supplements acts principally by suppressing endogenous PTH secretion, it should preferentially be given just before bedtime in order to compensate nocturnal serum calcium decrease and PTH increase. Suppression of PTH secretion results in suppression of bone remodelling by reducing the activation frequency of new remodelling loci. This tends to stabilize the skeleton and whilst this stabilization prevents further bone loss it leaves a situation in which capacity for increase in mass is also reduced.

Exercise

The value of physical activity in preserving bone mass is emphasized in several studies, showing that patients lost calcium while they were confined to bed-rest and that the loss did not subside until they were back on their feet. Mechanical stress not only preserves bone mass but also seems to enhance bone formation[46]. The goal of a prophylactic exercise programme should be to achieve the highest possible peak bone mass before old age and to maintain that peak as long as possible. Such a preventive programme might account for as much as 10% to 20% additional bone mass later on, and that difference might be 'crucial' in preventing injury and fractures from falls in the later years.

A relationship between muscle weight and bone mass in humans has been shown by Doyle *et al.*[47] in a necropsy study of the ash weight of the third lumbar vertebral body and the weight of the left psoas.

A positive effect of exercise on bone has been shown for the rat by Saville and White[48], for athletes by Nilsson and Westlin[49], for weightlifters and ballet dancers by Dalén and Olsson[50], and for tennis players by Huddleston *et al.*[51]. Aloia *et al.*[52] found an 11% higher total body calcium level after correction for age and body size in marathon runners and could record prevention of involutional bone loss by exercise in nine postmenopausal women[53]. Krϕlner *et al.*[54] published very recently positive results of a controlled trial in which the effect of physical exercise on vertebral bone loss was evaluated over an eight months period.

TREATMENT OF SYMPTOMATIC OSTEOPOROSIS

The so-called 'involutional', 'postmenopausal' or 'gerontoid' osteoporosis which may be diagnosed when women come to the clinic with symptoms due to bone failure, crush fracture of the spine or femoral neck fracture, are the manifestation of the end result of a heterogenous pathological process. Before embarking on any therapeutic programme, careful analysis of the underlying pathophysiology and bone turnover should be undertaken.

It is clear that diseases such as hyperparathyroidism, hyperthyroidism, Cushing's disease, osteomalacia and a malignant process such as myeloma, should be excluded first. Determination of serum levels of PTH, thyroxin, cortisol and 1,25-$(OH)_2$ D_3 are very useful, as is a simple serum protein electrophoresis, to eliminate the abovementioned curable or efficiently treatable conditions. The distinction between high or low turnover osteoporosis can best be established by quantitative bone histology on appropriately prepared samples of undecalcified bone biopsy specimens. However, the availability of this expertise is rare and other, more available, and maybe more conclusive, simple tests to decide on treatment are as follows.

The evaluation of symptomatic idiopathic osteoporosis, using currently available methods, can be made by serum estimation of calcium, phosphorus, alkaline phosphatase activity and 3-day consecutive 24-h urine collections divided into 2-h morning fasting specimens and 22-h creatinin, calcium and hydroxyproline estimation. Three consecutive day samples of urine are necessary because of important day-to-day variations in urinary calcium output even when the diet has been stopped. Provided that there are no major disturbances in PTH and vitamin D metabolites, a mean 24-h calcium excretion study of less than 50 mg/day indicates malabsorption of calcium or a very insufficient daily intake of calcium and a mean 24-h excretion of hydroxyproline of more than 50 mg/day indicates a high bone turnover with a negative bone balance. A high mean 24-h calcium excretion indicates a urinary loss of calcium despite a good intestinal calcium absorption. A low 24-h hydroxyproline excretion indicates a low bone turnover.

A high mean morning-fasting calcium/creatinine ratio of more than 0.15 indicates a negative calcium balance and a mean of 0.045 hydroxyproline/creatinine ratio a high bone turnover. An increased alkaline phosphatase level is always an indication of increased bone turnover but does not give information if the turnover is in a positive or negative balance. A low alkaline phosphatase level, a low fasting calcium/creatinine ratio and hydroxyproline/creatinine ratio in the presence of a normal 24-h calcium excretion is an indication of a low turnover. A low alkaline phosphatase level in combination with an increased-fasting calcium/creatinine ratio, or hydroxyproline/creatinine ratio, indicates a high turnover with a negative balance.

We found that in symptomatic vertebral crush fracture syndromes 39% had a high-fasting calcium/creatinine ratio, 84% a high-fasting hydroxyproline/creatinine ratio, 21% a high (for their age) 24-h calcium excretion of more than 200 mg/24 h, and 12% a low (less than 50 mg) calcium 24 h excretion (Table 1).

The treatment regimen depends on the results of the biochemical tests. Those who have a low, 24-h, calcium excretion are treated with vitamin D in order to increase their calcium absorption. Those with a high-fasting calcium/creatinine excretion are treated with oestrogen, with oestrogen alone if they no longer have their uterus and with oestrogen/progestogen if they still have their uterus. If they have objections to, or if there are contraindications for oestrogen treatment, then treatment with a progestogen or with an anabolic steroid may be considered. Those with a high calcium excretion over 24-h are treated with thiazides, which are known to reduce the excess calcium excretion by the kidney[55] and to reduce bone loss in men[56].

When the patient is hospitalized because of severe backache due to vertebral collapse, we usually give intravenous calcium infusion as suggested by Pak *et al.*[57]. Hypercalcaemia for several days suppresses PTH release and inhibits parathyroid activity for several months while at the same time the calcitonin excretion is stimulated[7]. It is our

Table 1 Abnormalities in urinary parameters in osteoporosis

Calcium/creatinine (2 h)	> 0.15	39%
Hydroxyproline/creatinine (2 h)	> 0.045	84%
Calcium (24 h)	> 200 mg	21%
Calcium (24 h)	< 50 mg	12%
Hydroxyproline (24 h)	> 50 mg	46%
Hydroxyproline (24 h)	< 25 mg	9%

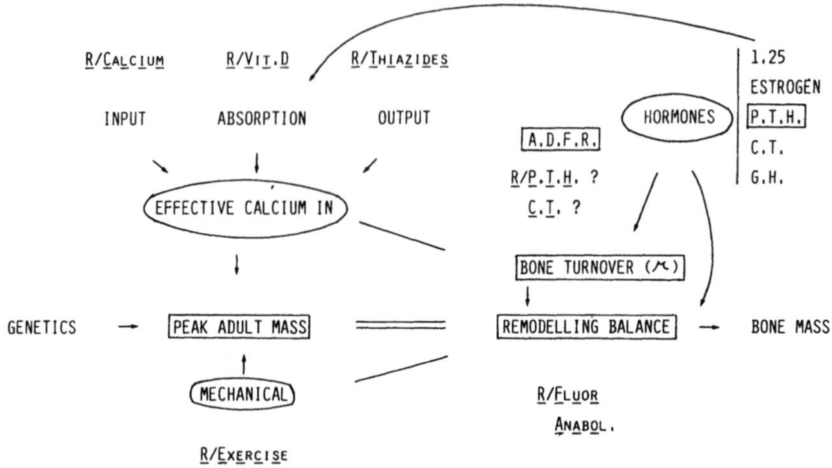

Figure 1 Factors involved in peak bone mass and bone remodelling and the place of action of a number of treatments
ADFR = Activate, Depress, Free and Repeat the cycle: CT = calcitonin; PTH = parathyroid hormone; GH = growth hormone

experience that this kind of treatment has a marked analgesic effect but it does not increase bone mass[58,59]. Futher therapeutic steps have to be taken according to the biochemical findings described above. (Figure 1).

Oestrogen treatment of osteoporosis

In patients with fractures, oestrogen treatment has been considered without much enthusiasm since it is only palliative, and since new bone cannot be generated and bone loss has already occurred to the extent that risk of fracture is high. However, recent data have shown that untreated patients with osteoporosis lose bone at a higher rate than do age-matched controls[60] and oestrogen administration markedly inhibits this bone loss[42]. Risk of further fractures can be decreased as well[61].

Elderly patients, sometimes severely disabled from many fractures, usually find that the management of vaginal bleeding 10 to 15 years after the menopause and follow-up visits to the gynaecologist, cause enough discomfort and inconvenience to outweigh the benefits derived from inhibiting bone loss. On the other hand, younger women who have had no more than one or two fractures may yet derive enough benefit from administration of oestrogens to make it worthwhile.

Calcium treatment of osteoporosis

Like oestrogen administration, calcium supplementation has not been enthusiastically recommended for patients who have already begun to suffer fractures from osteoporosis. It has generally been considered that these patients have already lost enough bone to render the skeleton excessively fragile and that since they tend to absorb calcium poorly no important benefit could be expected. Nevertheless, there are several arguments to make calcium administration a reasonable proposition for such patients. Firstly, calcium supplements do minimize bone loss in patients with osteoporosis[42]; secondly, bone loss in untreated osteoporosis is higher than previously thought and is greater than that in normal controls; and thirdly, the risk involved in the use of calcium supplements is minimal.

Positive calcium balance is almost invariably produced when an osteoporotic patient is given a calcium supplement, but this lasts for only a few months at best[43]. A temporary decrease of hydroxyproline in these patients is also observed during continuous calcium therapy[62]. The efficacy of calcium supplements in reducing bone loss seems slightly less than that of oestrogen. The combined effect of calcium and oestrogen supplements has been reported additionally to reduce the fracture rate. For example, Riggs and co-workers[61] found that calcium treatment reduced fracture rate by 50% and that oestrogen + calcium lowered the rate further to 25% of the rate in untreated women.

Anabolic steroids treatment of osteoporosis

Anabolic steroids have been tested in patients with osteoporosis. Androgens were once used in the treatment of this condition but have since been discarded because of their unwanted virilizing effect.

Anabolic steroids have effects on bones similar to those of oestrogens. Bone loss has been seen to stop during two or more years of observation and a slight gain in bone may occur, although the measurements of bone mass are not sensitive enough to be certain[63]. Chesnut *et al.*[64] made sequential measurements of total calcium in patients given methandienone (methandrostenolone) for up to two years, and found a modest gain in the mean total body calcium (2%) during the first year, with no further gains or loss thereafter. Although this gain was within the allowable error of the method, the final mean total body calcium of the treated group was significantly different from that of a control group, not given the drug, who continued to lose bone. This transient improvement in bone mass is explicable in terms of activity of the basic multicellular units (BMU) of bone, and the response to drugs (anabolic steroids and oestrogens) which suppress bone turnover by suppressing their birth rate[65]. From the time the drug is given the rate of appearance of new units (which always starts in a resorptive phase) decreases, but the activity of the pre-existing units continues unabated into their formative phase and to completion. This overlap between the activities of the more abundant old units, and the fewer new units, leads to a net gain of bone (formation unchanged, resorption reduced) which ends when the activity of all pre-existing units is exhausted. The duration of this transient gain of bone seems to be about 12 to 18 months[65]. No change was observed in the serum calcium concentration and there were insufficient data to establish whether the drug had a favourable effect on further fractures. Lindsay *et al.*[66] in a double-blind trial of a synthetic steroid (tibolone (OD 14), 2.5 mg daily), found over a two-year period that this steroid prevented bone loss in 33 postmenopausal women whereas a significant reduction in bone mineral content occurred in women taking a placebo.

There seems to be minimal risk associated with the use of anabolic steroids, although some have not been very widely used.

Vitamin D treatment of osteoporosis

Few would argue that vitamin D deficiency should be avoided if possible in all people, particularly in elderly postmenopausal women, whose exposure to sun and dietary intake may be marginal. Even mild deficiency will depress calcium absorption and cause negative calcium (bone) balance[67,68]. The bone loss is probably largely reversible if the deficiency is short-term. However, very long-term mild vitamin D deficiency may result in irreversible bone loss such as that seen in some patients many years after gastric or bowel surgery. Adequate levels of vitamin D should be guaranteed, both in healthy postmenopausal women and in those with osteoporosis, by administration of at least 400 units daily in the form of multivitamins or by exposure to a sun lamp for about 15 minutes daily. Measurement of serum 25-hydroxyvitamin D levels will allow documentation of adequate vitamin D status wherever there is doubt.

'Conventional' vitamin D, meaning vitamin D_2, has been used as a pharmacological agent rather empirically in patients with osteoporosis[69] in doses of up to 50 000 units daily. There is no good evidence that this will halt bone loss, stimulate new bone formation, or decrease the risk of fracture even when given along with calcium supplements, and there is substantial risk of vitamin D intoxication, especially when calcium supplements are added. Nordin *et al.*[42] suggest that pharmacological doses may even cause worsening of the bone loss. Because of the risk and weak evidence in favour of efficacy, conventional vitamin D in pharmacological doses is no longer indicated[70]. Further, it does not appear necessary as an adjunct to therapy with flouride as long as normal vitamin D nutrition is maintained[71].

Newer vitamin D agents, 1α-OHD_3 or 1,25-$(OH)_2D_3$

1α-OHD_3 is converted into 1,25-$(OH)_2D_3$ by the liver so that its behaviour is almost identical to that of orally administered 1,25-$(OH)_2D_3$. The rationale for the use of 1α-$(OHD)_3$ is based on the finding of a slightly lower 1,25-$(OH)_2$ vitamin D level in osteoporotics by Gallagher *et al.*[72] causing inefficient calcium absorption and poor renal conservation of calcium. Correction of the low level could then restore calcium economy to normal. A low level of serum 1,25-$(OH)_2D_3$ results in defective bone formation to the extent that the formation phase of BMU remodelling fails to fill completely the hole created by the resorption phase. The finding of low levels of 1,25-$(OH)_2D_3$ by Gallagher in postmenopausal women with osteoporosis was not confirmed in our series, neither was there a lower level of 25-$(OH)D_3$ or PTH[73].

The efficacy of 1α-vitamin D treatment in osteoporosis is not yet proved[42,74-76]. The results show generally that calcium absorption efficiency increases but urine calcium excretion also rises, which may offset the gain in absorption. Nordin *et al.*[42] and Christiansen *et al.*[76] have used 1α-OHD_3 in conjunction with oestrogens and have demonstrated inhibition of bone loss, decrease in fractures and perhaps a small gain in bone mass but similar results were also obtained with oestrogen treatment alone.

Fluoride treatment of osteoporosis

The notion of using fluoride as therapy for established osteoporosis arose from the observation that osteosclerosis was part of the clinical picture in patients with fluoride intoxication. Unfortunately, the studies on this plausible notion yielded different and inconclusive results. The field of research is only now beginning to emerge from a state of great chaos. Widely differing dosage regimens and supportive therapies have been employed; controls have been inadequate and methods of assessing efficacy less than universally acceptable. The dose is a particularly important aspect, for, unlike many of the other agents employed in this disorder, fluoride is a potent, toxic substance, for bone as well as for other tissues. Too high an exposure results in clearly abnormal osteoblastic activity and a histological picture with features of osteomalacia. Whether there is an appropriate therapeutic range, and whether dosage within that range can result in arrest or reversal of osteoporotic bone loss, is by no means decided. Available results, however, suggest that reversal of trabecular bone mass may well be possible in some cases.

The daily dose that has been employed in treatment of osteoporosis ranges from 13 mg to over 100 mg of fluoride ions/per day and in some published reports, therapy was continued for 10 years. Most reports indicate that treatment produces increased bone mass determined by histomorphometry. In one-third of patients no improvement of bone mass was noted[77].

There also appears to be a differential response in terms of bone mass between different parts of the skeleton; some parts gain bone and others lose it. The more central parts (vertebral bodies, pelvis), which are rich in trabecular bone, accumulate new bone[78]; the more peripheral parts (distal forearm, femur, metacarpal) lose compact bone or at least show no gains[79–82]. So what might be considered as advantageous for one part of the skeleton could be associated with deleterious effects on others.

Although there is some concern about the quality of bone that may be produced during fluoride treatment, recent studies have indicated actual reduction in fracture incidents[82,83] and Riggs and co-workers[61] reported that the combination of calcium, oestrogen and fluoride virtually abolished fractures after the first year of treatment.

An important aspect of fluoride therapy is the high incidence of unwanted side-effects[78,79,81,82]. The major toxic effects are gastric irritation and arthralgia, and they are often of sufficient severity to cause treatment to be stopped. As might be expected, the combination of fluoride with pharmacological doses of vitamin D was associated with hypercalcaemia[82] and such large doses of vitamin D should not be used. It is even questionable if vitamin D used as an adjunct to fluoride therapy is necessary as long as normal vitamin D in the nutrition is maintained.

Although fluoride therapy can be useful in vertebral crush fracture syndromes, fluoride cannot be recommended for general use and definitely not for treatment of femoral neck fracture cases.

Calcitonin treatment of osteoporosis

Calcitonin inhibits bone resorption by reducing the number and activity of osteoclasts, although this effect is probably not sustained in the long term. The results of studies of calcitonin in osteoporosis are varied, some showing benefit and others not. Jowsey *et al.*[84] found an increased bone resorption in patients treated with calcitonin due to secondary hyperparathyroidism induced by a small reduction in the serum calcium concentration. But the effect of the combined therapy calcitonin calcium on bone turnover was not different from that produced by oral calcium alone, neither treatment caused an improvement in bone mass, and bone mass may even have decreased[85]. Meunier *et al.*[86] gave porcine calcitonin to patients with postmenopausal osteoporosis for 12 months and observed no significant changes in bone turnover and bone mass and found, as might be expected, that vertebral fractures continued to occur.

At the present time there is no convincing evidence that calcitonin alone or in combination with oral calcium, exerts substantial and/or favourable effects in patients with established osteoporosis or that calcitonin reduces the risk of fractures. Inconvenience imposed by the need to give calcitonin parenterally is hardly outweighed by the advantages the treatment might have.

CURATIVE TREATMENT – RESTORATION OF SKELETAL MASS

To achieve restoration of skeletal mass within a reasonable time, the first requirement is to stimulate bone formation without stimulation of bone resorption. This uncoupling of resorption and formation is the goal based on the concept of basic multicellular units (BMU)[87]. The potential value of temporarily separating osteoclasts and osteoblasts from each other in time by administration and withdrawal of the drug could selectively focus its action on the desired cell line and free its opposite number of that effect. Frost called this approach: ADFR. ADFR represents Active, Depress, Free and Repeat the cycle as often as needed.

Three agents are known to stimulate bone formation: fluoride, growth hormone (somatomedin) and the human synthetic parathyroid hormone fragment h PTH (1-34). Growth hormone and h PTH (1-34) both appreciably increase bone turnover, but the average calcium balance changes little. Human parathyroid hormone fragment (1-34) has been tested in a small number of patients with osteoporosis[88]. The results were less than dramatic, and the increase in trabecular bone volume seemed to be at the expense of cortical bone.

One of the newest concepts in the treatment of osteoporosis – one that requires more study before it is used experimentally in humans – involves several steps, beginning with briefly activating bone resorption with agents such as parathyroid hormone[89]. This action in turn triggers increased formation; resorption is then acutely suppressed with calcitonin while the process of bone formation goes on for some time. In theory, at least, there is a net gain of bone mass and repetitions of the cycle should lead to sustained accretion.

References

1. Garn, S. M., Rohmann, C. G. and Wagner, B. (1967). Bone loss as a general phenomenon in man. *Fed. Proc.*, **26**, 1729
2. Dequeker, J. (1975). Bone and ageing. *Ann. Rheum. Dis.*, **34**, 100
3. White, M. P., Bergfeld, M. A., Murphy, N. A., Avioli, L. V. and Teitelbaum, S. L. (1982). Postmenopausal osteoporosis: A heterogeneous disorder as assessed by histomorphometric analysed of iliac crest bone from untreated patients. *Am. J. Med.*, **72**, 193
4. Frost, H. M. (1973). The spinal osteoporosis. *Clin. Endocrinol.*, **2**, 257
5. Lewis, A. F. (1981). Fracture of neck of the femur: changing incidence. *Br. Med. J.*, **283**, 1217
6. Albright, F. and Reifenstein, E. C. (1948). *The Parathyroid Glands and Metabolic Bone Desease*. (Baltimore: Williams and Wilkins)
7. Dequeker, J. (1972). *Bone Loss in Normal and Pathological Conditions*, p. 217. (Leuven: University Press)
8. Lindsay, R., Coutts, J. T. R. and Hart, D. M. (1977). The effect of endogenous oestrogen on plasma and urinary calcium and phosphate in oophorectomized women. *Clin. Endocrinol.*, **6**, 87
9. Heaney, R. P. (1981). Osteoporosis. In Bronner, F. and Cobum, J. W. (eds) *Disorders of Mineral Metabolism*, pp. 91–117. (New York: Academic Press)
10. Dequeker, J., Burssens, A., Creytens, G. and Bouillon, R. (1975). Ageing of bone. Its relation to osteoporosis in postmenopausal women. In van Keep, P.A. and Lauritzen, C. (eds) *Frontiers of Hormone Res.* Vol. 3, *Estrogens in the Post-Menopause*, pp. 116–130. (Basel: Karger)

11. Dequeker, J., Goris, P. and Uyttenhoeven, R. (1982). Osteoporosis and osteoarthritis (osteoarthrosis) anthropometic distinctions. *J. Am. Med Assoc.*, **249**, 1448
12. Roh, Y. S., Dequeker, J. and Mulier, J. C. (1973). Osteoarthrosis at the hand skeleton in primary osteoarthrosis of the hip and in normal controls. *Clin. Orthop. Rel. Res.*, **90**, 90
13. Roh, Y. S., Dequeker, J. and Mulier, J. C. (1974). Bone mass in osteoarthrosis, measured *in vivo* by photon absorption. *J. Bone Joint Surg.*, **56A**, 587
14. Roh, Y. S., Dequeker, J. and Mulier, J. C. (1974). Trabecular pattern of the upper end of the femur in primary osteoarthrosis and in symptomatic osteoporosis. *Belg. Tijdschr. Radiol.*, **57**, 89
15. Foss, M. V. L. and Byers, P. D. (1972). Bone density, osteoarthrosis of the hip and fracture of the upper end of the femur. *Ann. Rheum. Dis.*, **31**, 259
16. Frumar, A. M., Meldrum, D. R., Geola, F., Shamonti, I. M., Tataryn, I. V., Deftos, L. J. and Judd, H. L. (1980). Relationship of fasting urinary calcium to circulating estrogen and body weight in postmenopausal women. *J. Clin. Endocrinol. Metabol.*, **50**, 70
17. Dequeker, J. and Johnston, C. C. (1982). *Non-Invasive Bone Measurements: Methodological Problems.* (Oxford-Washington D.C.: IRL Press)
18. Rich, C., Bernstein, D. S., Gates, S., Heaney, R. P., Johnston, C. C., Rosenberg, C. A., Schnaper, H. W., Tewkburry, R. B. and Williams, G. A. (1966). Factors involved in an objective study of the efficacy of treatment of osteoporosis. *Clin. Orthop. Relat. Res.*, **45**, 63
19. Lindsay, R., Aitken, J. M., Anderson, J. B., Hart, D. M., MacDonald, E. B. C. and Clarke, A. C. (1976). Long-term prevention of postmenopausal osteoporosis by oestrogen. *Lancet*, **1**, 1038
20. Horsman, A., Gallagher, J. C., Simpson, M. and Nordin, B. E. C. (1977). Prospective trial of oestrogen and calcium in postmenopausal women. *Br. Med. J.*, **2**, 789
21. Recker, R. R., Saville, P. D. and Heaney, R. P. (1977). Effect of oestrogens and calcium carbonate on bone loss in postmenopausal women. *Ann. Intern. Med.*, **87**, 649
22. Christiansen, C., Christensen, M. S., McNair, P., Hagen, C., Stocklund, K. and Transbφl, I. (1980). Prevention of early postmenopausal bone loss: Controlled 2-year study in 315 normal females. *Eur. J. Clin. Invest.*, **10**, 273
23. Hutchinson, T. A., Polansky, S. M. and Feinstein, A. R. (1979). Post-menopausal oestrogens protect against fractures of hip and distal radius. A case-control study. *Lancet*, **2**, 705
24. Weiss, N. S., Ure, C. L., Ballard, J. H., Williams, A. R. and Daling, J. R. (1980). Decreased risk of fractures of the hip and lower forearm with postmenopausal use of estrogen. *N. Engl. J. Med.*, **303**, 1195
25. Dequeker, J. and Ferin, J. (1976). Effect of long-term estrogen therapy on bone remodelling in women with a natural menopause: cross-sectional and longitudinal study. In van Keep, P. A., Greenblatt, R. B. and Albeaux-Fernet, M. (eds) *Consensus on Menopause Research*, pp. 124-131. (Lancaster: MTP Press)
26. Lindsay, R., Fogelman, I. and Hart, D. M. (1982). Minimum effective dose of oestrogen for protection against postmenopausal bone loss (Abstract) *Calcif. Tiss. Int.*, **34** (Suppl.I), S-33
27. Thom, M. H., White, P. J., Williams, R. M., Sturdee, D. W., Paterson, M. E. L. and Wade-Evans, T. (1979). Prevention of endometrial disease in climacteric women receiving oestrogen therapy. *Lancet*, **2**, 455

28. Gambrell, R. D., Jr. (1982). Role of hormones in the etiology and prevention of endometrial and breast cancer. *Acta Obstet. Gynecol. Scand.*, **106**, 37
29. Lindsay, R., Hart, D. M., Maclean, A., Clarke, A. C., Kraszewski, A. and Garwood, J. (1978). Bone response to termination of oestrogen treatment. *Lancet*, **1**, 1325
30. Horsman, A., Nordin, B. E. C. and Crilly, R. G. (1979). Effect on bone of withdrawal of oestrogen therapy. *Lancet*, **2**, 33
31. Christiansen, C., Christensen, M. S. and Transbøl, I. (1981). Bone mass in postmenopausal women after withdrawal of oestrogen/gestagen replacement therapy. *Lancet*, **1**, 459
32. Lindsay, R., Hart, D. M., Purdie, D., Fergusson, M. M., Clarke, A. C. and Kraszewski, A. (1978). Comparative effects of oestrogen and progestogen on bone loss in postmenopausal women. *Clin. Sci. Mol. Med.*, **54**, 193
33. Dequeker, J., De Muylder, E. and Ferin, J. (1977). The effect of long-term lynestrenol treatment on bone mass in cycling women. *Contraception*, **15**, 717
34. Dequeker, J. and De Muylder, E. (1982). Long-term progestogen treatment and bone remodelling in perimenopausal women: a longitudinal study. *Maturitas*, **4**, 309
35. Gallagher, J. C. (1981). Biochemical effects of estrogen and progesterone on calcium metabolism. In De Luca, H. F., Frost, H. M., Jee, W. S. S., Johnston, C. C. and Parfitt, A. M. (eds) *Osteoporosis: Recent Advantages in Pathogenesis and Treatment*, pp. 231–238. (Baltimore: University Park Press)
36. Johnston, C. C., Norton, J. A., Khairi, R. A. and Longcope, C. (1979). Age-related bone loss. In Barzel, U.S. (ed.) *Osteoporosis II*, pp. 91–100. (New York: Grune and Stratton)
37. Stevenson, J. C., Abeyasekera, G., Hillard, C., Phang, K. G., MacIntyre, I., Campbell, S., Townsend, P. T., Young, O. and Whitehead, M. I. (1981). Calcitonin and the calcium-regulating hormones in postmenopausal women: effect of estrogens. *Lancet*, **1**, 693
38. Heaney, R.P. (1965). A unified concept of osteoporosis. *Am. J. Med.*, **39**, 877
39. Deftos, L. J., Weisman, W. H., Williams, G. W., Parthemore, J. G., Judd, H. L., Karpf, D. B., Frumar, A. M. and Davidson, B. J. (1980). Influence of age and sex on plasma calcitonin in human beings. *N. Engl. J. Med.*, **302**, 1351
40. Yoshioka, T., Sato, B., Matsumoto, K. and Ono, K. (1980). Steroid receptors in osteoblasts. *Clin. Orthop. Rel. Res.*, **148**, 297
41. Chen, T. L., Aronow, L. and Feldman, D. (1977). Glucocorticoid receptors and inhibition of bone cell growth in primary culture. *Endocrinology.*, **100**, 619
42. Nordin, B. E. C., Horsman, A., Crilly, R. G., Marshall, D. H. and Simpson, M. (1980). Treatment of spinal osteoporosis in postmenopausal women. *Br. Med. J.*, **280**, 451
43. Heaney, R. P., Recker, R. R. and Saville, P. D. (1978). Menopausal changes in calcium balance performance. *J. Lab. Clin. Med.*, **92**, 953
44. Matkovic, V., Kostial, K., Simonovic, I., Buzina, R., Brodarec, A. and Nordin, B. E. C. (1979). Bone status and fracture rates in two regions of Yugoslavia. *Am. J. Clin. Nutr.*, **32**, 540
45. Nordin, B. E. C., Horsman, A. and Gallagher, J. C. (1973). Effect of various therapies on bone loss in women. In Kuhlencordt, F. and Kruse, H. P. (eds) *Tenth European Symposium on Calcified Tissues*. pp. 451–454. (Berlin: Springer Verlag)
46. Dequeker, J. and Van Tendeloo, G. (1982). Metacarpal bone mass and upper-extremity strength in 18-year-old boys. *Invest. Radiol.*, **17**, 427
47. Doyle, F., Brown, J. and Lachance, C. (1970). Relation between bone mass and muscle weight. *Lancet*, **1**, 391

48. Saville, P. D. and White, M. P. (1969). Muscle and bone hypertrophy. Positive effect of running exercise in the rat. *Clin. Orthop.*, **65**, 81
49. Nilsson, B. E. and Westlin, N. E. (1971). Bone density in athletes. *Clin. Orthop.*, **77**, 179
50. Dalén, N, and Olsson, K. E. (1974). Bone mineral content and physical activity. *Acta Orthop. Scand.*, **45**, 170
51. Huddleston, A. L., Rockwell, D., Kulund, D. N. and Harrison, R. B. (1980). Bone mass in lifetime tennis athletes. *J. Am. Med. Assoc.*, **244**, 1107
52. Aloia, J. F., Cohn, S. H., Babu, T., Abesalis, C., Kalici, N. and Ellis, K. (1978). Skeletal mass and body composition in marathon runners. *Metabolism*, **27**, 1793
53. Aloia, J. F., Cohn, S. H., Ostuni, J. A., Cane, R. and Ellis, K. (1978). Prevention of involutional bone loss by exercise. *Ann. Intern. Med.*, **89**, 356
54. Krølner, B., Toft, B., Nielsen, S. P. and Tøndevold, E. (1983). Physical exercise as prophylaxis against involutional vertebral bone loss; a controlled trial. *Clin. Sci.*, **64**, 541
55. Lamberg, B. A. and Kuhlbäck, B. (1959). Effect of chlorothiazide and hydrochlorothiazide on the excretion of calcium in urine. *Scand. J. Clin. Lab. Invest.*, **11**, 351
56. Wasnich, R. D., Benfante, R. J., Yano, K., Heilbrun, L. and Vogel, J. M. (1983). Thiazide effect on the mineral content of bone. *N. Engl. J. Med.*, **309**, 344
57. Pak, C. Y., Zisman, E., Evens, R., Jowley, J., Delea, C. S. and Bartter, F. C. (1969). The treatment of osteoporosis with calcium infusions. *Am. J. Med.*, **47**, 7
58. Dudl, R. J., Ensinck, J. W., Baylink, D., Chesnut, C. H., Sherrard, D. and Nelp, W. B. (1973). Evaluation of intravenous calcium as therapy for osteoporosis. *Am. J. Med.*, **55**, 631
59. Walton, J., Dominguez, M. and Bartter, F. C. (1975). Effects of calcium infusions in patients with postmenopausal oesteoporosis. *Metab. Clin. Exp.*, **24**, 849
60. Dequeker, J., Verstraeten, A., Collee, G. and Gielen, J. (1981). Confrontation osteoarthrosis/osteoporosis: A cross-sectional and longitudinal study. In Peyron, J.G. (ed.) *Epidemiology of Osteoarthritis*, pp. 147–155. (Paris: Geigy Paris)
61. Riggs, B. L., Seeman, E., Hodgson, S. F., Taves, D. R. and O'Fallon, W. M. (1982). Effects of the fluoride/calcium regimen on vertebral fracture occurrence in postmenopausal osteoporosis. *N. Engl. J. Med.*, **306**, 446
62. Dequeker, J., Heylen, H., Van Steenkiste, J. and Vroninckx, R. (1972). Urinary total hydrocyproline, calcium and phosphorus excretion after adminstration of calcium and oestrogen to postmenopausal women. *Pharmacology*, **7**, 321
63. Chesnut, C. H., Nelp, W. B., Baylink, D. J. and Denney, J. D. (1977). Effect of methandrostenolone on postmenopausal bone wasting as assessed by changes in total bone mineral mass. *Metabolism*, **26**, 267
64. Chesnut, C. H., Ivey, J. L., Nelp, W. B. and Baylink, D. J. (1979). Assessment of anabolic steroids and calcitonin in the treatment of osteoporosis. In Barzel, U.S. (ed.) *Osteoporosis II*, pp. 135–150. (New York, San Francisco and London: Grune and Stratton)
65. Frost, H. M. (1973). The origin and nature of transients in human bone remodelling dynamics. In Frame, B., Parfitt, A. M. and Duncan, H (eds) *Clinical Aspects of Metabolic Bone Disease*, pp. 124–137. (Amsterdam: Excerpta Medica)
66. Lindsay, R., Hart, D. M. and Kraszewski, A. (1980). Prospective double-blind trial of synthetic steroid (Org. 0D14) for preventing postmenopausal osteoporosis. *Br. Med. J.*, **1**, 1207
67. Aaron, J. E., Gallagher, J. C. and Nordin, B. E. C. (1974). Seasonal variation of histological osteomalacia in femoral-neck fractures. *Lancet*, **2**, 84
68. Aaron, J. E., Stasiak, L., Gallagher, J. C., Longton, E. B., Nicholson, M.,

Anderson, J. and Nordin, B. E. C. (1974). Frequency of osteomalacia and osteoporosis in fractures of the proximal femur. *Lancet*, **1**, 229

69. Riggs, B. L., Jowsey, J., Kelly, P. J., Hoffman, D. L. and Arnaud, C. D. (1976). Effects of oral therapy with calcium and vitamin D in primary osteoporosis. *J. Clin. Endocrinol. Metab.*, **42**, 1139
70. Recker, R. R. (1981). Continuous treatment of osteoporosis: current status. *Orthop. Clin. North. Am.*, **12**, 611
71. Olah, A. J., Reutter, F. W. and Dambacher, M. A. (1978). Effects of combined therapy with sodium fluoride and high doses of vitamin D in osteoporosis. A histomorphometric study in the iliac crest. In Courvoisier, B., Donath, A. and Baud, C. A. (eds) *Fluoride and Bone*, pp. 242–246. (Geneva: Hans Huber)
72. Gallagher, J. C., Riggs, B. L., Eisman, J., Hamstra, A., Arnaud, S. B. and De Luca, M. F. (1979). Intestinal calcium absorption and serum vitamin D metabolites in normal subjects and osteoporotic patients. *J. Clin. Invest.*, **64**, 729
73. Geusens, P., Dequeker, J. and Verstraeten, A. (1983). Age-related blood changes in hip osteoarthritis patients: a possible indicator of bone quality. *Ann. Rheum. Dis.*, **42**, 112
74. Cohen, H. N., Farrah, D., Fogelman, I., Goll, C. C., Beastall, G. H., McIntosh, W. B., Fletcher, M. and Boyle, I, T. (1980). A low dose regime of 1α-hydroxy-vitamin D_3 in the management of senile osteoporosis. A pilot study. *Clin. Endocrinol.*, **12**, 537
75. Hoikka, V., Alhava, E. M., Aro, A., Karjalainen, P. and Rehnberg, V. (1980). Treatment of osteoporosis with 1-alpha-hydroxycholecalciferol and calcium. *Acta Med. Scand.*, **207**, 221
76. Christiansen, C., Christensen, M. S., Rødbro, P., Hagen, C. Transbøl, I. (1981). Effect of 1,25-dihydroxy-vitamin D_3 in itself or combined with hormone treatment in preventing postmenopausal osteoporosis. *Eur. J. Clin. Invest.*, **11**, 305
77. Briançon, D. and Meunier, P. J. (1981). Treatment of osteoporosis with fluoride, calcium and vitamin D. *Orthop. Clin. North Am.*, **12**, 629
78. Harrison, J.E., McNeill, K.G., Sturtridge, W.C., Bayley, T.A., Fornasier, V., Williams, C. and Tam, C. (1981). Three-year changes in bone mineral mass of postmenopausal osteoporotic patients based on neutron activation analysis of the central third of the skeleton. *J. Clin. Endocrinol. Metab.*, **52**, 751
79. Dambacher, M. A., Lauffenberger, T., Lammle, B. and Haas, H. G. (1978). Long term effects of sodium fluoride on osteoporosis. In Courvoisier, B., Donath, A. and Baud, C. A. (eds) *Fluoride and Bone*, pp. 238–246. (Bern, Stuttgart, Vienna: Hans Huber)
80. Ringe, J. D., Kruse, H. P. and Kuhlencordt, F. (1978). Long-term treatment of primary osteoporosis by sodium fluoride. In Courvoisier, B., Donath, A. and Baud, C. A. (eds) *Fluoride and Bone*, pp. 228–232. (Bern, Stuttgart, Vienna: Hans Huber)
81. Franke, J. (1978). Our experience in the treatment of osteoporosis with relative low sodium-fluoride doses. In Courvoisier, B., Donath, A. and Baud, C. A. (eds) *Fluoride and Bone*, pp. 256–262. (Bern, Stuttgart, Vienna: Hans Huber)
82. Riggs, B. L., Hodgson, S. F., Hoffman, D. L., Kelly, P. J., Johnson, K. A. and Taves, D. (1980). Treatment of primary osteoporosis with fluoride and calcium. *J. Am. Med. Assoc.*, **243**, 446
83. Reutter, F. W. and Olah, A. J. (1978). Bone biopsy findings and clinical observations in long-term treatment of osteoporosis with sodium fluoride and vitamin D_3. In Courvoisier, B., Donath, A. and Baud, C. A. (eds) *Fluoride and Bone*, pp. 249–255. (Bern, Stuttgart, Vienna: Hans Huber)
84. Jowsey, J., Riggs, B. L., Goldsmith, R. S., Kelly, P. J. and Arnaud, C. D.

(1971). Effects of prolonged administration of porcine calcitonin in postmenopausal osteoporosis. *J. Clin. Endocrinol.*, **33**, 752

85. Jowsey, J., Riggs, B. L., Kelly, P. J. and Hoffman, D. L. (1978). Calcium and salmon calcitonin in treatment of osteoporosis. *J. Clin. Endocrinol. Metab.*, **47**, 633
86. Meunier, P., Bressot, C., Vignon, E., Edouard, C., Alexandre, C., Courpron, P. and Laurent, J. (1978). Radiological and histological evolution of postmenopausal osteoporosis treated with sodium fluoride-vitamin D-calcium. In Courvoisier, B., Donath, A. and Baud, C. A. (eds) *Fluoride and Bone*, pp. 263–276. (Bern, Stuttgart, Vienna: Hans Huber)
87. Frost, H. M. (1973). *Bone Remodelling and its Relationship to Metabolic Bone Diseases*, Vol 3. (Springfield, Ill.: C. C. Thomas)
88. Reeve, J., Meunier, P. J., Parsons, J. A., Kleinerman, L., Neer, R. M., Renier, J., Slovik, D., Vismans, F. J., Bernat, M., Bijvoet, O. L., Courpron, P., Edouard, C, and Potts, J, T., Jr. (1980). Anabolic effect of human parathyroid hormone fragment on trabecular bone in involutional osteoporosis. A multicenter trial. *Br. Med. J.*, **280**, 1340
89. Rasmussen, H., Bordier, P., Marie, P., Auquier, L., Eisinger, J. B., Kuntz, D., Caulin, F., Argemi, B., Gueris, J. and Julien, A. (1980). Effects of combined therapy with phosphate and calcitonin on bone volume in osteoporosis. *Metab. Bone Dis. Relat. Res.*, **2**, 107

Chapter 18

Early diagnosis of osteoporosis

M. Notelovitz

Osteoporosis is referred to as a silent epidemic for two very good reasons; it is asymptomatic until an unsuspected fracture occurs, and it involves a large segment of the ageing postmenopausal population. It has been estimated that 150 000 osteoporosis-related hip fractures per year will occur in the USA and about 40 000 in the UK; some 10–15% of these women will die as a direct consequence of this event[1]. In addition, one-third of women who fracture their hips will require permanent nursing home care[2]. Over the age of 60, 25% of white women will have radiological evidence of vertebral crush fractures[3]. The cost in financial terms (in excess of two billion dollars), morbidity and mortality is thus self-explanatory.

Osteoporosis is not a specific disease entity. It is a clinical sign of a syndrome that results from an exaggeration of the physiological age-related bone loss to the point where the bone's structural integrity is impaired and fractures occur in the absence of significant trauma. The quality of the remaining bone is normal; there is just too little. The heterogeneity of osteoporosis is further illustrated by the differential bone loss pattern: more frequent in the axial skeleton in some and in the appendicular skeleton in others. The latter type of osteoporosis occurs more frequently in older individuals, and is sometimes referred to as senile osteoporosis. Depending upon its aetiology, certain types of osteoporosis, for example that related to the endocrine change of the menopause, may be preventable. This can only be achieved by early diagnosis and appropriate preventive measures – nutrition, exercise and judicious hormone therapy.

PHYSIOLOGY OF BONE[4,5]

Bone is a living organ. Older bone is constantly being removed (bone resorption) and replaced by new bone (bone formation). The bone remodelling cycle is usually in balance (coupled), with the amount of bone removed compensated by an equal amount of newly formed bone.

New bone formation is required for growth, for repair of the microscopic fractures resulting from everyday physical stress, and the replacement of worn-out bone. Each bone remodelling cycle begins with the breaking down and resorption of older bone by osteoclasts; this is followed by the filling in of the microscopic cavity and the laying down of a collagen matrix by newly differentiated cells known as osteoblasts. Mineralization of the bone matrix occurs thereafter, with the embedding of crystals of calcium and phosphorus in the framework of interlocking protein fibres. A number of other minerals are also present in bone – fluoride, magnesium, sodium and potassium – as well as a host of trace elements. These act as the 'mortar' holding the 'bricks' of calcium and phosphorus crystals together.

Bone has three surfaces, called envelopes. Each envelope has different anatomical features even though its cellular make-up is identical to the other two. The surface facing the marrow cavity is known as the endosteal envelope, the outer surface is the periosteal envelope, while the area in between is referred to as the intracortical envelope.

During childhood, new formation occurs on the periosteal envelope with a lesser amount of breakdown on the endosteal surface. The marrow cavity expands, but not at a cost of bone strength. During adolescence and early adulthood, bone formation occurs on both surfaces, leading to an overall gain in bone mass. Maximum bone mass (bone maturity) occurs at about age 35; from this point onward, everyone loses bone. This is characterized by a greater loss of bone on the endosteal surface than that laid down on the outer envelope[4,5].

There are two types of bone – trabecular and cortical. Trabecular bone – the spongy or cancellous bone found in the vertebral bodies of the spine and the ends of the long bones – has the most active bone remodelling cycle; 40% is 'turned over' per annum. Women lose about 0.19% of trabecular bone per year premenopausally (age 30 to 49 years). After the menopause this rate increases to about 1.01% per year[6]. The loss of trabecular bone occurs in a linear fashion[7]. As a result, approximately 30% of a woman's trabecular bone mass is lost between the ages of 30 and 80[6]. Because of this greater activity and bone loss, osteoporosis occurs at an earlier age and more frequently in the axial skeleton.

Cortical or compact bone, comprises 80% of the skeleton but is less active: about 10% of its mass is replaced per annum. Cortical bone loss has a biphasic pattern: women do not tend to lose cortical bone significantly before the menopause, but after age 50 lose bone at a rate of about 1% per year until age 65. The rate of bone loss slows down to an insignificant rate (0.18% per year) thereafter. The loss of cortical bone is especially pronounced during the first three to five years following the onset of the menopause. Approximately 25% of the cortical bone mass is normally lost over a 30 year span in women between 50 and 80 years of age[6]. Fractures of the distal radius and the neck of the femur are due primarily to cortical bone loss. The bone remodelling cycle lasts approximately three to four months and is repeated in a cyclic fashion[5].

A clinical distinction needs to be drawn between varying degrees of abnormal bone loss: osteopaenia refers to bone loss significantly lower (two standard deviations) than that of an age-matched individual, but without overt or radiologically detectable fractures. Osteoporosis is associated with clinical or radiological evidence of a fracture. Osteopaenia is potentially reversible, whereas the wedging or crush fracture of an osteoporotic vertebra, for example, results in permanent and irreversible distortion of the bone architecture.

Four practical points emerge from this very brief description of normal bone physiology that can aid in the early diagnosis of osteoporosis:

(1) Osteoporosis is a heterogeneic condition with many different aetiologies. This permits the development of certain 'at-risk' clinical profiles.

(2) Bone loss is normal. The early detection of osteopaenia will allow for corrective measures and the prevention of irreversible osteoporosis. The changes in the bone remodelling cycle are very subtle and sensitive techniques of bone mass measurement are

needed. Alternatively, tests representative of some biochemical constituents of bone (e.g. calcium and hydroxyproline) can be used as indirect measures of the bone mass status.

(3) Trabecular and cortical bone behave independently of one another, so that measuring the bone loss pattern in one, does not necessarily reflect a similar change in the other. Indeed, they may represent two types of osteoporosis with a separate aetiology, pathogenesis and treatment.

(4) Bone loss is slow and insidious and occurs over a prolonged period of time before it reaches a pathological state. Repeated measures to determine the annual rate of bone loss are just as important as the initial bone mineral content determination.

WHO WILL GET OSTEOPOROSIS?

The aetiology of osteoporosis can be subdivided into two main categories: secondary to diseases known to have an adverse effect on bone mass, and primary, where the cause is either not identifiable, is due to an aberration of the normal physiological bone loss pattern, or results from certain lifestyle practices that have a negative impact on bone metabolism. Primary (or idiopathic) osteopaenia/osteoporosis is more common.

A clinical profile can be developed that will allow for the identification of persons at higher risk (Table1). These can be subclassified into unavoidable and avoidable groups. *Unavoidable factors* include:

(1) Race. For reasons that are not completely defined, black women rarely develop osteoporosis. Women who are blond with fair complexions (especially of Northwestern European ethnic background) and oriental women, are at much higher risk.

(2) A family history of osteoporosis[8]. It is not clear whether this is a genetic factor or secondary to the environment and lifestyle of families subject to this condition.

(3) Every woman will experience the menopause. Except for those women who undergo a premature menopause (before age 40), it is not known what differentiates the 25% of naturally menopausal women who will develop osteoporosis from the majority who will not[9].

Table 1 Risk factors for developing osteoporosis*

1. *Primary or idiopathic*:		
A. *Unavoidable*:	Race – white and oriental	
	Family history	
	Menopause	
	Phenotype: petite; short	
B. *Avoidable*:	Nutritional factors	
	< Calcium	
	> Vitamin D	
	'Bone Robbers' –	caffeine >
		protein >
		fibre >
		acidifying foodstuffs
		salt >
		alcohol >
	Physical inactivity	
	Smoking	
2. *Secondary*:		
A. *Medical conditions*:	Chronic renal failure	
	Gastrectomy and intestinal bypass	
	Malabsorption syndromes	
B. *Endocrinopathies*:	Hyperparathyroidism	
	Hyperthyroidism	
	Adrenal–cortical >	
	Diabetes	
C. *Medications*:	Steroids	
	Anticonvulsants	
	Antacids (with aluminum)	
	Thyroid extracts – grains 3>/day	

*See text

(4) Phenotype. Women who are short and petite and who have a lighter skeleton are at greater risk[9]. Obesity is said to be protective for two main reasons; more endogenous oestrogen is metabolized by the peripheral conversion of androstenedione in fat cells; excessive weight provides a greater stress to the skeleton thereby stimulating new bone formation.

Lifestyle habits and practices can also influence the accretion and/or loss of bone mineral; these are controllable or *avoidable factors*. As noted previously, calcium is a major ingredient of mineralized bone. It has been established that the premenopausal woman requires 1000 mg of elemental calcium per day to remain in balance. The respective values for peri- and the untreated postmenopausal woman are 1200 and 1400 mg respectively[10]. The average intake of calcium among white American women is 450–500 mg per day. Thus, the majority of women at risk of developing osteoporosis are in chronic negative balance – often throughout their lifetime.

Even in the presence of a normal calcium intake, abuse of the so-called 'bone robbers' may negate the achievement of normal bone nutrition. Included in this category are: excess intake of caffeine-containing beverages (five or more cups of coffee per day)[11]; high animal protein intake[12]; vegetables and other foodstuffs that bind calcium and prevent or retard its absorption, e.g. spinach and asparagus (oxalates), and the outer husks or cereal grains (phytates); alcohol abuse and, according to some, a high consumption of acidifying foods such as soda drinks[12]. Salt has also been implicated; as little as one teaspoonful per day (2000 mg) may be too much[13]. Vitamin D is essential for normal calcium absorption, but only 400 IU per day or exposure to fifteen minutes of sunshine per day is needed by the healthy adult[14]. An excessive intake of vitamin D – greater than 1000 IU per day – may have the opposite effect and enhance bone loss.

Physical activity is one of the more clearly defined determinants of new bone formation. Conversely, immobility, even in healthy young adults, is associated with an acute measurable increase in urinary calcium excretion, that persists with the duration of inactivity. The amount of daily gravitational exercise is probably one of the most important factors to consider[15].

Although there is no consensus, smoking is found more frequently among osteoporotic than non-osteoporotic women. It is not clear whether smoking reduces bone mass by direct affect on bone metabolism; by the induction of an earlier menopause, or because smokers usually weigh less[16].

Secondary factors refer to certain medical conditions and/or the associated treatment[17]. Long-term drug therapy with steroids (for asthma); aluminium-containing antacids (for ulcer disease), certain anticonvulsants (e.g. dilantin) and overenthusiastic replacement therapy for hypothyroidism (thyroid grains 3 or more) all have negative effects on bone mass, but may be necessary for the general well-being of the individual.

Medical conditions that interfere with the normal mechanism of calcium metabolism and absorption are highly associated with osteopaenia and osteoporosis. Examples include chronic renal failure (including patients on dialysis and postrenal transplant); a history of previous gastrectomy or intestinal bypass procedures and the various malabsorption syndromes. Non-reproductive endocrinopathies, for example, hyperparathyroidism, hyperthyroidism, adrenal–cortical overactivity and diabetes, are all potential secondary inducers of increased bone loss[17].

Neoplastic disease – multiple myeloma and metastatic carcinoma – may present with a clinical and/or radiological picture suggestive of osteoporosis, but are not causes of impaired bone metabolism[17].

No one has yet equated the above risk factors with a 'weighted score' that should make some of the factors clinically more significant than others. Empiric observations suggest that the unavoidable factors (race, family history, phenotype and menopause) should be regarded as the predisposing initiators and the avoidable factors (diet, exercise, etc.) as the accelerators of bone loss.

SCREENING FOR OSTEOPOROSIS: INDIRECT MEASURES

Screening for osteopaenia/osteoporosis by indirect measures, can be equated to the assessment of glucosuria for the detection of diabetes. Both serve as practical, but relatively insensitive and inconsistent indicators of the primary disorder.

A number of biological parameters have been associated with clinical osteoporosis[18] (Table 2). Of these, only urinary calcium and hydroxyproline excretion have been uniformly accepted as being representative of bone mineral and matrix status, respectively.

Calcium has a diurnal storage and nocturnal release pattern[19]. In normal postmenopausal women, the natural loss of calcium increases from about 1 to approximately 2 mmol/8 hours. If there is no short-

Table 2 Indirect methods of screening for osteoporosis

Urine tests:[19–21]:	24 hour calcium excretion	20–30 mg = osteomalacia
		200 mg > secondary causes
	Fasting calcium/creatinine (> 0.16)	
	Fasting hydroxyproline/creatinine (> 0.017)	
	Free cortisol (24 hour sample)	
Blood:[19,28]	Calcium/phosphorous <	
	Alkaline phosphatase >	
	Progesterone < 0.5 mg/ml	
	Androstenedione <	
	Calcitonin < (after calcium infused)	
	1,25-vitamin D <	
	Oestrogens: oestrone < 30 pg/mi	
	oestradiol (total) < 10 pg/ml	

time calcium storage during the day, this calcium has to come from the stable bone mineral pool and is an indirect measure of osteoclast (bone resorption/loss) activity. The most convenient means of assessing the degree of loss is by measurement of the urinary calcium/creatinine ratio, after an overnight fast. Patients are instructed to discard the first voided urine sample (after a 12-hour overnight fast) and to drink about 200 ml of distilled water. The second voided urine sample is assayed for calcium and creatinine. A ratio in excess of 0.16 is indicative of exaggerated osteoclast activity. Similarly, an increase of the hydroxyproline/creatinine ratio (< 0.017) is indicative of increased bone matrix resorption. Increased fasting calcium/creatinine and hydroxyproline/ creatinine ratios have been well correlated with the vertebral crush fracture syndrome, and therefore serve as simple and practical means of monitoring the degree of bone loss[20,21]. The calcium/creatinine ratio may also be used to assess the efficacy of therapy. Studies comparing differing dosages of oestrogen replacement and methods of bone mineral assessment (CT scanning and calcium/ creatinine ratios) have provided the same effective clinical dose reponse for the inhibition of bone loss (0.625 mg of conjugated oestrogen)[22,23].

To exclude secondary causes of osteoporosis and certain associated conditions, e.g. osteomalacia, a biochemical profile that measures fasting levels of plasma calcium, phosphorus, alkaline phosphatase, glucose, creatinine/BUN, proteins and certain electrolytes, should be included in any primary screening programme. If normal, they need not be repeated.

DIRECT MEASUREMENT

Non-invasive bone measurement is a preferable way of diagnosing osteopaenia and can be compared to the detection of hyperglycaemia as a means of diagnosing diabetes. It assesses the aberrant clinical sign diagnostic of the disease but does not help with the elucidation of its aetiology.

Of the various methods that have been described (Table 3) only five are actually available and practical for clinical usage.

Radiogrametry

Based on the physiological loss of bone from the endosteal envelope and new bone formation on the periosteum, alterations in the total

Table 3 Non-invasive direct measures of bone mass evaluation

X-ray:	Radiogrametry
	Radiographic densitometry
	Magnification radiogrametry
	Lateral spinal X-ray
Photonabsorptiometry:	Single: single point
	rectilinear
	Dual
Computerized tomography:	
Other:	Compton scattering
	Neutron activation

mass of tubular bones can be readily assessed from radiographs taken of the hand. A high quality postero-anterior X-ray of the non-dominant hand taken on a fine grain industrial film, is all that is required. Using very fine Vernier X-ray calipers, the midpoint of the second metacarpal is defined, and measurement is made of both the medullary and the cortical diameters. Within-observer variation for the outer measurement (1.2%) is very similar to that of between-observer assessments (1.5%). The respective errors for inner diameters are 4.8% and 6.5% of the overall mean value. The degree of variability can be significantly reduced by including the measurement of the second, third and fourth metacarpals. The precision improves from 5–10% with single measurements to 1–3% with multiple measurements of a number of metacarpal bones.

In order to correct for individual differences in bone size, the cortical thickness is sometimes expressed as a percentage of the total width at the midshaft of the metacarpal (metacarpal index). The measure of cortical area correlates better with the amount of bone present than the cortical width alone.

Radiogrametry has been widely used in cross-sectional studies. With longitudinal studies, the coefficient of variation of this technique for replicate measurements is 1–3%, necessitating a change of greater than 6% between two measurements before a real change can be determined. Measurements every three months are recommended.

Radiogrametry is easy to perform, exposes the patient to minimal radiation and is the least expensive method available. The metacarpal index correlates well with regional and systemic osteoporosis. It is primarily a measure of cortical bone and allows for the assessment of changes in the endosteal and periosteal surfaces. It does have some, albeit fairly poor, correlation with vertebral compression fractures[24,25].

Magnification radiogrametry allows for the better assessment of the intracortical porosity associated with renal dysfunction, certain endocrinopathies and other metabolic disorders.

Radiographic photodensitometry

This technique involves the taking of a standardized X-ray of the hand together with an aluminium step-wedge that has similar absorption characteristics of bone, and which is placed adjacent to the phalanges. Once again, the non-dominant hand is used. Comparison of the density of the bone and step-wedge by special computer analysis allows for the calculation and estimation of the bone mineral content of the bone[26]. Although contrary opinions have been expressed, the results are reflective mainly of cortical bone.

A precision of 3 – 4% has been recorded by measuring larger areas of the phalanges, thus reducing problems associated with repositioning. Because of radiation scattering in thicker parts of the body and the preferential attenuation of the softer energies from the polychromatic X-ray beam as it passes through the body (beam hardening), this technique can only be utilized in areas with less than 5 cm of soft tissue cover[26].

The taking of the X-ray is inexpensive and provides little radiation exposure. The cost of the computer analysis of the bone density is, however, relatively expensive, and limits the practical clinical usefulness of this technique, especially when compared with other more specific and sensitive methods.

Single photondensitometry

This method is based on a well-collimated beam (5 mm) of monoenergetic radiation (usually ^{125}I), that is used to scan a peripheral part of the skeleton. A limb, usually the arm, is placed between a sealed radioactive isotope below and a scintillation detector above. The limb is either immersed in water or covered by some tissue-equivalent material to ensure equal soft-tissue coverage. The amount of bone mineral present is proportional to the change in beam intensity over the bone. Bone mass expressed in g/cm can be estimated by appropriate mathematical calculations and comparison with known standards[24–26].

The usual sites measured are the distal and midshaft areas of the non-dominant radius. The midportion of the radius is mostly cortical bone, while the distal radius has between 25 and 70% of trabecular bone depending upon the point of measurement. The more proximal this measurement, the lesser will be the contribution of trabecular bone. One of the main problems associated with this technique is accurate repositioning (and hence reproducibility) especially of the distal radius. This has been overcome in part by the introduction of rectilinear scanning: with this technique approximately 1 cm of bone is scanned in 2 mm step-wise increments, thereby reducing the chance of missing the previously measured location[26].

With commercially available instruments, the use of specially designed armholders, and insistence on detail with repeated measurements, single photondensitometry has been found to have a precision of 1–2%. Accuracy is enhanced by doing multiple measurements.

Measurement of the bone mineral content by this technique can be used to differentiate effectively low-bone from high-bone mass populations. With longitudinal evaluation, not only should measurements be made fairly often (three to four months), but assessment must be based on the bone density (as opposed to the bone mineral content) at each point measured. This is obtained by dividing the bone mineral content by the bone width (BMC/BW); the result is expressed in g/cm^2. With this measurement, different rates of bone loss from the midshaft and distal radius in the same individual have been noted, thereby permitting the simultaneous assessment of cortical and trabecular bone response to a given therapy or management programme.

An additional advantage of this technique is that the instrument is portable, and allows for the screening of populations far removed from medical centres[27]. Figure 1 reflects the results of a cross-sectional evaluation of the bone mineral content of randomly selected black and white women (over age 60) from a low socio-economic rural area. The mean bone mineral content of the black women was significantly greater than the whites at each age point; on individual assessment, 15% of the blacks and 45% of the white women had a bone mineral content value below an empirically derived fracture threshold (0.65 g/cm). Thus, in very much the same way that a Pap smear is used to screen for cervical disease, so single photonabsorptiometry can be utilized for the community screening of asymptomatic osteopaenia. An incidental finding of interest in the previously mentioned study, was the identical rate of bone loss in the black and white subjects.

Advantages of single photonabsorptiometry include: low radiation (1/100 of a standard X-ray); easy to perform (takes approximately

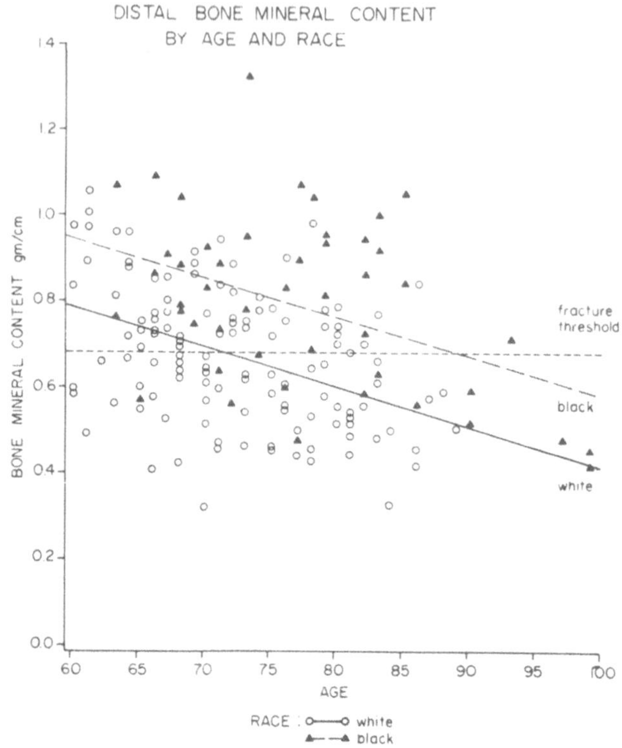

Figure 1 Bone mineral content measured by single photonabsorptiometry as part of a rural osteoporosis programme. Black women, ▲ – – –, had the same rate of bone loss as whites, o———, but had a greater bone mineral content (see text)

10 minutes); good correlation between the cortical bone mass measured in the radius and other cortical sites elsewhere (neck of the femur); excellent correlation in radial bone mass and total body calcium (as measured by neutron activation) in normals but less so in women with osteoporosis; established accuracy and precision in numerous published clinical trials[25]; and potential availability at a moderate cost per test[27].

Disadvantages are: the initial cost of the instrument ($20 000); problems with repositioning and hence its variability for assessing trabecular bone loss; inability to measure specific changes on the endosteal and periosteal envelopes.

Dual photonabsorptiometry

One of the major advantages of this method is the dual energy of the radioactive isotope (usually ^{153}gadolinium) which eliminates the need for a constant thickness of soft tissue around the bone, and so permits the evaluation of deeper structures, e.g. the vertebrae and the femoral neck[26].

Most of the instruments available utilize a rectilinear mode of scanning. About 20–30 minutes are needed to scan the lumbar vertebrae. It is associated with a very low amount of radiation – 5–15 mrem. Dual photonabsorptiometry of the vertebrae is a measure of both the trabecular and cortical bone and may thus be limited to a certain degree in its ability to monitor only trabecular bone loss. Its advantage, and proven sensitivity in clinical practice, however, is based on the fact that fractures of the vertebrae and the femur are the result of *both* cortical and trabecular bone loss, and this may therefore serve as an advantage over other techniques that only measure loss of the softer cancellous bone.

Much more expertise is needed with dual photonabsorptiometry. Reports at this time indicate that it has a reproducibility coefficient of 2–3% – about the same as single photonabsorptiometry. Although some overlap in the bone mineral content measurement occurs between normal controls and patients with osteoporosis, this is reported to be less than that which occurs when single photonabsorptiometry of the forearm is used[7,26].

At this time, instruments are rather expensive and are not generally available. Because of its relative specificity for trabecular bone measurement, the combined use of dual and single photonabsorptiometry should provide a practical and cost-effective means of evaluating the axial and appendicular skeleton.

Computed tomography

Computed axial tomography (CT) has been successfully adapted to measure bone in both the axial and appendicular skeleton. The advantage of CT scanning is that it combines a quantitative approach with very clear imaging and thus allows for precise regional localization to a certain part of the bone. Cancellous bone can be clearly separated from cortical bone[22].

CT scanning has been used to measure changes in the trabecular areas of the radius and the spine, but requires sophisticated calibration and positioning techniques.

Intensive research in the area has lead to the development of standardized techniques and soft-ware, that allow for the modification of most existing CT scanners to measure accurately the trabecular bone mineral content of individual vertebrae. Patients are positioned using a CT localization system so that the midplane of the bodies of these vertebrae are obtained with image analysis soft-ware. A similar approach is used to obtain a lateral scout view of the spine. The midplanes of four vertebrae are obtained and a single 1 cm slice measured at each level, yielding four separate values to quantify and average. The mineral content of the midportion of the upper lumbar is usually measured. This site is chosen because there is a close correlation between the bone mineral content in adjacent vertebrae, and because the volume of cancellous bone at this point is large thereby avoiding the incorporation of the dense vertebral end plates. The lower lumbar vertebrae frequently have degenerative disease with reactive sclerosis, and this too may affect the measurement.

The precision with *in vivo* vertebral mineral determination using the CAT scan is 1.6% when special soft-ware and calibrating techniques are used. This increases to 3–4% if a simpler external localization technique is used[22].

With CT scanning, much greater losses in bone mass have been noted in certain high-risk populations – e.g. women who have recently undergone a surgical menopause – than was previously recognized. In one study, the bone mineral loss measured by CT over a two-year period was 17.4 ± 9.86% compared with 3.86 ± 3.8% at the radial diaphysis using single photonabsorptiometry and 2.44 ± 2.8% with radiogrametry (combined cortical thickness)[22].

The vertebral body is a mixture of haemopoietic marrow, fat and bone in varying amounts. Critics of CT scanning maintain that the fat, and to a lesser extent the marrow, confounds the CT measurement, and that much of the 'bone loss' is due to alterations in the soft tissue content. One way of overcoming this potential disadvantage is by the use of dual-energy CT scanning[26].

According to Genant *et al.*[22], patient time on the scanner is only 10–15 minutes and the total radiation to the upper abdomen 100–200 mrem. At the present time, CT scanning is not readily available for large scale osteopaenia/osteoporosis screening because of the relative inaccessibility of the instrument for non-urgent preventive health care screening. Added to this is the relatively high cost of the procedure. With time, CT scanning technology is bound to improve to the point where it will, indeed, become available and cost-effective for the population at large.

CONCLUSION

There is a progressive and absolute increase in the incidence of osteoporosis other than that accounted for by the ageing of most populations. During the decade 1968–1977, there was a 66% net increase in fractures of the neck of the femur in the UK[1]. The proportion of beds needed to care for these patients in trauma and orthopaedic departments, rose from 13.3% to 18.3% and at a cost of forty million pounds annually[1]. Much of this pathology can be prevented. To achieve this goal, early diagnosis is mandatory.

Retrospective evaluation of an older population with established osteoporosis has indicated that women with a propensity to multiple fractures have certain characteristics – early menopause and a decrease in the bone mineral content of the distal radius as measured by single photonabsorptiometry[29]. But what is really needed is much earlier evaluation of populations at risk, so that the detection of low bone mass profiles can be corrected by appropriate preventive measures.

Two main approaches are necessary: educating consumers about the existence of this condition and its potential consequence if ignored; the establishment of osteoporosis screening centres where individuals can have their bone mineral content and other relevant factors assessed[17]. A suggested protocol includes initial screening of at-risk populations at 35 years of age with a combination of single and dual photonabsorptiometry: this measurement (if the bone mass is normal) should be repeated at three to five years intervals until the advent of the menopause. For the next one to two years, these tests should be repeated at three to four monthly intervals until a reliable rate of bone loss can be established. If it is less than 1% per annum, less frequent analysis will be needed. With this approach, two of the more important variables that determine whether an individual will develop osteoporosis – bone mineral content and rate of bone loss – can be objectively measured and followed. By combining dual and single photonabsorptiometry the differential bone loss rate in trabecular and cortical bone can be defined and monitored.

Non-expensive tests such as initial biochemical plasma profile (see before) and regular fasting urinary calcium/creatinine ratios will add to the accuracy of the screening programme and enhance the efficacy of monitoring an individual's bone mass status.

The little old lady deformed by a Dowager's hump and the fracture of the hip attributed to 'old age' can and should be relegated to the past. Both conditions are indicative of a pathological event (osteoporosis) and are not a part of normal ageing.

References

1. Lewis, A. F. (1981). Fracture of neck of the femur: changing incidence. *Br. Med. J.*, **283**, 1217
2. Keene, J. S. and Anderson, C. A. (1982). Hip fractures in the elderly. Discharge predictions with a functional rating scale. *J. Am. Med. Assoc.*, **284**, 564
3. Heaney, R. P. (1976). Estrogens and postmenopausal osteoporosis. *Clin. Obstet. Gynecol.*, **19**, 791
4. Sharpe, W. D. (1979). Age changes in human bone: an overview. *Bull. N. Y. Acad. Med.*, **55**, 757
5. Courpron, P. (1981). Bone tissue mechanisms underlying osteoporoses. *Orthop. Clin. North. Am.*, **12**, 513
6. Nagant de Deuxchaisnes, C. (1981). The pathogenesis and treatment of involutional osteoporosis. In Dixon, A. St. J., Russel, R. G. G. and Stamp, T. C. B. (eds) *Osteoporosis: A Multidisciplinary Problem*, pp. 291–333. (London: Academic Press)
7. Riggs, B. L., Wahner, H. W., Dunn, W. L., Mazess, R. B., Offord, K. P. and Melton, L. J. (1981). Differential changes in bone mineral density of the appendicular and axial skeleton with aging. *J. Clin. Invest.*, **67**, 328
8. Møller, M., Horsman, A., Harvald, B., Hauge, M., Henningsen, K. and Nordin, B. E. (1978). Metacarpal morphometry in monozygotic and dizygotic elderly twins. *Calcif. Tiss. Res.*, **25**, 197
9. Lane, J. M. and Vigorita, V. J. (1983). Current concepts review: osteoporosis. *J. Bone Joint Surg. Am.*, **65-A**, 274
10. Heaney, R. P., Recker, R. R. and Saville, P. D. (1977). Calcium balance and calcium requirements in middle-aged women. *Am. J. Clin. Nutr.*, **30**, 1603
11. Heaney, R. P., and Recker, R. R. (1982). Effects of nitrogen, phosphorous and caffeine on calcium balance in women. *J. Lab. Clin. Med.*, **99**, 46
12. Bresnan, J. T. and Bresnan, M. E. (1982). Dietary protein, metabolic acidosis, and calcium balance. *Adv. Nutr. Res.*, **4**, 77
13. Goulding, A. (1980). Effects of dietary NACl supplements on parathyroid function, bone turnover and bone composition in rats taking restrictive amounts of calcium. *Mineral Electrolyte Metab.*, **4**, 203
14. DeLuca, H. F. (1982). New developments in the Vitamin D endocrine system. *J. Am. Diet. Assoc.*, **80**, 231
15. Editorial (1983). Osteoporosis and activity. *Lancet*, **1**, 1365
16. Williams, A. R., Weiss, N. S., Ure, C. L., Ballard, J. and Daling, J. R. (1982). Effect of weight, smoking, and estrogen use on the risk of hip and forearm fractures in postmenopausal women. *Obstet. Gynecol.*, **60**, 695
17. Notelovitz, M. and Ware, M. (1982). *Stand Tall. The Informed Woman's Guide to Preventing Osteoporosis.* (Gainesville: Triad Publishers)

18. Upton, G. V. (1982). The perimenopause. Physiologic correlates and clinical management. *J. Reprod. Med.*, **27**, 1
19. Parfitt, A. M. (1981). The integration of skeletal and mineral homeostasis. In DeLuca, H. F., Frost, H. M., Jee, W. S. S., Johnson, C. C. and Parfitt, A. M. (eds) *Osteoporosis: Recent Advances in Pathogenesis and Treatment*, p. 115. (Baltimore: University Park Press)
20. Gallagher, J. C., Riggs, B. L. and DeLuca, H. F. (1980). Effect of estrogen on calcium absorption and serum vitamin D metabolites in postmenopausal osteoporosis. *J. Clin. Endocrinol. Metab.*, **51**, 1359
21. Crilly, R., Horsman, A., Marshall, D. H. and Nordin, B. E. C. (1979). Prevalence, pathogenesis and treatment of post-menopausal osteoporosis. *Aust. N.Z. J. Med.*, **9**, 24
22. Genant, H. K., Cann, C. C. and Faul, D. D. (1982). Quantitative computed tomography for assessing vertebral bone mineral. In Dequeker, J. and Johnston, C. C. (eds) *Non-Invasive Bone Measurements: Methodological Problems*, pp. 215–249. (Oxford: IRL Press Ltd.)
23. Geola, F.L., Frumar, A.M., Tataryn, I.V., Lu, K.H., Hershman, J.M., Eggena, P., Sambhi, M.P. and Judd, H.L. (1980). Biological effects of various doses of conjugated equine estrogens in post-menopausal women. *J. Clin. Endocrinol. Metab.*, **51**, 620
24. Recker, R, R. (1982). Non-invasive measurements of bone loss. In Dequeker, J. and Johnston, C. C. (eds) *Non-Invasive Bone Measurement: Methodological Problems*, pp. 1–13. (Oxford: IRL Press Ltd.)
25. Johnston, C. C. (1983). Non-invasive methods for quantifying appendicular bone mass. In Avioli, L. V. (ed.) *The Osteoporotic Syndrome. Detection, Prevention and Treatment*, pp. 73–84. (New York: Grune and Stratton)
26. Mazess, R. B. (1983). Non-invasive methods for quantifying trabecular bone. In Avioli, L. V. (ed.) *The Osteoporotic Syndrome. Detection, Prevention and Treatment*, pp. 85–114. (New York: Grune and Stratton)
27. Notelovitz, M., Rector, C., March, J. and Lambert, T. Screening for osteoporosis in rural communities. Unpublished data
28. Laufer, L. R., Davidson, B. J., Ross, R. K., Lagasse, L. D., Siiteri, P. K. and Judd, H. L. (1983). Physical characteristics and sex hormone levels in patients with osteoporotic hip fractures or endometrial cancer. *Am. J. Obstet. Gynecol.*, **145**, 585
29. Jensen, G. F., Christiansen, C., Boesen, J., Hegedüs, V. and Transbøl, I. (1982). Epidemiology of postmenopausal spinal and long bone fractures. *Clin. Orthop. Related Res.*, **166**, 75

Chapter 19

Interrelation of oestrogen and the major calcium regulating hormones

J. C. Stevenson

The loss of ovarian function at the menopause presents a particular challenge to calcium homoeostasis and bone. It is well established that loss of ovarian function at any age leads to loss of bone[1-3] (Figure 1).

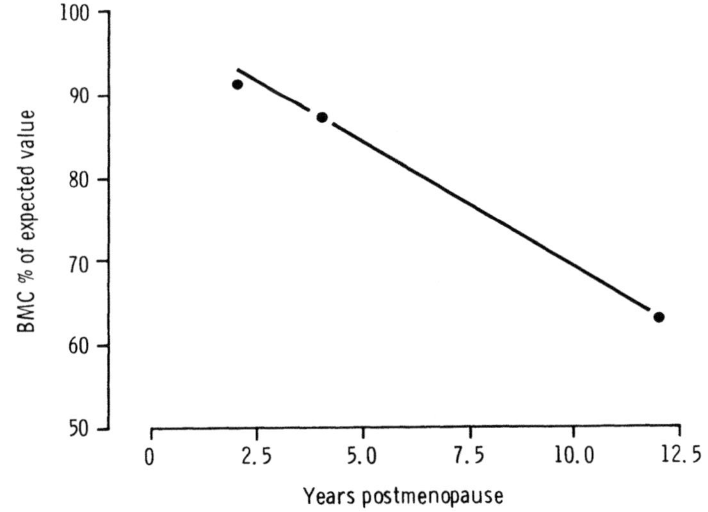

Figure 1 Bone mineral content of distal forearm, expressed as a percentage of expected value for age, plotted against years postmenopause in 3 young women with premature menopause

This bone loss is most rapid in the early postmenopause and particularly affects trabecular bone[4]. In some women, the reduction in skeletal mass is such that it predisposes to fractures – osteoporosis.

Although there is a general decline of bone mass with age in both sexes, due to decreasing bone formation, the accelerated bone loss following the menopause appears largely due to increased resorption[5,6]. This postmenopausal bone loss can be prevented by administration of exogenous oestrogen[7,8] but recurs when such treatment is withdrawn.

The underlying pathogenesis of this increased bone resorption has been the subject of much controversy, but recent advances in hormone measurement have led to a clearer understanding. It had long been thought that the increased resorption of bone was secondary to impairment of intestinal calcium absorption[9], with bone calcium being homoeostatically mobilized to maintain plasma levels. This assumption was based on the fact that a form of osteoporosis could be produced in various laboratory animals by withholding calcium from their diet. Of course, the bones of growing animals are hardly a suitable model for the bones of postmenopausal osteoporotics. However, measurements of intestinal calcium absorption in women with postmenopausal osteoporosis do indeed show that there is some impairment. If the hypothesis is correct, plasma calcium levels would tend to be on the lower side of normal and homeostatic increases in the calcium-elevating hormones, parathyroid hormone (PTH) and 1,25-dihydroxyvitamin D, would be observed. In fact, the opposite is found. Plasma calcium levels rise at the menopause[10] but fall again with oestrogen replacement[11]. Levels of PTH, as measured by radioimmunoassay recognizing the biologically active *N*-terminal portion of the molecule, are slightly lower in postmenopausal than in premenopausal women (Figure 2)[12,13]. These levels rise with oestrogen administration, presumably as a homeostatic response to the fall in plasma calcium[14,15]. It is interesting to observe that these changes in PTH secretion are reflected and indeed magnified in postmenopausal osteoporotics[16,17].

It thus appears that increased bone mobilization in postmenopausal women is not primarily due to an increase in PTH causing enhanced resorption. Of course, a change in skeletal sensitivity to the resorptive action of PTH could allow an increase in bone mobilization even in the face of small falls in the circulating levels of the hormone.

Similar to PTH, lower levels of 1,25-dihydroxyvitamin D are found

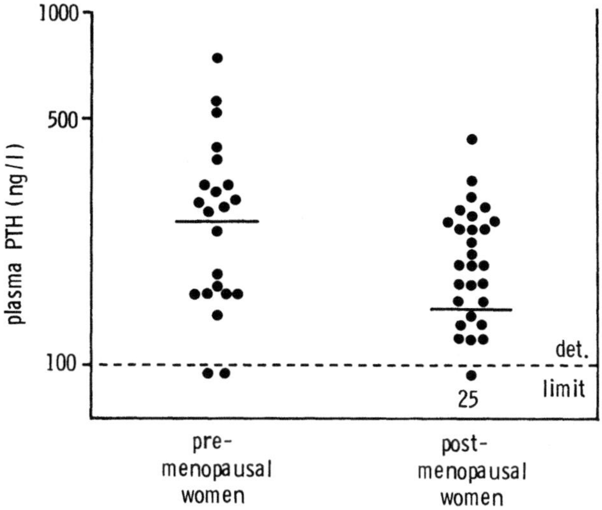

Figure 2 Plasma PTH levels (ng/l) in premenopausal and postmenopausal women. (Reproduced with permission of Wetenschappelijke uitgeverij Bunge)

in postmenopausal compared to premenopausal women (Figure 3)[12,13]. Furthermore, postmenopausal osteoporotics have even lower levels compared to controls, and this is reflected by a lower intestinal calcium absorption[18]. Although 1,25-dihydroxyvitamin D is a most potent bone-resorbing agent, it does not seem that postmenopausal bone mobilization is due to an elevation in circulating levels of the hormone. Again, this does not preclude a change in skeletal sensitivity to its actions. Oestrogen replacement therapy causes a small increase in both 1,25-dihydroxyvitamin D levels and intestinal calcium absorption in postmenopausal osteoporotics[17] although such an effect has not been observed in women during the early postmenopause[15,19]. It is thus apparent that the lowered intestinal absorption of calcium seen in postmenopausal women, and particularly in osteoporotics, is secondary to the lower levels of 1,25-dihydroxyvitamin D. Any primary intestinal defect impairing calcium absorption in postmenopausal osteoporotics is most unlikely; such women increase their absorption to normal with physiological 1,25-dihydroxyvitamin D replacement[17].

The question then arises as to whether the lower circulating 1,25-dihydroxyvitamin D levels are due to a primary renal defect of production, or secondary to both the increased postmenopausal bone mobilization and changes in PTH and oestrogen. It was suggested by one study that elderly osteoporotics had deficient production of

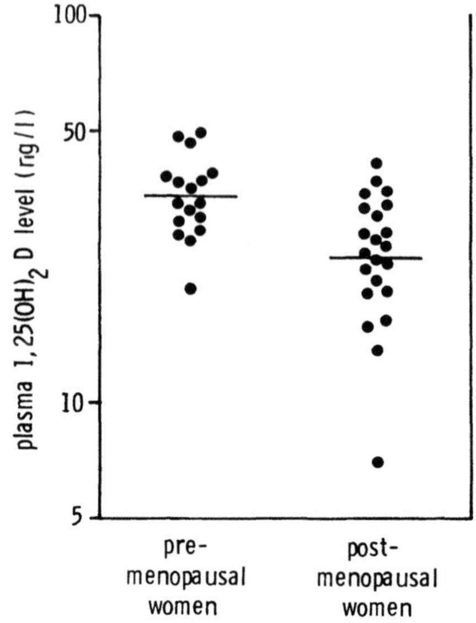

Figure 3 Plasma 1,25-dihydroxyvitamin D levels (ng/1) in premenopausal and postmenopausal women. (Reproduced with permission of Wetenschappelijke uitgeverij Bunge)

1,25-dihydroxyvitamin D[20]. However, this study used young, and hence inappropriate, controls, thereby neglecting any age-related decline in hormone production. Another study assessed renal 1α-hydroxylase reserve in postmenopausal osteoporotics and compared them to age-matched non-osteoporotic controls[21]. No difference between the two groups was found. In summary, the changes seen in plasma calcium, PTH and 1,25-dihydroxyvitamin D following the menopause are secondary to the increased bone mobilization caused by loss of oestrogen secretion; they are the effects, not the cause.

Lack of oestrogen leads to increased bone resorption and oestrogen replacement therapy prevents it. It is not established, however, that this is a direct effect of oestrogen on bone, especially since oestrogen receptors have not been demonstrated in bone[22,23]. Could the anti-resorptive effects of oestrogen be indirect? Calcitonin is a hormone whose function in humans is to oppose osteoclastic bone resorption[24]. There is a sex difference in its levels, being lower in women than in men. The finding that this sex difference was abolished by the combined oral contraceptive pill first raised the suggestion that gonadal steroids might influence calcitonin secretion in humans [25]. It was then shown that oestrogen replacement in postmenopausal women caused an increase in calcitonin secretion[15,26] but these levels fell again when treatment was withdrawn. Circulating levels of calcitonin are normally very low, and there is also an age-related decline in secretion [27,28]. Thus changes in calcitonin levels at the menopause would normally be difficult to demonstrate because of the necessity of obtaining sex- and age-matched controls. However, by studying calcitonin secretion in young women with early menopause, preliminary results have shown that their calcitonin secretion is markedly impaired compared to age-matched premenopausal controls[29]. The onset of the menopause thus accelerates the age-related decline of calcitonin secretion, leaving postmenopausal women with particularly low levels. Furthermore, even lower calcitonin secretion has been demonstrated in postmenopausal osteoporotics compared to non-osteoporotic age-matched controls[30].

Until recently, decreased levels of calcitonin were thought to be without clinical significance. This is because no immediately apparent bone disorder was seen in patients who were totally thyroidectomized. However, it is now becoming clear that this concept is incorrect. Of course, since calcitonin can also be produced in the thymus and lung as well as in the thyroid in man, totally thyroidectomized patients may not be completely deficient in circulating calcitonin[31]. There is no doubt, though, that their levels are low and this is reflected by a reduced bone mass[32]. In a patient with complete calcitonin deficiency, severe osteoporosis was found[33]. It is therefore most likely that the low calcitonin levels and increased bone loss in postmenopausal women are causally related. In an analogous situation in males, men with hypogonadism have both lowered calcitonin levels and lowered bone density[34]. The concept is further strengthened by the fact that studies using direct and accurate assessments of bone mass show a positive effect of calcitonin therapy in postmenopausal osteoporosis[35–37].

In the light of this recent information, the interrelation of oestrogen and the major calcium regulating hormones can be summarized. Loss of oestrogen secretion at the menopause leads to mobilization of bone. This is due, at least in part, to a fall in calcitonin secretion. The removal of this antiresorptive factor permits an increase in bone resorption, without concomitant increases in bone-resorbing hormones being necessary. The release of bone calcium into the circulation leads to the small, homeostatic falls in PTH and 1,25-dihydroxyvitamin levels, the latter in turn causing a decline in the intestinal absorption of calcium.

Not surprisingly, all these changes are most marked in postmenopausal osteoporotics. Therapies aimed at the prevention and treatment of this distressingly common disease should be rationalized according to this pathogenesis. Attempts to reverse only the changes secondary to increased bone mobilization are always likely to prove unsuccessful.

Acknowledgements

It is a pleasure to acknowledge my colleagues in the Endocrine Unit, Royal Postgraduate Medical School, and in the Academic Unit of Obstetrics and Gynaecology, King's College Hospital Medical School, London, UK, for their involvement in some of the studies mentioned above. I am also most grateful to Miss Jacqueline Pennock and Professor Frank Doyle, Department of Academic Radiology, Royal Postgraduate Medical School, for bone density measurements. Support from Laboratoires Besins Iscovesco is also gratefully acknowledged.

References

1. Lindsay, R., Hart, D. M., Aitken, J. M., MacDonald, E. B., Anderson, J. B. and Clarke, A. C. (1976). Long-term prevention of postmenopausal osteoporosis by oestrogen. *Lancet*, **1**, 1038
2. Horsman, A., Gallagher, J. C., Simpson, M. and Nordin, B. E. C. (1977). Prospective trial of oestrogen and calcium in postmenopausal women. *Br. Med. J.*, **2**, 789
3. Christiansen, C., Christensen, M. S., McNair, P., Hagen, C., Stocklund, K. and Transbøl, I. (1980). Prevention of early postmenopausal bone loss: controlled 2-year study in 315 normal females. *Eur. J. Clin. Invest.*, **10**, 273
4. Krølner, B. and Nielsen, S. P. (1982). Bone mineral content of the lumbar spine in normal and osteoporotic women: cross-sectional and longitudinal studies. *Clin. Sci.*, **62**, 329
5. Heaney, R. P., Recker, R. R. and Saville, P. D. (1978). Menopausal changes in bone remodelling. *J. Lab. Clin. Med.*, **92**, 964
6. Nordin, B. E. C., Aaron, J., Speed, R. and Crilly, R. G. (1981). Bone formation and resorption as the determinants of trabecular bone volume in postmenopausal osteoporosis. *Lancet*, **2**, 277
7. Lindsay, R., Hart, D. M., Forrest, C. and Baird, C. (1980). Prevention of spinal osteoporosis in oophorectomised women. *Lancet*, **2**, 1151
8. Christiansen, C., Christensen, M. S. and Transbøl, I. (1981). Bone mass in postmenopausal women after withdrawal of oestrogen/gestagen replacement therapy. *Lancet*, **1**, 459
9. Nordin, B. E. C. (1960). Osteomalacia, osteoporosis and calcium deficiency. *Clin. Orthop.*, **17**, 235
10. Aitken, J. M., Hart, D. M. and Smith, D. A. (1971). The effect of long-term mestranol administration on calcium and phosphorus homeostasis in oophorectomized women. *Clin. Sci.*, **41**, 233

11. Whitehead, M. I., Lane, G., Townsend, P. T., Abeyasekera, G., Hillyard, C. J. and Stevenson, J. C. (1982). Effects in postmenopausal women of natural and synthetic estrogens on calcitonin and calcium-regulating hormone secretion. *Acta Obstet. Gynecol. Scand. (Suppl.)*, **106**, 27
12. Stevenson, J. C. (1983). Vitamin D in postmenopausal women. In Duursma, S. A. and vd Sluys Veer, J. (eds) *Vitamine D*, pp. 43–55. (Utrecht: Wetenschappelijke uitgeverij Bunge)
13. Stevenson, J. C., Abeyasekera, G., Hillyard, C. J., Phang, K. G., MacIntyre, I., Campbell, S., Lane, G., Townsend, P. T., Young, O. and Whitehead, M. I. (1983). The regulation of calcium-regulating hormones by exogenous sex steroids in early postmenopause. *Eur. J. Clin. Invest.*, **13**, 481
14. Riggs, B. L., Jowsey, J., Goldsmith, R. S., Kelly, P. J., Hoffman, D. L. and Arnaud, C. D. (1972). Short- and long-term effects of estrogen and synthetic anabolic hormone in postmenopausal osteoporosis. *J. Clin. Invest.*, **51**, 1659
15. Stevenson, J. C., Abeyasekera, G., Hillyard, C. J., Phang, K. G., MacIntyre, I., Campbell, S., Townsend, P. T., Young, O. and Whitehead, M. I. (1981). Calcitonin and the calcium-regulating hormones in postmenopausal women: effect of oestrogens. *Lancet*, **1**, 693
16. Riggs, B. L., Jowsey, J., Kelly, P. J. and Arnaud, C. D. (1976). Role of hormonal factors in the pathogenesis of postmenopausal osteoporosis. *Isr. J. Med. Sci.*, **12**, 615
17. Gallagher, J. C., Riggs, B. L. and Deluca, H. F. (1980). Effect of estrogen on calcium absorption and serum vitamin D metabolites in postmenopausal osteoporosis. *J. Clin. Endocrinol. Metab.*, **51**, 1359
18. Gallagher, J. C., Riggs, B. L., Eisman, J., Hamstra, A., Arnaud, S. B. and Deluca, H. F. (1979). Intestinal calcium absorption and serum vitamin D metabolites in normal subjects and osteoporotic patients. *J. Clin. Invest.*, **64**, 729
19. Christiansen, C. (1982). Osteoporosis and vitamin D metabolites. A status report. In Norman, A. W., Schaefer, K., Herath, D. V. and Grigoleit, H. G. (eds) *Vitamin D. Chemical, Biochemical and Clinical Endocrinology of Calcium Metabolism*, pp. 915–920. (Berlin: Walter de Gruyter)
20. Slovik, D. M., Adams, J. S., Neer, R. M., Holick, M. F. and Potts, J. T. (1981). Deficient production of 1,25-dihydroxyvitamin D in elderly osteoporotic patients. *N. Engl. J. Med.*, **305**, 372
21. Riggs, B. L., Hamstra, A. and Deluca, H. F. (1981). Assessment of 25-hydroxyvitamin D 1α-hydroxylase reserve in postmenopausal osteoporosis by administration of parathyroid extract. *J. Clin. Endocrinol. Metab.*, **53**, 833
22. Nutik, G. and Cruess, R. L. (1974). Estrogen receptors in bone. An evaluation of the uptake of estrogen into bone cells. *Proc. Soc. Exp. Biol. Med.*, **146**, 265
23. Chen, T. L. and Feldman, D. (1978). Distinction between alpha-fetoprotein and intracellular estrogen receptors: evidence against the presence of estradiol receptors in rat bone. *Endocrinology*, **102**, 236
24. Stevenson, J. C., Hillyard, C. J., MacIntyre, I., Cooper, H. and Whitehead, M. (1979). A physiological role for calcitonin: protection of the maternal skeleton. *Lancet*, **2**, 769
25. Hillyard, C. J., Stevenson, J. C. and MacIntyre, I. (1978). Relative deficiency of plasma-calcitonin in normal women. *Lancet*, **1**, 961
26. Morimoto, S., Tsuji, M., Okada, Y., Onishi, T. and Kumahara, Y. (1980). The effect of oestrogens on human calcitonin secretion after calcium infusion in elderly female subjects. *Clin. Endocrinol.*, **13**, 135
27. Samaan, N. A., Anderson, G. D. and Adam-Mayne, M. E. (1975). Immuno-

reactive calcitonin in the mother, neonate, child and adult. *Am. J. Obstet. Gynecol.*, **121**, 622

28. Deftos, L. J., Weisman, M. H., Williams, G. W., Karpf, D. B., Frumar, A. M., Davidson, B. J., Parthemore, J. G. and Judd, H. L. (1980). Influence of age and sex on plasma calcitonin in human beings. *N. Engl. J. Med.*, **302**, 1351
29. Stevenson, J. C., MacIntyre, I. and Whitehead, M. I. (1982). Impaired calcitonin secretion after premature menopause. *Calcif. Tiss. Int.*, **34** (Suppl. 1), S21
30. Taggart, H. McA., Chesnut, C. H., Ivey, J. L., Baylink, D. J., Sisom, K., Huber, M. B. and Roos, B. A. (1982). Deficient calcitonin response to calcium stimulation in postmenopausal osteoporosis? *Lancet*, **1**, 475
31. Silva, O. L., Wisneski, L. A., Cyrus, J., Snider, R. H., Moore, C. F. and Becker, K. L. (1978). Calcitonin in thyroidectomized patients. *Am. J. Med. Sci.*, **275**, 159
32. McDermott, M. T., Kidd, G. S., Blue, P., Ghaed, V. and Hofeldt, F. D. (1983). Reduced bone mineral content in totally thyroidectomized patients: possible effect of calcitonin deficiency. *J. Clin. Endocrinol. Metab.*, **56**, 936
33. Stevenson, J. C., White, M. C., Joplin, G. F. and MacIntyre, I. (1982). Osteoporosis and calcitonin deficiency. *Br. Med. J.*, **285**, 1010
34. Foresta, C., Busnardo, B., Ruzza, G., Zanatta, G. and Mioni, R. (1983). Lower calcitonin levels in young hypogonadic men with osteoporosis. *Horm. Metab. Res.*, **15**, 206
35. Wallach, S., Cohn, S. H., Ellis, K. J., Kohberger, R., Aloia, J. F. and Zanzi, I. (1977). Effect of salmon calcitonin on skeletal mass in osteoporosis. *Curr. Ther. Res. Clin. Exp.*, **22**, 556
36. Rasmussen, H., Bordier, P., Marie, P., Auquier, L., Eisinger, J. B., Kuntz, D., Caulin, F., Argemi, B., Gueris, J. and Julien, A. (1980). Effect of combined therapy with phosphate and calcitonin on bone volume in osteoporosis. *Metab. Bone Dis. Relat. Res.*, **2**, 107
37. Chesnut, C. H., Baylink, D. J., Roos, B. A., Gruber, H. E., Ivey, J. L., Matthews, M., Nelp, W. B. and Sisom, K. (1981). Calcitonin and postmenopausal osteoporosis. In Pecile, A. (ed.) *Calcitonin 1980. Chemistry, Physiology, Pharmacology and Clinical Aspects*, pp. 247–255. (Amsterdam: Excerpta Medica)

Chapter 20

Risks of endometrial and mammary cancer morbidity and mortality in long-term oestrogen treatment

C. Lauritzen and F. Meier

INTRODUCTION

The possible syncarcinogenic activity of oestrogens has been the subject of worldwide discussion again since 1975 when the results of two case–control studies, in which were observed an increased incidence of endometrial cancer in women who had used oestrogens, were published[1,2]. Later studies confirmed these findings although mostly lower and more realistic risk ratios were given[3–6]. The limits and pitfalls of retrospective studies were discussed by Horwitz and Feinstein[7].

In European studies[8–12] an increase in the risk of endometrial cancer could not be shown in studies dealing with long-term oestrogen users. However, indications, doses, preparations, mode of administration and additional use of progestogens were completely different in the USA and Europe. In Europe the doses usually given were lower and treatment was always cyclical, never continuous. Whenever possible progestogen was added to the oestrogen in the second phase of the treatment cycle. Oestriol was a frequently used oestrogen.

With regard to breast cancer, a correlation between the use of oestrogens and an increased relative risk of the development of this tumour has not been shown so far in most studies[11,13-15]. In only one study was a small increase found with higher doses, and this after treatment for more than 10 years[16]. In two other studies, in which a moderate increase of the relative risk was noted, inappropriate control groups were used[17,18].

Against this background, and with the aim of reviewing our own therapeutic procedures in oestrogen substition over the last 14 years, we performed a retrospective study of all patients in our practice who had received, between 1968 and the present, oestrogens for climacteric complaints for longer than one year.

MATERIAL AND METHODS

We studied a total of 458 patients who had received oestrogens in my own and my colleague's (Dr. Knörr) private practice. All had been treated according to the same principles of hormone therapy. The mean duration of treatment was 5.3 years (2 – 15 years) or 2786 woman years. These oestrogen-treated patients were compared with an equal number of women who had never received oestrogens and who presented themselves for routine gynaecological check-ups only. In neither group were there any patients who had had a hysterectomy. All were postmenopausal, most of them after a natural menopause. In both groups there was about the same low percentage (4%) of patients who had had an oophorectomy. They were of comparable age and body weight, parity and social status and were of the same nationality and race. The duration of supervision was also approximately the same, i.e. 5.3 (1 – 15) years of medication in the treated patients and 4.9 years in the control cases. All patients were personally interviewed in order not to miss any relevant disease in the medical history (Table 1). Patients with severe contraindications for oestrogens and with serious diseases in their personal history were not allotted to the control group.

Of the patients taking oestrogens, 28% had taken conjugated oestrogens orally and cyclically, 26% had taken oestrogen + a progestogen orally (for 10 days each cycle), 29% received oestriol or oestriol succinate or polyoestriol phosphate-depot-injections, and 17% had injections of oestradiol valerate + dehydroepiandrosterone enantate or testosterone enantate (Table 2). The doses used were for conjugated oestrogens 0.625 mg per day in 31% of patients and 1.25 mg per day in 69%. Higher doses were not used. When treatment with

Table 1 Duration of oestrogen therapy in 458 patients. (Mean treatment: 5.3 (2–15 years) representing 2786 woman-years). Retrospective study carried out by the University of Ulm Department of Obstetrics and Gynecology, 1968–1981

Duration (year)	*Number of takers*	*Woman-years*
2	20	33
3	53	139
4	96	348
5	69	303
6	38	224
7	31	214
8	25	208
9	27	253
10	21	229
> 10	78	835
	n = 458	2786

Table 2 Types of oestrogens used in 458 patients for treatment of climacteric complaints. (Mean age: 55 years, women-years: 2786). Study carried out by the University of Ulm Department of Obstetrics and Gynecology, 1968–1981

Preparations used	*Number of patients*	*%*
Oral:		
Conjugated oestrogens*	127	28
Conjugated oestrogen + progestogen	47 }	26
Oestradiol valerate + progestogen	75 }	
Oestriol, oestriol succinate	118 }	
Injection:	}	29
Oestriol polyphosphate	16 }	
Oestradiol + dehydroepiandrosterone	52	12
Oestradiol + testosterone-oenanthate	23	5
	n = 458	100

*Cyclical only

oestriol was given, 2 mg daily was prescribed in 38% of cases, 4 mg in 46%, and 6 mg in 16% as a maintainance dose. The relative risk was calculated by the method of Mantel and Haenszel[19].

RESULTS

Thromboembolism

There was no significant difference between oestrogen-treated patients and the control cases (Table 3) with regard to the incidence of thrombophlebitis, deep venous thrombosis and pulmonary embolism.

Table 3 Vascular diseases in 458 long-term oestrogen treated patients (2786 women-years) as compared with matched controls. Study carried out by the University of Ulm Department of Obstetrics and Gynecology, 1968–1981

	With oestrogen		*Without oestrogen*		*Significance*
	n	%	*n*	%	
Thrombophlebitis	12	2.6	6	1.7	n.s.*
Pulmonary embolism	3	0.7	4	1.1	n.s.
Myocardial infarction	6	1.3	11	3.1	$p < 0.01$
Cerebrovascular accident	6	1.3	9	2.5	n.s.

* n.s. = not significant

Myocardial infarction

Oestrogen-treated patients had a lower incidence of myocardial infarction than non-treated control patients. The difference was significant ($p < 0.01$).

Cerebrovascular accidents

The number of strokes or other cerebrovascular accidents was not significantly different in the two groups (Table 3).

Other internal diseases

There was no increase in gall-bladder disease, liver disease or pancreatitis (Table 4) in the oestrogen-takers compared to the controls.

Endometrial cancer

The relative risk was computed for the duration of treatment (2–4, 5–10 years and more than 10 years) and separately for each of the preparations used (Table 5). For conjugated oestrogens the total

Table 4 Gall-bladder, liver and pancreas diseases in 458 long-term oestrogen treated women (2786 woman-years) as compared to a non-treated control group. Study carried out by the University of Ulm Department of Obstetrics and Gynecology, 1968–1981

	With oestrogen		*Without oestrogen*		*Significance*
	n	%	*n*	%	
Gall-bladder diseases	41	9.2	35	9.2	n.s.*
Liver dysfunction	9	1.3	2	2.2	n.s.
Pancreatitis	1	0.2	8	0.6	n.s.

* n.s. = not significant

Table 5 Relative risk for endometrial cancer in 458 long-term oestrogen treated patients (2786 women-years). Study carried out by the University of Ulm Department of Obstetrics and Gynecology, 1968 – 1981

Preparations	*Total*	*Duration of treatment*			*Woman-years*
		2 – 4	5 – 10	≤ 10	(2786)
Conjugated oestrogens	0.78	0.60	0.81	0.93	693
Oestradiol valerate	0.73	0.71	0.79	0.86	338
Oestriol and its succinate	0.34	0.27	0.39	0.35	578
Oestrogen + progestogen	0.21	0.20	0.24	0.22	859
Oestradiol + androgen	0.55	0.56	0.47	0.60	318

Note: the difference between unopposed conjugated oestrogens or unopposed oestradiol valerate on the one hand and oestriol or oestrogen + progestogen on the other is significant ($p < 0.01$)

relative risk was 0.78. This increased from 0.60 at 1 – 3 years to 0.93 after more than 10 years. For oestradiol valerate the total risk was 0.73. There was an increase from 0.71 after 1 – 3 years to 0.86 at more than 10 years. The overall risk for oestriol was as low as 0.34. For this oestrogen there was no significant increase of the risk in relation to the duration of the treatment. Oestradiol valerate + progestogen showed a low risk of 0.21 with no increase observed with the progress of time. Also for the oestrogen – androgen preparations the risk was lower than for oestrogens alone, namely 0.55. Again, with the passing of time no significant increase was observed at any stage.

Breast cancer

The incidence of breast cancer was lower in patients on oestrogens than in women not taking hormones (Table 6). Patients who had received

Table 6 Incidence and relative risk of mammary cancer in 458 patients under long-term oestrogen substitution (2786 woman-years) as compared to untreated controls (matched pairs). University of Ulm Department of Obstetrics and Gynecology, 1983

Medication groups	*Incidence 100 000^{-1}* year^{-1}		
Oestrogens	123		
Oestrogen + progestogen	109		
No hormones	154		
	Relative risk (± 95% reliability)		
Duration of medication (years)	2 – 4	5 – 10	> 10
Oestrogens	1.13	0.92	1.23
	(0.5 – 1.6)	(0.4 – 1.2)	(0.3 – 3.4)
Oestrogen + progestogen	0.88	0.98	1.10
	(0.4 – 1.3)	(0.5 – 1.2)	(0.4 – 2.6)
Significance	no	no	no

oestrogen + progestogen had an even lower incidence, which was significant on the 0.05 level compared to 'oestrogens only' and 'no hormones'.

The relative risk was about 1.1 in oestrogen users and showed a small but insignificant increase with time. The addition of a progestogen lowered the risk significantly ($p < 0.05$) in the first 5 year period. In later years the differences were not so pronounced. However, after more than ten years, the risks were lower in oestrogen + progestogen users than in oestrogen-only users.

Mortality

During oestrogen medication there were 24 deaths in 2786 woman-years. In the untreated control group the number of deaths was greater, namely 35 in 2770 woman-years. The difference is statistically significant on the 95% level. Vascular deaths occurred more often in the control group than in oestrogen-takers. Similarly deaths from endometrial and breast cancer were more frequent in non-treated controls than in oestrogen-takers, although the differences were small. There were no significant differences between the two groups with regard to all other cancers (Table 7).

Table 7 Mortality in 458 patients under long-term oestrogen substitution (2786 woman-years) as compared to untreated matched control groups (2770 woman-years). University of Ulm Department of Obstetrics and Gynecology, 1983

		2786 woman-years	*2770 woman-years*
		With oestrogens	*Without oestrogens*
Patients who died during the period of observation		n = 24	n = 35
Diseases	Coronary thrombosis	2	4
	Thromboembolism	1	3
	Cerebrovascular accident	1	3
	Other internal diseases	6	9
	After hip surgery	0	1
Cancer cases	Breast cancer	4	5
	Endometrial cancer	2	3
	Cervical cancer	0	1
	Ovarian cancer	0	1
	Other cancers*	4	3
	Accidents	4	2

*Intestinal, pancreas, liver, gall-bladder

Progestogen addition to the oestrogen

The addition of a progestogen to the oestrogens may reduce the risk of hyperplasia of the oestrogen target organs and even of cancer. However, the question arises whether the addition of the progestogen might not induce other risks for the patient, especially the risk of vascular disease. We have therefore studied separately the 122 cases of oestrogen + progestogen users (Table 8). The mean duration of treatment in these cases was 4.2 years or 521 woman-years in total. A comparison with the 336 oestrogen-only cases (1642 woman-years) showed no significant increase in vascular symptoms or disease which might be attributed to the addition of the progestogen. However, the number of cases and of woman-years may be too small to allow definitive conclusions.

DISCUSSION

We believe that the two study groups of hormone users and the control group were comparable as the population from which both were drawn was homogenous. The matching was possible with very satisfying results; to our knowledge the groups differed only in respect of the taking or not taking of oestrogens and combinations of oestrogens with other hormones.

We would not wish to overemphasize the value of these data, but they would seem to suggest that *there is no indication that long-term oestrogen treatment will increase the risk of morbidity of vascular disease or of endometrial*

Table 8 Side-effects of long-term oestrogen – progestogen medication in 122 patients compared with 336 patients taking unopposed oestrogens. University of Ulm Department of Obstetrics and Gynecology, 1968 – 1981

	Oestrogen-treated women: $n = 458$	
Diseases	*With additional progestogen*: $n = 122$ (%)	*Without progestogen*: $n = 336$ (%)
Cardiovascular	0	3.2
Cerebrovascular	0	1.7
Hypertension	4.8	9.8
Thrombophlebitis	2.4	3.2
Phlebothrombosis	11.3	25.3
Pulmonary embolism	0.8	0.5

or mammary carcinoma. Our results correspond with those of other European studies[9-12]. Also our own earlier investigations[8] showed no increase of risk for endometrial cancer in oestrogen users when we repeated the calculating procedure of Smith *et al.*[1] taking women with other gynaecological cancers as the control group and when we repeated the procedure of Dunn and Bradbury[20] taking postmenopausal bleeding patients as a sample which was then stratified according to histological diagnosis and oestrogen use. Thus, with very different methods we came to the same conclusion on the basis of data obtained from our European patients.

The observed, decreased risk and perhaps even prophylactic effect of the addition of a progestogen to oestrogen on the incidence of endometrial and perhaps mammary carcinoma corresponds with the results of Gambrell[21] and those of Nachtigall[22]. We observed the same in women taking oestriol; this has so far not been observed by others but findings concerning mortality are about equal to those of Nachtigall[22], Burch *et al.*[23] and Cowan and Bush[24] who found lowered mortality in oestrogen users compared to controls. This is in agreement with the low risk of oestrogen users for vascular complications as shown by several groups of investigators[13,25,26].

Our explanation of the differences reported in the US and the European studies is as follows: the doses of oestrogen given in the USA were mostly higher than those administered in Europe, where in general 0.625 mg up to 1.25 mg of conjugated oestrogen or 1–2 mg oestradiol valerate were prescribed and higher doses were avoided. In the USA medication was mostly continuous and in Europe cyclical. The addition of a progestogen was unusual in the USA and quite accepted in Europe. Oestriol, which in the usual once-a-day dose does not cause proliferation of the endometrium, is often prescribed in Europe, seldom or never in the USA. Thorough checking for indications and contraindications was apparently more usual in the old world.

We consider unnecessarily high dosage, administration of oestrogens only, uninterrupted administration and omitting to combine oestrogen therapy with a progestogen, as serious mistakes. We think that the treatment cycle should be as similar to the normal cycle as possible. Therefore the results of the American studies may show what could happen under the worst conditions when the basic rules of female sexual hormone substitution have been so badly neglected for such a long time.

SUMMARY

We submit a retrospective study of 458 patients on long-term oestrogen treatment and an identical number of matched controls. Our results seem to indicate that there is no increase of cardiovascular complications in oestrogen users as compared to appropriate controls. Also the risk for endometrial and mammary carcinoma seems not to increase when the basic rules of treatment are properly observed. There is a tendency towards a slight increase of risk of cancer of the endometrium and the breast with the duration of medication. However, this is not so where oestriol, oestrogen–progestogen or oestrogen–androgen combinations are administered. The total risk of both cancers is lower for oestrogen–progestogen and for oestriol than for conjugated oestrogens or oestradiol valerate alone. Our relative risk ratios do not usually rise above one.

Thus, according to our results, the prescribing doctor who treats his patients with oestrogens for a long time need not fear that he may cause harm to the patients or that possible risks may not justify the expected benefits, provided he proceeds according to the established rules of hormone medication.

References

1. Smith, D. C., Prentice, R., Thompson, D. J. and Herrmann, W. L. (1975). Association of exogenous estrogen and endometrial cancer. *N. Engl. J. Med.*, **293**, 1164
2. Ziel, H. K. and Finkle, W. D. (1976). Association of estrone with the development of endometrial carcinoma. *Am. J. Obstet. Gynecol.*, **124**, 735
3. Antunes, C. M. F., Stolley, P. D., Rosenshein, N. B., Davies, J. L., Tonascia, J. A., Brown, C., Burnett, L., Rutledge, A., Pokempner, M. and Garcia, R. (1979). Endometrial cancer and estrogen use. *N. Engl. J. Med.*, **300**, 9
4. Gray, L. H., Christopherson, W. M. and Hoover, R. N. (1977). Estrogens and endometrial cancer. *Obstet. Gynecol.*, **49**, 385
5. Jick, H., Watkins, R. N., Hunter, J. R., Dinan, B. J., Madsen, S., Rothman, K. J. and Walker, A. M. (1979). Replacement estrogens and endometrial cancer. *N. Engl. J. Med.*, **300**, 218
6. McDonald, T. W., Annegers, J. F., O'Fallon, W. M., Dockerty, M. B., Malkasian, G. D. and Kurland, L. T. (1977). Exogenous estrogen and endometrial carcinoma: Case-control and incidence study. *Am. J. Obstet. Gynecol.*, **127**, 572
7. Horwitz, R. I. and Feinstein, A. R. (1980). The clinical epidemiology of breast and uterine cancer. In Pasetto, N., Paoletti, B. and Ambrus, J. L. (eds) *The Menopause and Postmenopause*, pp. 195–205. (Lancaster: MTP Press)
8. Lauritzen, C., Wolf, A. S. and Strabl, M. (1978). A retrospective study concerning postmenopausal estrogen therapy and endometrial cancer. In Brush, M. G.,

King, R. J. B. and Taylor, R. W. (eds) *Endometrial Cancer*, pp. 39–46. (London: Baillière Tyndall)

9. Rauramo, L. (1978). Oestrogen replacement therapy and endometrial carcinoma. In Brush, M. G., King, R. J. B. and Taylor, R. W. (eds) *Endometrial Cancer*, pp. 81–87. (London: Baillière Tyndall)
10. Pfleiderer, A. and Paessler, U. (1978). Risk factors for endometrial cancer. In Brush, M. G., King, R. J. B. and Taylor, R. W. (eds) *Endometrial Cancer*, pp. 10–16. (London: Baillière Tyndall)
11. Völker, W. (1980). Estrogen and estrogen–progestagen compounds. Is there a risk for the development of endometrial and breast cancer in the perimenopausal woman? In Pasetto, N., Paoletti, R. and Ambrus, J. L. (eds) *The Menopause and Postmenopause*, pp. 273–288. (Lancaster: MTP Press)
12. Uyttenbroeck, F. and Wauters, H. (1977). L'influence des contraceptifs oraux, des progestagènes et des oestrogènes dans la genèse des lésions précancéreuses et cancéreuses de l'appareil génital et du sein. *Verhandeling Koninglijke Vlaamse Akademie voor Geneeskunde van België*, **39**, 159
13. Boston Collaborative Drug Surveillance Program (1974). Surgically confirmed gallbladder disease, venous thromboembolism and breast tumors in relation to postmenopausal estrogen therapy. *N. Engl. J. Med.*, **290**, 15
14. Sartwell, P. E., Arthes, F. G. and Tonascia, J. A. (1977). Exogenous hormones, reproductive history and breast cancer. *J. Natl. Cancer Inst.*, **59**, 1589
15. Bland, K. J., Buchanan, J. B., Weissberg, B. F. and Gray, L. A. (1980). Exogenous estrogen therapy in the menopause: Influence on mammary cancer risk. In Pasetto, N., Paoletti, R. and Ambrus, J. L. (eds) *The Menopause and Postmenopause*, pp. 245–254. (Lancaster: MTP Press)
16. Hoover, R., Gray, L. A., Cole, P. and MacMahon, B. (1976). Menopausal estrogens and breast cancer. *N. Engl. J. Med.*, **295**, 401
17. Casagrande, J., Gerkins, J., Henderson, B. E., Mack, T. and Pike, M. C. (1976). Exogenous estrogens and breast cancer in women with natural menopause. *J. Natl. Cancer Inst.*, **56**, 839
18. Mack, T. M., Pike, M. C., Henderson, B. E., Pfeffer, R. I., Gerkins, V. R., Arthur, M. and Brown, S. E. (1976). Estrogens and endometrial cancer in a retirement community. *N. Engl. J. Med.*, **294**, 1262
19. Mantel, N. and Haenszel, W. (1959). Statistical aspects of the analysis of data from retrospective studies of disease. *J. Natl. Cancer Inst.*, **22**, 719
20. Dunn, L. J. and Bradbury, J. T. (1967). Endocrine factors in endometrial cancer. *Am. J. Obstet. Gynecol.*, **97**, 465
21. Gambrell, R. D., Jr. (1980). Rate of estrogens and progestagens in the etiology of breast and endometrial neoplasia. In Pasetto, N., Paoletti, R. and Ambrus, J.L. (eds) *The Menopause and Postmenopause*, pp. 298–304. (Lancaster: MTP Press)
22. Nachtigall, L. E. (1977). *The Nachtigall Report*. (New York: Putman)
23. Burch, J. C., Byrd, B. F. and Vaughn, W. K. (1978). The effects of long-term estrogen administration to women following hysterectomy. In van Keep, P. A. and Lauritzen, C. (eds) *Estrogens in the Postmenopause*, pp. 208–214. (Basel: Karger)
24. Cowan, L. and Bush, T. (1982). Paper presented at the 22nd Conf. Cardiovascul. Epidemiol., Am. Heart Assoc., San Antonio, Texas
25. Hammond, C. B., Jelovsek, F. R., Lee, K. L., Creasman, W. T. and Parker, R. T. (1979). Effects of long-term estrogen replacement therapy. I. Metabolic effects. *Am. J. Obstet. Gynecol.*, **133**, 525
26. Ross, R. K., Paganini-Hill, A., Mack, T. M., Arthur, M. and Henderson, B. M. (1981). Menopausal estrogen therapy and protection from death from ischaemic heart disease. *Lancet*, **1**, 858

Chapter 21

Cardiovascular impact of therapy and risks

M.-A. Limouzin-Lamothe

The consistently lower incidence of cardiovascular disease and atherosclerotic manifestations in premenopausal women compared to that of age-matched men has been recognized for a long time and generates increasing interest. Globally, the male–female ratio has been reported to range from 6 to 2 in developed countries[1,2]. However, this sex difference in Coronary Heart Disease (CHD) incidence declines after the age of 50 and almost disappears in the higher age group, as a consequence of increased frequency of accidents in women after the menopause. The hypothesis that oestrogen secretion might play a major part in this sex-related protection has been extensively discussed.

Several observations[3–5] and two longitudinal population studies[1,6] have demonstrated an association between premature menopause and increased incidence of CHD (Figure 1). There is also an increased frequency of stroke in women who have undergone surgical castration[7]. This established sex difference in CHD incidence, together with sex differences in general risk factors for vascular disease (i.e. abnormal lipoprotein spectrum, high blood pressure, decreased glucose tolerance), and the fact that in animal models oestrogens appear capable of preventing atherogenesis[8] provided the rationale for trying oestrogens to avoid the recurrence of atherosclerotic manifestations. The results were frustrating as an increased recurrence of cardiovascular accidents was observed[9,10].

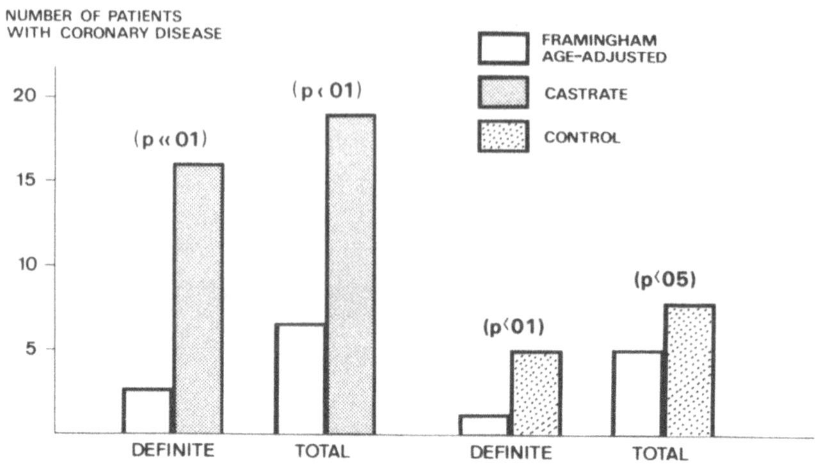

Figure 1 Coronary disease in castrate and non-castrate (control) women vs expected prevalence. (Adapted from Robinson *et al.*[5])

Extensive case–control studies and several large prospective studies[11,12] have clearly demonstrated that the use of oral contraceptives is a risk factor for morbidity and mortality from CHD and thromboembolism. On the other hand information concerning the influence of postmenopausal exogenous hormonal replacement therapy remains scanty and some of the results obtained should be regarded as inconclusive.

Rosenberg *et al.*[13] found a 0.39 crude risk ratio for current oestrogen use in women of over 50. These data would suggest that women under oestrogen influence have a lower cardiovascular morbidity and mortality. However, most of the apparently protective effect disappeared after adjusting for other risk factors. While Ross *et al.*[14] suggest that oestrogen replacement therapy in postmenopausal women may protect against death from ischaemic heart disease, his interpretation does not take into account the fact that hypertension appears as the main risk factor. Moreover, he comes to the strange conclusion that antihypertensive treatment is more important as a risk factor than high blood pressure and that antihyperglycaemic treatment leads to a higher risk than diabetes. Although these are retrospective studies, the group of patients who have undergone oestrogen replacement therapy may very well not be representative of the general population. Since practitioners have been warned against hazardous

Table 1 Risk factors of cardiovascular mortality in women of 50–59 years of age

	Myocardial infarction	*Controls*
Diabetes	7%	2%
Hypertension	27%	17%
Hyperlipidaemia	4%	2%
Smoking habit	22%	20%

Adapted from Adam *et al.*[15]

effects of oral contraceptives in women over the age of 40, especially in those with risk factors such as high blood pressure or impaired lipid metabolism, it can be assumed that hormonal replacement therapy has been avoided in women already under treatment for hypertension (Table 1).

Nachtigall's report of her work[16] supports this hypothesis. While a lower incidence of myocardial infarction over a 10 year period was found in the oestrogen-treated group (1.2% vs 3.7%), she stated that women showing signs of hypertension prior to treatment were excluded from the trial.

In women over the age of 70, current or previous oestrogen use leads globally to a 1.74% increment of cerebrovascular accidents (Table 2) Pfeffer *et al.* showed that hypertension and diabetes are the main risk factors which increase even more with oestrogen use, especially in the younger age group[17] (Table 3).

Table 2 Oestrogens and risk of cerebrovascular disease in women of 70–79 years of age

	Cerebrovascular disease	*Control*	*Total*
With oestrogens	40	154	194
Without oestrogens	63	422	485
Total	103	576	679
			Relative risk: 1.74

Adapted from Pfeffer, R.I. *et al.* (1976). *Am. J. Epidemiol.*, **103**

Table 3 Evaluation of the cerebrovascular risk in postmenopausal women

Age	*Hypertension*	*Oestrogenic treatment*	*Relative risk*
58–69	–	–	1.00
	–	+	0.89
	+	–	1.92
	+	+	2.15
70–79	–	–	1.00
	–	+	1.47
	+	–	3.91
	+	+	4.06

Adapted from Pfeffer *et al.*[17]

WHAT METABOLIC CHANGES OCCUR AT THE MENOPAUSE? ARE THEY LIKELY TO MODIFY THE RISK FOR CARDIOVASCULAR AND ISCHAEMIC HEART DISEASE?

The risk factors for CHD and thromboembolic accidents are well known. They include total cholesterol, specific distribution of cholesterol within the lipoprotein classes characterized by high LDL- and low HDL-cholesterol levels[18], higher than normal blood pressure and diabetes. Abnormal clotting factors and fibrinolytic activity are also involved in thromboembolic accidents. After the age of 50, LDL-cholesterol levels do not appear to be the most determinant factor[19] while a major risk of myocardial infarction is related to an increased proportion of cholesterol within the VLDL fraction as well as higher VLDL triglycerides[20]; arterial diseases relate also to low HDL levels[21]. A rise in blood pressure carries a risk which increases with age.

Suppression of the ovarian function is followed within a few months by profound changes in the lipoprotein pattern: triglycerides show a significant increase[22] while there is a redistribution of the cholesterol within the lipid fractions, characterized by a tendency towards a drop in the HDL/LDL ratio even though there are but slight changes in HDL levels.

Though there is no specific proof that oestrogen deprivation has a direct influence on blood pressure or on the renin–aldosterone system, it has been noted that arterial blood pressure usually rises in women after the age of 40 while it remains stable in age-matched men. In younger age groups males have higher blood pressure than females. While hypertension is more frequent in men than in women until the age of 45, later on, due to an increase of frequency of hypertension in women, the sex ratio is around 1. A considerable increase in the incidence of hypertension is observed in women within the first years following the menopause.

Finally, it has been shown that glucose tolerance decreases with age. An abnormal response to the gluco-tolerance test increases spontaneously after the age of 50. Deterioration of this response, however, could be merely a consequence of age; Silverstone considers it as secondary to a progressive diminution of active body mass. If hormonal changes were not involved, the impairment of glucose tolerance would probably be similar in age-matched groups of both sexes, or even less pronounced in women who spontaneously have a higher insulin secretion than men. Conversely, diabetes appears to be more frequent in women[23] within five years after the menopause, when the percentage of diabetes in women increases dramatically from 4.5% to 11%[24].

Work on animal models supports the hypothesis that oestrogen deprivation plays a major role in glucose tolerance deterioration. In castrated female rats blood glucose levels increase 40%, while insulin secretion decreases and histology shows a diminution of pancreatic β cells[25]. Natural oestrogens have a direct effect on the pancreatic islets, increasing both the number of cells and their ability to secrete insulin.

Thus oestrogen deprivation carries the risk of cardiovascular accidents through several mechanisms. As a consequence, the detrimental or beneficial effects of oestrogen and progestogen treatment on the incidence of cerebral vascular accidents or on myocardial infarction should be taken into account before any decision is made on which treatment should be chosen.

Regarding the therapy, there are two theoretical possibilities. The first is that those women free from any metabolic risk would be the only ones to benefit from the advantages of hormonal therapy. Bearing in mind the percentage of hypertension, hyperlipaemia and the frequency of diabetic or prediabetic status in this age group, then almost 60% of women would be excluded from treatment. Moreover, strict, time-consuming and expensive supervision throughout treatment would be necessary to monitor the metabolic parameters. Only very few women would then qualify for hormonal replacement therapy.

The alternative possibility is that research should be aimed towards therapeutic regimens which, even over long periods of time, would not provoke any undesirable metabolic manifestations. The need for thorough evaluation of the metabolic effects of sex steroids is now obvious. There has been a tendency to focus interest on oestrogens, but since it is now widely accepted that replacement therapy should combine both steroids, more studies should be directed towards the effects of progestogens and of the various oestrogen–progestogen combinations.

First we shall consider the effects of these hormones on the risk factors for atherosclerosis: how do they tend to raise blood pressure and disturb the lipid profile; then we shall examine the changes oestrogen and progestins may induce in the clotting–fibrinolysis balance which play a role in cerebral–vascular accidents.

HOW DO OESTROGENS AND PROGESTOGENS INFLUENCE BLOOD PRESSURE?

Oral contraceptive use in young women is known to raise blood pressure[26]. However, in the younger age group definite hypertension is rare and it can seldom be claimed that hypertension in a particular user was induced by the oestrogen–progestogen combination[27] since there would also be personal or family risk factors to be taken into account. In such circumstances oral contraceptives may be considered as having revealed a problem rather than having caused it. Similarly a few studies have come to the conclusion that the administration of oestrogens to postmenopausal women did not induce hypertension despite the fact that an increase in diastolic blood pressure was observed[28,29], particularly with conjugated oestrogens rather than with oestradiol. These studies can be criticized in the same way as those mentioned earlier.

Even though the use of oral contraceptives is not very likely to induce hypertension in younger women, one should keep it in mind that with increasing age the risk of hypertension also increases, to the extent that over 40% of 'normal' postmenopausal women are spontaneously hypertensive.

If a study is aimed at choosing amongst the available treatments and establishing those that are less likely to provoke hypertension, then one should first consider the mechanisms involved in blood pressure regulation and understand the manner in which exogenous sex hormones are likely to interfere with this regulation.

The hypertensive effect of oestrogens is thought to be related to alterations of the renin – angiotensin system. The first step is the induction of increased synthesis of plasma – renin – substrate (PRS) by the liver. This occurs both in normotensive and hypertensive patients. As PRS is the limiting factor for the renin – substrate reaction, a rise in PRS will provoke a rise in plasma – renin – angiotensin (PRA) and consequently a rise in angiotensin II (A II). If the feedback mechanism responds normally, renin secretion will drop in reply to the high circulating levels of A II and a new balance is found. While PRS remains high (as seen during oral contraceptive use)[29] renin excretion will drop and PRA levels will go back to normal. This has been demonstrated both in animals and humans[30,31]. However, the regulation and the balance of this system is often impaired or limited.

As far as the sex steroids are concerned, the less their capacity to increase PRS synthesis by the liver, the less will be their ability to unbalance the system (and eventually to provoke hypertension).

Menard[31] confirms this by showing, in both animal and human studies, that there is a correlation between the other well-known effects of oestrogens on the liver and PRS induction. As for other hepatic proteins, PRS elevation induced by oestrogens is dose-related. Mestranol, known to be more toxic, has a greater effect than ethinyloestradiol, while oestradiol given subcutaneously induces only a slight change[31]. With Enovid (an oral contraceptive), oestradiol benzoate, oestrone and conjugated oestrogens[32–34] PRS-PRA and A II have been found to rise. Geola *et al.*[35], in a six weeks trial with Premarin, found a dose – response curve strictly correlated with TBG changes and confirmed the dose relationship between PRS increase and an abnormal increase in hepatic protein synthesis (Figure 2). Elkik *et al.*[36] studied 18 postmenopausal women who were given either conjugated oestrogens or percutaneous oestradiol at equipotent doses. A considerable increase in angiotensin was found in the conjugated oestrogen users, while no change was observed following the use of percutaneous oestradiol. We have shown earlier[37] a two- to three-fold increase in angiotensin synthesis using *oral* micronized oestradiol while no significant change was observed when equivalent doses of oestradiol were administered percutaneously.

More recently Mashchak described an increase in angiotensinogen plasma levels in women treated with a daily dose of 2 mg of oral

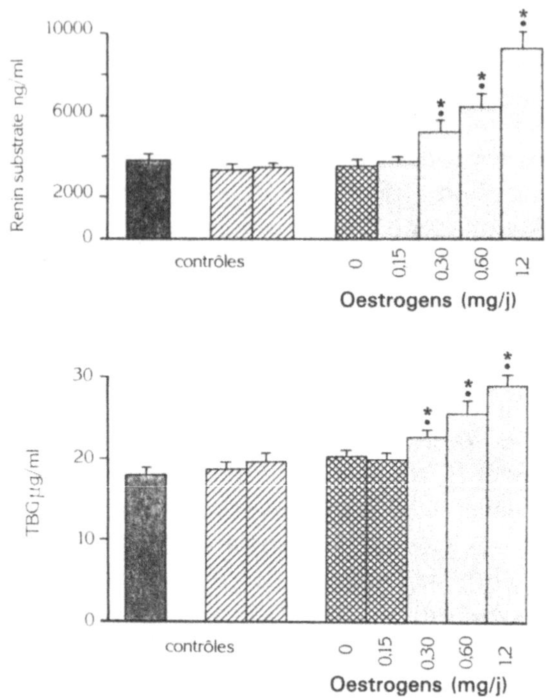

Figure 2 Oral conjugated oestrogens administered per os during 6 weeks. (Adapted from Geola *et al.*[35])

oestradiol[38]. Roy *et al.*[39] comparing several oral contraceptive users with women using vaginal rings loaded with norgestrel and oestradiol found no increase in angiotensin in women using the rings (Table 4).

Other effects of oestrogens in blood pressure control, such as a local vascular response to stress, could be discussed. By focusing on the angiotensin–renin system it can be inferred from these results that oestradiol is less likely to impair blood pressure than synthetic or conjugated oestrogens. Also, the route of administration seems to be of major importance.

Progestogens, particularly the 19-nor-derivatives may have a direct hypertensive effect; a clear relationship has been demonstrated between the dose either of norethisterone or of norgestrel and the incidence of hypertension[21,40].

Oestrogens have a positive effect on the water and sodium balance. In menstruating women, progesterone secretion, through its natriuretic effect[41], antagonizes this effect of oestrogens.

When oestrogens alone are given to postmenopausal women, weight

Table 4

	Daily *dose* (mg)	*Angiotensinogen*	
Percutaneous oestradiol	3	=	Elkik *et al.*[36]
Vaginal oestradiol		=	Roy *et al.*[39]
Micronized oestradiol	2	↗	Mashchak *et al.*[38]
Conjugated oestrogens	0.625	↗	Geola *et al.*[35]
	1.25	↗	Elkik *et al.*[36]
			Mashchak *et al.*[38]
Piperazine oestrone sulphate	2.5	↗	Mashchak *et al.*[38]

gain and bloating is often observed as a result of water retention; this can contribute to the onset of hypertension. Synthetic progestogens derived from progesterone or nortestosterone have no effect on sodium balance[42]. Only norgestrel has been reported to exert a slight natriuretic effect[43].

Conversely, Corvol *et al.*[44] reported recently that micronized progesterone, given orally at the usual therapeutic dosage, is capable of antagonizing the mineralocorticoid effect of 9α-fluorohydrocortisone.

Up to now, there has been no definite proof that progesterone would exert an antihypertensive effect. However, some of its properties favour this hypothesis. Progesterone shares some effects with other compounds known to have an antihypertensive action. It is known to be a calcium antagonist, and it reduces the number of receptors in smooth muscle cells[45]; both the above effects should lead to peripheral vasodilation. Pilot studies have been undertaken in order to examine this possibility.

Because some progestogens may have a provocative effect, care in the choice of the progestogen in postmenopausal replacement therapy might help to prevent any alteration of blood pressure.

SEX STEROIDS AND LIPID CHANGES

Extensive literature reports on the effects of sex steroids upon serum lipids and lipoproteins. Due consideration has not always been given to the fact that oestrogenic and progestogenic components may have different, and sometimes opposite, metabolic effects.

Oestrogens

The most consistent effect of oral oestrogen is an increase in plasma triglyceride concentration. This is reported of ethinyloestradiol[46-50] and of conjugated oestrogens[51-53]. The increase is constant and dose-related[35,51]. With piperazine oestrone sulphate, oestradiol valerate and orally administered micronized oestradiol, results are more conflicting. Though most authors observed increased concentrations of triglycerides[54-56] some did not[57-59].

The first hypothesis was that synthetic 17C-alkylated oestrogens would increase serum triglycerides while non-alkylated (i.e. natural) oestrogens would not. But whether natural oestrogens might or might not increase triglycerides is still much a matter of discussion. Tikkanen observed a non-significant increase in triglycerides in women treated with 2 mg of oestradiol valerate[56]. Fåhraeus obtained similar results using 2 mg oestradiol in a micronized form[57] but triglyceride elevation occurred when the daily dosage was increased to 4 mg. It should be pointed out, however, that in both cases the tendency was towards a rise in triglycerides while in the first report the increase was significant in those patients who had a normal plasma triglyceride level before starting on the therapy. Though Pystynen *et al.*[52] saw no increase from baseline levels in early postmenopausal women receiving 4 mg oestradiol valerate, a significant decrease was observed in control patients.

The elevation in plasma triglyceride corresponds to a rise in VLDL lipoprotein and apo-lipoprotein[60] and is probably mediated through an increased lipoprotein synthesis in the liver.

Routes of administration that bypass the liver show opposite changes; a decrease in triglycerides has been observed with oestradiol given percutaneously[61-63], even at high dosage, and by injection[46], while no change was observed in vaginal ring users[64].

A study comparing oral micronized oestradiol, oestradiol valerate, and percutaneous oestradiol[65] showed a clear difference in the triglyceride content of VLDL between the oral and percutaneous groups (Figure 3). Finally Basdevant[66] noticed in hyperlipidaemic postmenopausal patients treated by percutaneous oestradiol a definite, significant decrease in total triglycerides.

It appears clear that an appropriate oestrogen replacement therapy is capable of preventing the spontaneous rise in triglyceride levels, secondary to oestrogen privation.

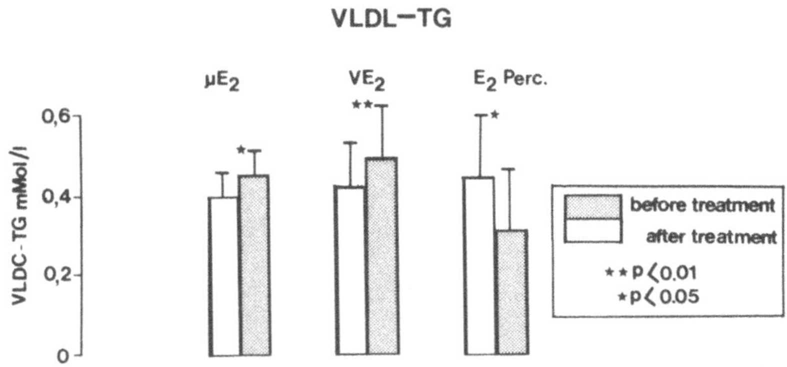

Figure 3 Adapted from Basdevant and Guy-Brand$_{66}$. μE_2 = micronized oestradiol 2 mg/d oral; VE_2 = oestradiol valerate 2 mg/d oral; E_2Perc = oestradiol 3 mg/d percutaneous application

According to most authors, total plasma cholesterol levels are not generally influenced by any of the usual oestrogen treatments[56,57,59]. However, a redistribution of cholesterol among the lipoprotein fraction has been described combining a reduction in LDL-C values with an increase in HDL-C during therapy with oestradiol or micronized oral oestradiol[56,57]. A slight, but non-significant rise was induced by percutaneous oestradiol. As Fåhraeus pointed out, the HDL rise was limited to HDL_2 fraction. This change could be considered beneficial in relation to cardiovascular risk. Such conclusions are, however, debatable since this HDL rise is observed also with ethinyloestradiol in a dose-related manner[59,67], while epidemiological studies have also shown that increasing doses of ethinyloestradiol correlate with a higher risk of cardiovascular accidents. Furthermore, Punnonen and Rauramo using supraphysiological doses of oestradiol observed a rise in HDL 10 days after injection, but two weeks later the HDL levels returned to pretreatment values although the systemic oestrogen effect persisted[68].

If an HDL rise induced by oestrogen should be considered beneficial, even though HDL levels do not decrease significantly with oestrogen deprivation, then it would be logical to infer that the best treatment regarding cardiovascular prevention would be that which induces the greatest rise in HDL. Following this idea, ethinyloestradiol or mestranol, given at the highest possible dosage, should appear the most beneficial. However, all epidemiological studies on cardiovascular risk firmly contradict such evidence. One may therefore question the 'beneficial' effect of any iatrogenic HDL rise.

The increase of HDL and especially HDL_2 may very well be related to changes in its catabolism which involves hepatic lipase and/or to perturbations in HDL formation related to VLDL catabolism by lipoprotein lipase[69].

More work is necessary in this area, including measurement of post-heparin lipolytic activity during oestradiol treatment, in order to clarify the metabolic implications of HDL increase induced by oestrogens.

Progestogens

The most striking effect of progestogens on the lipid pattern is its influence on cholesterol. Simple measurement of total cholesterol does not reflect the wide changes in its repartition within the different lipoprotein classes. The administration of norethisterone leads to an increase in IDL-total lipids and LDL-C while norgestrel administration has been shown to have no effect on LDL-C but decrease LDL-triglycerides. Studies on MPA show either no effect or a small increase in LDL-C levels[59]. Most studies have confirmed the lowering effect of norgestrel on triglycerides which was observed long ago in oestrogen–progestogen combinations. However, Silfverstolpe *et al.*[56] did not confirm any significant decrease. This is surprising since increased catabolic rate of triglycerides, transformation from VLDL to LDL by steroids with androgen-like effect, is a common finding and could account for the rise in LDL.

An inverse correlation is frequently noted between triglycerides and LDL. The capacity of synthetic progestogens to lower HDL-C is linked to their androgenic properties. HDL-C reduction is more pronounced with norethisterone, levo-norgestrel, and ethynodiol diacetate than with 17α-hydroxyprogesterone derivatives. This effect is also dose-dependent. MPA has little influence on HDL when administered orally, while patients receiving depot MPA have lower levels than IUD controls.

When postmenopausal women were randomly given either norgestrel or oral progesterone (3000 mg), a definite reduction of HDL-C in the HDL_2 fraction was observed in the norgestrel group[57]. Interestingly desogestrel does not appear to induce changes similar to those induced by levo-norgestrel.

Non-oral routes of administration for progestogens do not appear to modify their effect on HDL. Reports on vaginal ring users[64] show a decrease in HDL-C when the ring was loaded with either norethisterone, norgestrel or MPA. The marked stimulation of post-heparin lipase activity, together with the simultaneous change in HDL-lipid concentration suggests a role for hepatic lipase in the degradation of this lipoprotein.

HDL-C reduction might have serious clinical implications since the incidence of total arterial disease has been reported to correlate with HDL reduction and to relate to the dosage of norethisterone or norgestrel[70].

From a theoretical point of view, since the HDL reduction is selectively limited to the HDL_2 fraction, progestogens which would provoke HDL reduction cannot be considered as devoid of hazardous side-effects and may increase cardiovascular risk. Thus progestogens with androgen-like activity should not be considered appropriate for hormonal replacement therapy.

HAEMOSTASIS AND COAGULATION

Reports of thromboembolic cases among young women, the absence of atherosclerotic lesions in several well-documented cases of myocardial infarction, and the fact that these accidents may occur within a few weeks following the start of treatment, suggest that early development of atherosclerosis may not explain some of the thromboembolic events observed in female patients undergoing hormonal therapy. Therefore changes in clotting, fibrinolysis and alterations within vessel walls secondary to sex steroids should be considered.

Oestrogens, both synthetic and conjugated, and even oestriol are known to provoke increased coagulation by raising the levels of clotting factors (mainly VII and X). Lately interest has focused on anti-thrombin III (AT III) since repeated thromboembolic episodes have been observed in congenital AT III-deficient people.

Whilst first studies of AT III levels in oral contraceptive users showed conflicting results, technical improvement now allows more reliable measurements and the latest studies carried out in postmenopausal women showed that ethinyloestradiol, even given at low dose, decreases AT III[71]. Oestradiol valerate and oestradiol aministered orally also decrease AT III levels and AT III activity[72,73]. No such change was observed in a comparative study when oestradiol was applied percutaneously[23,66] (Table 5).

Alterations in platelet function can also predispose to thrombosis. During oestrogen treatment changes may occur within the first week. Platelet aggregation induced by ADP is enhanced by mestranol,

Table 5

	Antithrombin III	
	Plasma	*Serum activity*
E_2 Percut. (3 mg)	=	=
E_2 Valerate (2 mg)	↘	↘
E_2 Micron. (2 mg)	↘ ($p < 0.05$)	↘ ($p < 0.01$)

Adapted from Conard *et al.*[73]

ethinyloestradiol, and conjugated equine oestrogens whereas only the synthetic oestrogens alter the electrophoretic response[74].

Decreased fibrinolysis resulting from low plasminogen or increased concentration of inhibitors (such as α2-antiplasmin) may also be involved. In this respect, reports concerning oestrogens are somewhat puzzling, since plasminogen was found to rise with ethinyloestradiol alone[72], or combined[75], whereas global antifibrinolytic activity was consistently increased.

The balance between clotting and fibrinolysis may also be altered. Ethinyloestradiol, but not oestriol, has been reported to reduce the fibrinolysis activators concentration within the vessel walls. The finding that fibrinolytic activity of the vessel walls decreased in postmenopausal women receiving ethinyloestradiol is of particular interest, especially since the same author found no such modification when using the natural 17β-oestradiol, even orally and at supraphysiological doses. In view of this the physiological hormone should be preferred, even though no definite explanation can be proposed.

For many years, oestrogens were blamed for cardiovascular accidents in young pill users. However, since de Gennes reported the same type of accidents in patients using progestogens alone, studies should focus on the effect of progestogens on haemostatic mechanisms.

No consistent alterations in clotting factors have been reported[73,76,77]. Most of the progestogens, chlormadinone acetate[78], norethisterone[78], ethynodiol diacetate[76], norgestrienone[79] and progesterone itself[80] do not modify AT III levels or activity. In contrast, lynestrenol was found to decrease AT III[81] and Conard *et al.*[79] report a further decrease when norethisterone is combined with ethinyloestradiol.

Fibrinolysis is more often impaired. Poller *et al.*[77] found the dilute clot lysis time to be slightly reduced with chlormadinone acetate;

plasminogen levels decreased with MPA but not with ethynodiol diacetate or chlormadinone acetate[82]. Finally, platelet behaviour is not disturbed, ADP-induced aggregation is normal with chlormadinone acetate[77] and PGI_2 production is not modified by norgestrel, lynestrenol or norethisterone[83].

Even though changes in haemostatic variables are minimal, most of the synthetic progestogens have been shown to alter at least one factor and they cannot be considered as totally devoid of thromboembolic risk. Furthermore, since replacement therapy involves both hormones, attention should be paid to the effects of the different associations. Progestogens may in some cases enhance the oestrogenic side-effects, but when using natural hormones no tendency towards enhanced haemostasis was found[80].

VASCULAR ANATOMICAL AND PHYSIOLOGICAL ALTERATIONS

Whenever histological studies have been performed on women who have died from thrombotic accidents and who had been using sex hormones, multifocal lesions, independent of the atherosclerotic process, were found on both arteries and veins.

Changes were seen in the different layers of the vessel walls. The thickening of the intima was characterized by proliferation of the muscular cells and increased connective tissue while endothelial proliferation was also observed. These changes have been described as closely related to the dose and duration of use of the pill[84]. Such lesions can be reproduced experimentally by injection of ethinyloestradiol and chlormadinone acetate, separately or combined[85]. No further studies have been published concerning the effects of other oestrogens, especially those used in the postmenopause, and their combination with progestogens. Nevertheless, at a time in life when spontaneous changes of the vessel walls are frequent, it would appear obvious that any risk of provoking further disorders should be avoided. Whilst awaiting other studies, both ethinyloestradiol and chlormadinone acetate should not be recommended.

CONCLUSION

In order to evaluate the beneficial or deleterious effects of hormone replacement therapy in relation to cardiovascular risk, it should be kept in mind that spontaneous heightening of risk in the postmenopausal years correlates with spontaneous metabolic changes.

Any replacement therapy which would eliminate or diminish these risk factors, i.e. lower the blood pressure, improve glucose tolerance, re-establish the feminine lipid profile, would appear ideal.

Conversely, any compound provoking metabolic disorders would lead to increased cardiovascular risk. Treatment that might induce specific changes implying supplementary risk factor, such as changes in vessel walls, should be avoided. Consequently, ethinyloestradiol should not be considered for replacement therapy. If we consider oestrogens alone, most of the changes are related to modification of protein synthesis within the liver (VLDL, angiotensin etc.) in regard to which both the molecule and the administration route play a part. When oestrogens are given orally, the hepatic receptors are over-stimulated; the more closely the molecule is related to oestradiol the less the perturbations are induced. Ethinyloestradiol provokes more significant changes than the so-called natural oestrogens. However, we should bear in mind that 'it seems that there is no dose of orally administered conjugated equine oestrogens which will provide precise physiological replacement and also avoid potentially harmful side-effects'[35]. Use of oestradiol might appear to be the right choice. But even though the side-effects are limited, they are not eliminated (angiotensin, triglycerides increase) and an increase in cardiovascular risk cannot be totally excluded.

Routes of administration of natural oestrogen other than oral should be preferred – whether percutaneous or vaginal (or other). The prerequisite must be to avoid over-concentraiton of the steroid within the liver.

The metabolic toxicity of the nor-steroid progestogens has been described and should lead to suppression of their use in replacement therapy. Progesterone derivatives have hardly any potential side-effects. If studies would confirm the antihypertensive action of progesterone, this should be considered as beneficial.

If treatments were prescribed with regard to all the above-mentioned factors, usinbg hormones identical or closely related to the endogenous steroids, and an appropriate administration route, then and only then might hormone replacement therapy be devoid of any deleterious effect and even be potentially beneficial regardings cardiovascular risk.

References

1. Lindquist, O. (1979). *Influence of the Menopause on Ischaemic Heart Disease and its Risk Factors and Bone Mineral Content*. Diss. University of Göteborg, Sweden

2. Ryan, K. J. (1976). Estrogens and atherosclerosis. *Clin. Obstet. Gynecol.*, **19**, 805
3. Johansson, B. W., Kaij, L., Kullander, S., Lenner, H. C., Svanberg, L. and Åstedt, B. (1975). On some late effects of bilateral oophorectomy in the age range 15–30 years. *Acta Obstet. Gynecol. Scand.*, **54**, 449
4. Parrish, H. M., Carr, C. A., Hall, D. G. and King, T. M. (1967). Time interval from castration in premenopausal women to development of excessive coronary atherosclerosis. *Am. J. Obstet. Gynecol.*, **99**, 155
5. Robinson, R. W., Higano, N. and Cohen, W. D. (1959). Increased incidence of coronary heart disease in women castrated prior to the menopause. *Arch. Int. Med.*, **104**, 908
6. Gordon, T., Kannel, W. B., Hjortland, M. C. and McNamara, P. M. (1978). Menopause and coronary heart disease. *Ann. Intern. Med.*, **89**, 157
7. Ask-Upmark, E. (1962). Life and death without ovaries. *Acta Med. Scand.*, **172**, 129
8. Pick, R., Stamler, J. and Katz, L. N. (1959). Influence of estrogens on lipids and atherosclerosis in experimental animals. In Pincus, G. (ed.) *Hormones and Atherosclerosis*, p. 229. (London: Academic Press)
9. Oliver, M. F. and Boyd, G. S. (1961). Influence of reduction of serum lipids on prognosis of coronary heart disease. A five-year study using oestrogen. *Lancet*, **2**, 499
10. Stamler, J. (1977). The Coronary Drug Project. Findings with regard to estrogen, dextrothyroxine, clofibrate and niacin. *Adv. Exp. Med. Biol.*, **82**, 52
11. Mann, J. I., Vessey, M. P., Thorogood, M. and Doll, R. (1975). Myocardial infarction in young women with special reference to oral contraceptive practice. *Br. Med. J.*, **2**, 241
12. Vessey, M. P. and Mann, J. I. (1978). Female sex hormones and thrombosis. Epidemiological aspects. *Br. Med. Bull.*, **34**, 157
13. Rosenberg, L., Armstrong, B. and Jick, H. (1976). Myocardial infarction and estrogen therapy in post-menopausal women. *N. Engl. J. Med.*, **294**, 1256
14. Ross, R. K., Paganini-Hill, A., Mack, T. M., Arthur, M. and Henderson, B. E. (1981). Menopausal oestrogen therapy and protection from death from ischaemic heart disease. *Lancet*, **1**, 858
15. Adam, S., Williams, V. and Vessey, M. P. (1981). Cardiovascular disease and hormone replacement treatment: a pilot case–control study. *BR. Med. J.*, **282**, 1277
16. Nachtigall, L. E., Nachtigall, R. M., Nachtigall, R. D. and Beckman, R. H. (1979). Estrogen replacement therapy: II. A prospective study in the relationship to carcinoma and cardiovascular and metabolic problems. *Obstet. Gynecol.*, **54**, 74
17. Pfeffer, R. I., Whipple, G. H., Kurosaki, T. T. and Chapman, J. M. (1978). Coronary risk and estrogen use in post-menopausal women. *Am. J. Epidemiol.*, **107**, 479
18. Kannel, W. B., Castelli, W. P., Gordon, T. and McNamara, P. M. (1971). Serum cholesterol, lipoproteins and the risk of coronary heart disease. *Ann. Intern. Med.*, **74**, 1
19. Kannel, W. B., Hjortland, M. C., McNamara, P. M. and Gordon, T. (1976). Menopause and risk of cardiovascular disease. *Ann. Int. Med.*, **85**, 447
20. Carlton, M., Simons, L. A. and Gibson, J. C. (1980). Vascular disease risk factors in women with premature menopause. *Horm. Metab. Res.*, **12**, 208
21. Kay, C. R. (1980). The happiness pill? *J.R. Coll. Gen. Pract.*, **30**, 8
22. Wahl, P. W., Warnick, G. R., Albers, J. J., Hoover, J. J., Walden, C. E., Bergelin, R. O., Ogilvie, J. T., Hazzard, W. R. and Knopp, R. H. (1981).

Distribution of lipoprotein triglyceride and lipoprotein cholesterol in an adult population by age, sex and hormone use. *Atherosclerosis*, **39**, 111

23. Basdevant, A. and Hautecouverture, M. (1979) Effets des estrogènes sur le métabolisme des lipides et des glucides. *Rev. Prat.*, **29**, 1769
24. Hammond, C. B., Jelovsek, F., Lee, K. L., Creasman, W. T. and Parker, R. T. (1979). Effects of longterm estrogen therapy. I. Metabolic effects. *Am. J. Obstet. Gynecol.*, **133**, 525
25. Bailey, C. J. and Ahmed-Sorour, H. (1980). Role of ovarian hormones in the long-term control of glucose homeostasis. *Diabetologia*, **19**, 475
26. Corvol, P., Breminer, J., Foliot, A. and Menard, J. (1973). Rôle physiologique (direct ou indirect) des hormones sexuelles dans le contrôle des métabolismes de l'eau et du sodium. *Endocrinology*, **93**, 747
27. Corvol, P., Menard, J. and Milliez, P. (1979). Estrogènes et risque vasculaire. *Rev. Prat.*, **29**, 1755
28. Utian, W. H. (1978). Effect of postmenopausal estrogen therapy on diastolic blood pressure and bodyweight. *Maturitas*, **1**, 3
29. Weinberger, M. H., Collins, R. D., Dowdy, A. J., Nokes, G. W. and Luetscher, J. A. (1969). Hypertension induced by oral contraceptives containing estrogen and gestagen. *Ann. Int. Med.*, **71**, 891
30. Cain, M. D., Walters, W. A. and Catt, K. J. (1971). Effects of oral contraceptive therapy on the renin – angiotensin system. *J. Clin. Endocrinol. Metab.*, **33**, 671
31. Menard, J. and Catt, K. J. (1973). Effects of estrogen treatment on plasma renin parameters in the rat. *Endocrinology*, **92**, 1382
32. Helmer, O. M. and Griffith, R. S. (1952). Effect of administration of estrogens on renin – substrate (hypertensinogen) content of rat plasma. *Endocrinology*, **51**, 421
33. Pallas, K. G., Holzwarth, G. J., Stern, M. P. and Lucas, C. P. (1977). The effect of conjugated estrogens on the renin – angiotensin system. *J. Clin. Endocrinol. Metab.*, **44**, 1061
34. Zakheim, R. M., Molteni, A., Mattioli, L. and Mullis, K. B. (1976). Angiotensin I – converting enzyme and angiotensin II levels in women receiving an oral contraceptive. *J. Clin. Endocrinol. Metab.*, 42, 488
35. Geola, F. L., Frumar, A. M., Tataryn, I. V., Lu, K. H., Hershman, J. M., Eggena, P., Sambhi, M. P. and Judd, H.L. (1980). Biological effects of various doses of conjugated equine estrogens in postmenopausal women. *J. Clin. Endocrinol. Metab.*, **51**, 620
36. Elkik, F., Guyenne, P. N., Gompel, A., Corvol, P., Mercier-Bodard, C., Mauvais-Jarvis, P. and Kuttenn, F. (1982). Effects of percutaneous estradiol and conjugated estrogens on the level of plasma proteins and triglycerides in postmenopausal women. *Am. J. Obstet. Gynecol.*, **143**, 888
37. Taurelle, R., Corvol, P. and Limouzin-Lamothe, M. A. (1982). Influence of the route of administration of oestradiol on angiotensinogen hepatic synthesis. In van Keep, P. A., Utian, W. H. and Vermeulen, A. (eds) *The Controversial Climacteric*, p. 36. (Lancaster: MTP Press)
38. Mashchak, C. A., Lobo, R. A., Dozono-Takano, R., Eggena, P., Nakamura, R. M., Brenner, P. F. and Mishell, D. R. (1982). Comparison of pharmacodynamic properties of various estrogen formulations. *Am. J. Obstet. Gynecol.*, **144**, 511
39. Roy, S., Mishell, D. R., Jr., Gray, G., de Quattro, V., Shaw, S. T., Dozono-Takano, R., Brenner, P. F. and Eide, I. (1980). Comparison of metabolic and clinical effects of four contraceptive formulations and a contraceptive vaginal ring. *Am. J. Obstet. Gynecol.*, **136**, 920

40. Meade, T. W., Greenberg, G. and Thompson, S. G. (1980). Progestogens and cardiovascular reactions associated with oral contraceptives and a comparison of the safety of 50 μg and 30 μg estrogen preparations. *Br. Med. J.*, **280**, 1157
41. Landau, R. L., Bergenstal, D. M., Lugibihl, K. and Kascht, M. E. (1955). Metabolic effects of progesterone in man. *J. Clin. Endocrinol. Metab.*, **15**, 1194
42. Soveri, P. and Fyhrquist, F. (1977). Plasma renin activity and angiotensin II during oral contraception. *Ann. Clin. Res.*, **9**, 346
43. Oelkers, W., Schöneshöfer, M. and Blümel, A. (1974). Effects of progesterone and four synthetic progestagens on sodium balance and the renin–aldosterone system in man. *J. Clin. Endocrinol. Metab.*, **39**, 882
44. Corvol, P., Elkik, F., Feneant, M., Oblin, M. E., Michaud, A., Claire, M. and Menard, J. (1983). *Effect of Progesterone and Progestins on Water and Salt Retention.* (New York: Raven Press)
45. Williams, L. T. and Lefkowitz, R. J. (1977). Regulation of rabbit myometrial alpha adrenergic receptors by estrogen and progesterone. *J. Clin. Invest.*, **60**, 815
46. Donde, U. M. and Virkar, K. (1975). Effect of contraceptive steroids on serum lipids. *Am. J. Obstet. Gynecol.*, **123**, 736
47. Gustafson, A. and Svanborg, A. (1972). Gonadal steroid effects on plasma lipoproteins and individual phospholipids. *J. Clin. Endocrinol. Metab.*, **35**, 203
48. Hazzard, W. R., Notter, D. T., Spiger, M. J. and Bierman, E. L. (1972). Oral contraceptives and triglyceride transport: Acquired heparin resistance on the mechanism for impaired post-heparin lipolytic activity. *J. Clin. Endocrinol. Metab.*, **35**, 425
49. Spellacy, W. N., Buhi, W. C. and Birk, S. A. (1974). Norgestrel and carbohydrate–lipid metabolism: glucose, insulin and triglyceride changes during six months time of use. *Contraception*, **9**, 615
50. Wynn, V. and Doar, J. W. (1966). Some effects of oral contraceptives on carbohydrate metabolism. *Lancet*, **2**, 715
51. Furman, R. H., Alaupovic, P. and Howard, R. P. (1967). Effects of androgens and estrogens on serum lipids and the composition and concentration of serum lipoproteins in normolipemic and hyperlipidemic states. *Prog. Biomed. Pharmacol.*, **2**, 215
52. Pystynen, P., Pyykkö, K., Jokela, H., Niemelä, A. and Saarikoski, S. (1980). Effects of 4 mg estradiol valerianate on serum lipids in newly oophorectomized women. *Maturitas*, **2**, 95
53. Stern, M. P., Brown, B. W., Haskell, W. L., Farquhar, J. W., Wehrle, L. and Wood, P. D. (1976). Cardiovascular risk and use of estrogens or estrogen–progestagen combinations. *J. Am. Med. Assoc.*, **235**, 811
54. Isaacs, A. J. and Havard, C. W. H. (1977). Effect of piperazine oestrone sulphate on serum lipids and lipoproteins in menopausal women. *Acta Endocrinol.*, **85**, 143
55. Paterson, M. E. L., Sturdee, D. W., Moore, B. and Whitehead, T. P. (1980). The effect of various regimes of hormone therapy on serum cholesterol and triglyceride concentrations in postmenopausal women. *Br. J. Obstet. Gynaecol.*, **87**, 552
56. Silfverstolpe, G., Johnson, P., Samsioe, G., Svanborg, A. and Gustafson, A. (1981). Lipid metabolic studies in oophorectomized women. Effects of exogenous sex steroid. *Atca Endocrinol.*, **96**, 527
57. Fåhraeus, L., Larsson-Cohn, U. and Wallentin, L. (1982). Lipoproteins during oral and cutaneous administration of oestradiol 17β to menopausal women. *Acta Endocrinol.*, **101**, 597
58. Lagrelius, A. (1981). Treatment with oral estrone sulphate in the female climacteric. *Acta Obstet. Gynecol. Scand.*, **60**, 481

59. Wallentin, L. and Varenhorst, E. (1978). Changes of plasma lipid metabolism in males during estrogen treatment for prostatic carcinoma. *J. Clin. Endocrinol. Metab.*, **47**, 596
60. Titov, U. N., Sanfirona, V. M. and Hodakova, T. D. (1980). Lipoprotein metabolism disturbances induced by oral contraceptives. *Farmakol. Toksikal.*, **43**, 345
61. Dorangeon, P., Cosson, R. and Leutenegger, M. (1980). Incidence sur l'équilibre lipidique de deux modalités d'estrogénothérapie de la ménopause. *Rev. Fr. Endocrinol. Clin.*, **21**, 19
62. Lagroua Weill-Halle, M. A. (1981). Estrogénothérapie percutanée de la ménopause. *Rev. Fr. Gynécol.*, **72**, 283
63. Loeper, J., Loeper, J., Ohlghiesser, C., de Lignières, B. and Mauvais-Jarvis, P. (1977). Influence de l'oestrogénothérapie sue les triglycérides. *Nouv. Presse Méd.*, **6**, 2747
64. Ähren, T. (1982). *Contraceptive Vaginal Rings.* (Uppsala: Acta Universitatis Uppsaliensis)
65. Basdevant, A., de Lignières, B. and Guy-Grand, B. (1983). Differential lipemic and hormonal responses to oral and parenteral 17β-estradiol in postmenopausal women. *Am. J. Obstet. Gynecol.*, **147**, 77
66. Basdevant, A. and Guy-Grand, B. (1982). Effets de l'administration percutanée d'estradiol 17β chez les femmes ménopausées hyperlipidémiques. *J. Gynécol. Obstét. Biol. Reprod.*, **11**, 277
67. Wallace, R. B., Hoover, J., Barrett-Connor, E., Rifkind, B. M., Hunninghake, D. B., MacKenthun, A. and Heiss, G. (1979). Altered plasma lipid and lipoprotein levels associated with oral contraceptive and oestrogen use. *Lancet*, **2**, 111
68. Punnonen, R. and Rauramo, L. (1980). The effect of castration and estrogen therapy on serum high-density lipoprotein cholesterol. *Int. J. Gynaecol. Obstet.*, **17**, 434
69. Nikkilä, E. A., Kuusi, T., Harno, K., Tikkanen, M. and Taskinen, M. R. (1980). Lipoprotein lipase and hepatic endothelial lipase are key enzymes in the metabolism of plasma high density lipoproteins, particularly of HDL_2. In Gotto, A. M., Smith, J. R. and Allen, L. C. (eds) *Atherosclerosis V. Proceedings of the Fifth International Symposium on Atherosclerosis*, pp. 387–392. (New York, Hildeberg, Berlin: Springer Verlag)
70. Kay, C. R. (1982). Progestogens and arterial disease. Evidence from the Royal College of general practitioners' study. *Am. J. Obstet. Gynecol.*, **142**, 762
71. Davies, T., Fieldhouse, G. and McNicol, G. E. (1976). The effects of therapy with estriol succinate and ethinyl estradiol and the haemostatic mechanism in post menopausal women. *Thromb. Haemostasis*, **35**, 2
72. Åstedt, B. (1971). Low fibrinolytic activity of veins during treatment with ethinyloestradiol. *Acta Obstet. Gynecol. Scand.*, **50**, 279
73. Conard, J. and Samama, M. (1983). The effects of progestins on coagulation. In Wayne Bardin, C., Milgröm, E. and Mauvais-Jarvis, P. (eds) *Progesterone and Progestins*, pp. 447–452. (New York: Raven Press)
74. Elkeles, R. S., Hampton, J. R. and Mitchell, J. R. (1968). Effect of oestrogens on human platelet behaviour. *Lancet*, **2**, 315
75. Ygge, J., Brody, S., Korsan-Bengtsen, K. and Nilsson, L. (1969). Changes in blood coagulation and fibrinolysis in women receiving oral contraceptives. *Am. J. Obstet. Gynecol.*, **104**, 87
76. Howie, P. W., Prentice, C. R. and Mallinson, A. C. (1970). Effect of combined oestrogen–progestogen oral contraceptives, oestrogen and progestogen on antiplasmin and antiothrombosis activity. *Lancet*, **2**, 1329

77. Poller, L., Thompson, J. M., Tabiowo, A. and Priest, C. M. (1969). Progesterone oral contraception and blood coagulation. *Br. Med. J.*, **1**, 554
78. Larsson-Cohn, U., Johansson, E. D. B., Wide, L. and Gemzell, C. (1972). Effects of continuous daily administration of 0.1 mg of norethindrone on the plasma levels of progesterone and on the urinary excretion of LH and total oestrogens. *Acta Endocrinol.*, 71, 551
79. Conard, J., Cazenave, B., Samama, M., Horellou, M. H., Zorn, J. R. and Neau, C. (1980). Antithrombine-III content and antithrombin activity in oestrogen–progestogen and progestogen-only treated women. *Thromb. Res.*, **18**, 675
80. Fenichel, P., Balarac, N., Isetta, M., Melandri, E., Tran, D. K., Bayle, J. and Gillet, J. Y. (1982). Effet d'une association estradiol percutané – progestérone micronisée orale sur l'hémostase en période de périménopause. *Rev. Fr. Gynécol. Obstét.*, **77**, 93
81. Bounameaux, H., Duckert, F., Walter, M. and Bounameaux, Y. (1978). The determination of antithrombin-III. Comparison of six methods. Effect of oral contraceptive therapy. *Thromb. Haemostas.*, **39**, 607
82. Nilsson, I. M., Kullander, J. and Åstedt, B. (1970). Coagulation and fibrinolytic studies during continuous low doses gestagen. *Acta Endocrinol.*, **65**, 111
83. Ylikorkala, O., Puolakka, J. and Viinikka, L. (1981). Oestrogen containing oral contraceptives decrease prostacycline production. *Lancet*, **1**, 42
84. Irey, N. S., McAllister, H. A. and Henry, J. M. (1978). Oral contraceptives and stroke in young women: a clinicopathologic correlation. *Neurology*, **28**, 1216
85. Gammael, E. B. (1976). Intimal thickening in arteries of rats treated with synthetic sex hormones. *Br. J. Exp. Pathol.*, **57**, 248

Chapter 22

Perimenopausal oestrogen therapy and breast cancer

P. Ide

The possible rôle of peri- and postmenopausal oestrogen therapy in the development of breast neoplasia has been suspected. The presence of oestrogen receptors in some tumour tissue and the effects of tumour treatment with an anti-oestrogen has been well documented. It has been established that an average of 10 years is necessary for the growth of the neoplasia to reach a detectable level[1]. Because of this latency period only long-term follow-up studies can show the oestrogen-associated breast cancer risk. In general, it can be said that an increase in relative risk (RR) of breast carcinoma is found with the length of the treatment period. In a first evaluation of the morbidity in their large sample of oestrogen-treated women Burch and Byrd[2] found the same incidence of breast tumours as might be expected in untreated women. In a later evaluation Burch *et al.*[3] found a slight increase in oestrogen-treated women over the age of 55 years. Hoover *et al.*[4] found an increasing relative risk to 2.0 after 1.5 years of follow-up. The latter team also found a dose–response relationship with a relative risk of 2.7 for those women using more than 0.625 mg of conjugated oestrogens (CE) per day over a period of more than 10 years. This latter finding was confirmed by Ross *et al.*[5] in a statistically reliable study. The relative risk increased to 2.5 in women using a large dose of CE (1.25 mg/day over 3 years). This was shown to be the case only in women with intact ovaries. In contrast, Hoover *et al.*[6] found a relative risk of 3.7 in postmenopausal women who had had a bilateral oophorectomy and were on large doses of CE.

In addition, in women using high dosages of oestrogens, the relative risk seemed higher for multiparous women, for those who had had a first child at a young age, for those without benign breast disease and for those with a family history of breast cancer. Apart from the last factor the others are normally considered as being associated with a lower relative risk of breast cancer.

In considering oestrogen-associated breast cancer risk one should mention the various subgroups of women with known risk factors. Ross *et al.*[5] found that a history of surgically confirmed breast disease raised the risk to 5.7 relative to non-users without previous benign breast disease. Hoover *et al.*[6] found the highest relative risk in those women with a family history of breast cancer (3.9) and Black and Leis[7] found increased oestrogen-associated breast cancer risk only among nulliparous patients.

Obesity and overweight have been associated with breast cancer [5,8,9]. This is explained by a greater oestrogen production from aromatization of precursors such as androstenedione[10]. Sherman *et al.*[11] found a relationship between the exogenous oestrogen use and excess weight. The relative risk was 0.41 for women whose weight was less than the median, compared with 1.29 for those whose weight exceeded the median.

It is possible that overweight and oestrogen use result in a more intense oestrogenic environment by the addition of the endogenous oestrogen production and the exogenous oestrogen intake. In the same study (case–control) the mean age of the breast cancer patients using oestrogens was 58.1 years. This is significantly lower than in non-users (63 years). Oestrogen-treated women in the lowest tertile of body weight had had the diagnosis of breast cancer made seven years earlier than those in the highest tertile of weight. Possibly higher[11] oestrogen concentrations are obtained by oestrogen therapy in women with smaller body size.

Irrespective of whether the hormonal preparation used is conjugated oestrogens or oestradiol valerate, the result is an increase in the circulating level of oestrone rather than of oestradiol[12]. Moreover, patients using CE have extremely high blood levels of equilin, a potent oestrogen that remains detectable in the body for a long time after treatment is discontinued[12,13].

It has been estimated that a woman who has experienced a natural menopause at the age of 50 and who has been receiving 1.25 mg of conjugated oestrogens daily for three years will have a life time probability of contracting breast cancer that is 10% greater than that of a comparable, non-treated woman[5].

Thus it would appear that the benefits of oestrogen therapy at this high dosage level would need to be extremely great to warrant such risk. At lower dosage levels (0.625 mg CE) the relative risk is more favourable, although the impact on breast cancer risk is still unclear[4-6].

A statistically significant relationship has been calculated by Janzon *et al.*[14] and Buchanan *et al.*[15] between the Wolfe Mammographic Parenchym Pattern (WMPP)[16] and known risk factors for breast cancers such as age ($p < 0.0002$), parity ($p < 0.0002$), age at birth of first child ($p < 0.0014$), family history ($p < 0.0970$) and a previous breast biopsy ($p < 0.0066$).

The original classification of the WMPP is based on the relative amounts of fat, epithelial and connective tissue densities, and prominent ducts observed on the mammogram. The classification is as follows:

N_1: lowest risk: parenchyma composed primarily of fat with, at most, small amounts of 'dysplasia'. No ducts visible.

P_1: low risk: parenchyma briefly flat with prominent ducts in anterior portion up to one-fourth of volume of the breast.

P_2: high risk: severe involvement with prominent duct pattern occupying more than one-fourth of volume of the breast.

DY: highest risk: severe involvement with dysplasia. It often obscures an underlying prominent duct pattern. N_1 and P_1 are considered as essentially normal and low risk, whereas P_2 and DY are considered as high risk for subsequent breast cancer development.

Wolfe *et al.*[17] found that in 2731 consecutive prevalent breast cancers, 55% presented a P_2 or DY parenchym pattern. Over a six-year period of follow-up in the incidence series, 88% of 332 cases were classified in P_2 and DY WMPP. Of the 332 patients with incidence breast cancer 186 patients were aged over 50. This group runs the relative risk for subsequent breast cancer development compared with the N_1 group, 1.85 for P_1, and 52.24 for the DY group. Krook *et al.*[18] found similar differences, but of a lesser magnitude comparing the different mammographic parenchym patterns with the rate of development of breast cancer in a screening group of 10 035 women. P_2 and DY mammographic parenchym patterns are still very common over the age of 50. In a screened population of 12 308 women, 45.5% were in the P_2 and DY groups[14].

CONCLUSION

Not every woman may need the same oestrogen or the same dose. Obese women for example have a higher endogenous oestrone production and consequently may be less prone to hip fractures and osteoporosis and more prone to breast cancer. In some subgroups of women the use of conjugated oestrogens is associated with an increased breast cancer risk: the mammographic parenchym pattern can be very helpful in identifying such women as being at risk. In these cases overstimulation of breast tissue with oestrogens must be avoided. Probably the use of oestriol is preferable, because oestriol is very effective in the treatment of the climacteric syndrome[19].

References

1. Tubiana, M., Chauvel, P., Renaud, A. and Malaise, E. (1975). Vitesse de croissance et histoire naturelle du cancer du sein. *Bull. Cancer*, **62**, 341
2. Burch, J. and Byrd, J. (1971). Effects of long-term administration of estrogen on the occurrence of mammary cancer in women. *Ann. Surg.*, **174**, 414
3. Burch, J., Byrd, J. and Vaughn, W. (1974). The effects of long-term estrogen on hysterectomized women. *Am. J. Obstet. Gynecol.*, **118**, 778
4. Hoover, R., Gray, L., Cole, P. and Macmahon, B. (1976). Menopausal estrogens and breast cancer. *N. Engl. J. Med.*, **295**, 401
5. Ross, R., Paganini-Hill, A., Gerkins, V., Mack, T. M., Pfeffer, R., Arthur, M. and Henderson, B. (1980). A case control study of menopausal estrogen therapy and breast cancer. *J. Am. Med. Assoc.*, **243**, 1635
6. Hoover, R., Glass, A., Finkle, W., Azevedo, D. and Milne, K. (1981). Conjugated estrogens and breast cancer risk in women. *J. Natl. Cancer Inst.*, **67**, 815
7. Black, M. and Leis, H. P. (1972). Mammary carcinogenesis. *N.Y. State J. Med.*, **72**, 1601
8. Brinton, L. A., Williams, R. R., Hoover, R. N., Stegens, N. L., Feinleib, M. and Fraumeni, J. F., Jr. (1979). Breast cancer risk factors among screening program participants. *J. Natl. Cancer Inst.*, **62**, 37
9. De Waard, F. and Baanders-van Halewijn, E. (1974). A prospective study in general practice of breast cancer risk in postmenopausal women. *Int. J. Cancer*, **14**, 153
10. Judd, H. (1976). Hormonal dynamics associated with the menopause. *Clin. Obstet. Gynecol.*, **19**, 775
11. Sherman, B., Wallace, R. and Bean, J. (1983). Estrogen use and breast cancer. *Cancer*, **51**, 1527

12. Whittaker, P. G., Morgan, M., Dean, P., Cameron, E. H. D. and Lind, T. (1980). Serum equilin, oestrone, and oestradiol levels in postmenopausal women receiving conjugated equine oestrogens (Premarin). *Lancet*, **1**, 14
13. Hammond, C. and Maxson, W. (1982). Current status of estrogen therapy for the menopause. *Fertil. Sterii.*, **37**, 5
14. Janzon, L., Andersson, I. and Petersson, H. (1982). Mammographic patterns as indicators of risk of breast cancer. *Radiology*, **143**, 417
15. Buchanan, J., Weisberg, B., Sandoz, J., Gray, L. and Bland, K. (1981). Selected prognostic variables for mammographic parenchym patterns. *Cancer*, **47**, 2135
16. Wolfe, J. (1976). Breast patterns as an index of risk for developing breast cancer. *Am. J. Roentgenol.*, **126**, 1130
17. Wolfe, J., Albert, S., Belle, S. and Salane, M. (1982). Breast parenchymal patterns: analysis of 332 incident breast carcinoma's. *Am. J. Roentgenol.*, **138**, 113
18. Krook, P., Carlile, T., Bush, W. and Hall, M. H. (1978). Mammographic parenchymal patterns as a risk indicator for prevalent and incident cancer. *Cancer*, **41**, 1093
19. Tzingounis, V., Aksu, M. F. and Greenblatt, R. B. (1980). The significance of oestriol in the management of the post-menopause. *Acta Endocrinol. (Suppl.)*, **233**, 45

Chapter 23

Effects of postmenopausal treatment on lipoproteins

A. Volpe, E. Zirilli, F. Barbieri, M. Baraldi, V. Boraldi, F. Facchinetti and A. R. Genazzani

INTRODUCTION

The menopause, whether induced surgically or occurring spontaneously, is accompanied by increases in serum cholesterol and triglycerides[1], changes in lipoprotein distribution[2-4] and heightened risk of cardiovascular disease[5].

Therapy in the postmenopause can modify blood levels of lipoproteins. Until a few years ago oestrogens were thought to be the only agents responsible for these changes. Some data, however, conflict with this presumption[6-11].

Since the risk of cardiovascular disease increases in women using oral contraceptives after the age of 35, patients undergoing oestrogen therapy during the postmenopause would therefore be expected to be at greater risk. This has not been confirmed, however[12]. The differing results between women using oral contraceptives and those treated with oestrogens during the postmenopause may be due to various factors :

(1) A qualitative difference between the oestrogens taken by the two groups (natural oestrogens in the postmenopause, synthetic ones during the fertile years);
(2) Different dosages of oestrogens in the two groups;

(3) Absence of, or only low doses of, progestogens in postmenopausal pateints.

The difference between the two groups may well depend on this last factor alone.

Oestrogen therapy in women in an early menopause (either surgical or spontaneous) has been shown to change the lipid balance and may reduce the associated risk of vascular disease[13,14]. Recent clinical data would seem to demonstrate that administration of high doses of progestogens is correlated with greater risk of cardiovascular disease[6,8,9,15]. As cardiovascular disease more frequently affects women over 50 years of age it may be due to increased low density lipoprotein-cholesterol (LDL-C) levels[2,3].

It is therefore important in climacteric therapy to select particularly oestrogen–progestogen combinations which do not change lipoprotein levels. Several previous studies have shown that it is possible to minimize the lipoprotein changes induced by oestrogen–progestogen by carefully balancing the doses of the two components[6].

MATERIAL AND METHODS

Eighteen postmenopausal women were studied divided into three groups. The average age of the patients, the number of years since the onset of the menopause, plasma basal levels of total cholesterol, high density lipoprotein-cholesterol (HDL-C), LDL-C and total triglycerides were similar in the three groups.

All patients suffered from marked climacteric symptoms, particularly hot flushes, and showed high FSH levels and low E_2 levels

Table 1 Clinical features of the patients who underwent therapy with norethisterone acetate or medroxyprogesterone acetate and conjugated oestrogens (CO)

GROUP	N° PAT.	AGE	ONSET OF MENOPAUSE	WEIGHT	FSH (mUI/ml)	LH (mUI/ml)	E_2 (pg/ml)	COL. TOT. (mmol/l)	HDL-c (mmol/l)	TG (mmol/l)
1° (CO)	8	52.3±3.4	49.5±1.9	59.4±5.7	80.1±13.2	72.2±19.8	23.4±5.7	5.6±1.4	1.59±0.3	0.84±0.2
2° A+B	5	54.8±2.7	50.3±2.8	57.8±6.1	75.7±15.5	75.7±15.6	19.3±6.5	6.1±0.5	1.66±0.46	0.77±0.54
3° B+A	5	53.6±2.8	49.7±2.6	57.4±4.8	84.7±16.8	73.3±21.4	21.3±7.8	6.8±1.43	1.55±0.37	0.88±0.21

A= CONJUGATED OESTROGENS (0.625 mg/day x 21 days) + NORETHISTERONE ACETATE (10 mg/day from 12th to 21st day x two cycles)

B= CONJUGATED OESTROGENS (0.625 mg/day x 21 days) + MEDROXYPROGESTERONE ACETATE (10 mg/day from 12th to 21st day x two cycles)

(Table 1). The patients had not received any hormone therapy or other treatment capable of influencing lipid metabolism for at least three months before the study. None of them had a history of excessive tobacco or alcohol consumption or previous cardiovascular disease or current renal, hepatic or thyroid conditions, as shown by laboratory and clinical tests before treatment was started.

Group I (8 women) received only 0.625 mg/day conjugated oestrogens (CO) during four 21-day cycles.

Group II (5 women) received during four cycles of three weeks 0.625 mg conjugated oestrogens (CO) plus, for the first two cycles, norethisterone acetate (NET) (10 mg/day) from day 12 to day 21 and for the remaining two cycles, plus medroxyprogesterone acetate (MAP) (10 mg/day) from day 12 to day 21.

Group III (5 women) received CO (0.625 mg/day) for 21 days plus, for the first two cycles, medroxyprogesterone acetate (MAP) (10 mg/day) from day 12 to day 21 and plus norethisterone acetate (NET) (10 mg/day) from day 12 to day 21, for the two last cycles (Table 1).

Prior to therapy, after two cycles, and again after treatment, weight, blood pressure, subjective symptoms were checked and total cholesterol (C), triglycerides (TG), HDL-C and LDL-C plasma levels were measured in the three groups during or after treatment. Blood sampling was performed between 8 a.m. and 9 a.m. each day after fasting all night. Total cholesterol and triglycerides were measured by enzymatic assay[9,10]; HDL-C was measured by the CHOD-PAP method after precipitation and centrifugation[10,11]. LDL-C was calculated as the difference between total cholesterol and HDL-C plus very low density lipoprotein-cholesterol (VLDL-C), also assayed after precipitation and centrifugation by the CHOD-PAP method[10,11]. FSH, LH and E_2 were measured by radioimmunoassay.

RESULTS

No significant variations in total cholesterol were observed in any of the patients studied. A slight, not significant, increase in triglycerides was observed in each of the groups, more evidently in the patients undergoing only conjugated oestrogen therapy. In those patients treated with conjugated oestrogens plus norethisterone a decrease in plasma HDL-C levels of over 10% with respect to basal values ($p < 0.05$) was observed (Figure 1). This decrease was not correlated with initial

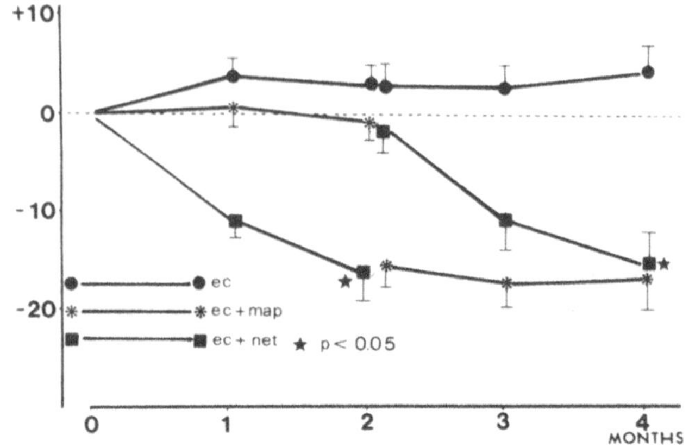

Figure 1 Percentage of change in HDL-cholesterol during treatment with conjugated oestrogens alone, conjugated oestrogens plus medroxyprogesterone acetate, conjugated oestrogens plus norethisterone acetate. ec = conjugated oestrogens; map = medroxyprogesterone acetate; net = norethisterone acetate

values. In the other two groups no significant variations in plasma HDL-C were observed.

Treatment with conjugated oestrogens plus norethisterone acetate also resulted in significant increase ($p < 0.05$) in LDL-C levels (Figure 2), while treatment with oestrogens alone or progestogens plus MAP did not significantly modify LDL-C levels.

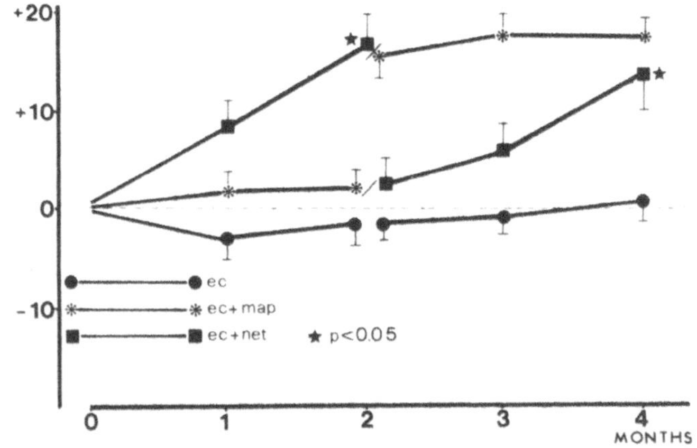

Figure 2 Percentage of change in LDL-cholesterol during treatment with conjugated oestrogens alone, conjugated oestrogens plus medroxyprogesterone acetate, conjugated oestrogens plus norethisterone acetate. ec = conjugated oestrogens; map = medroxyprogesterone acetate; net = norethisterone acetate

DISCUSSION

Our data show that conjugated oestrogens alone do not significantly modify lipid metabolism. Previous reports on the effects of using conjugated oestrogens on postmenopausal women are conflicting. Whilst most authors report little or no effect on cholesterol levels[16-20], significant cholesterol depression has also been observed[21]. Similarly, conjugated oestrogens have been variously reported as increasing triglycerides[20,22,23] and of having an effect on lipid metabolism[17,18].

Failure of micronized 17β-oestradiol to alter either cholesterol or triglycerides after three months' treatment is consistent with the reports of Wallentin and Larsson-Cohn[24] and Paterson *et al.*[20]. However, Utian[16] and Pyörälä[25] both reported reductions of cholesterol with oestradiol valerate treatment.

It does seem that, generally speaking, oestrogens have a beneficial effect on lipid metabolism by raising HDL-C levels and lowering those of LDL-C[2,7,10,24,26].

As oestrogen treatment not balanced by a progestogen increases the risk of endometrial adenocarcinoma[27], progestogens are usually added for a period[28] to each cycle of oestrogen treatment. Unfortunately, progestogens may increase the risk of heart disease and of atherosclerotic complications[29].

It would seem that this negative effect that progestogens have on lipid metabolism is much greater in the case of compounds with androgenic activity[11,30-33]. Our data confirm this hypothesis. In fact, norethisterone acetate induced a significant increase in LDL-C in both groups treated with it, while MAP, a progestogen with weak androgenic activity, did not induce any significant variation in lipoprotein levels.

There is a positive correlation between LDL-cholesterol and the risk of coronary heart disease[34]. A possible inverse relation between HDL-cholesterol and coronary heart disease has received even more attention[35]; thus it would appear that hormone preparations that simultaneously raise LDL-C levels and lower HDL cause the most concern.

Hirvonen *et al.*[8] report that androgenic progestogens of the 19-nortestosterone series reverse the beneficial effect of postmenopausal oestrogen treatment on HDL-cholesterol, whereas the hydroxyprogesterone derivative, medroxyprogesterone acetate, has no such effect[30]. Even in women using a combined oral contraceptive the lipoprotein levels vary with the type and the dose of the component steroids. Wahl *et al.*[30] observed the highest LDL-C and lowest HDL-C mean values in users of oral contraceptives containing progestogens with androgenic activity such as norgestrel and norethisterone acetate.

Samsioe[9] reports a weaker effect on lipoproteins on the part of oral contraceptives containing desorgestrel than that of those with levonorgestrel.

In general it seems that HDL-C levels increase with increasing doses of oestrogens and decrease with increasing doses or potency of progestogens[10,7]. Thus it is advisable, particularly in treating postmenopausal women, to choose a progestogen with weak and androgenic activity or none at all. Alternatively one can use oestrogen–progestogen combinations to minimize the effects on lipoprotein levels. It is also possible to supplement oestrogen treatment with an intrauterine progesterone contraceptive delivery system. The progesterone released by the device does not alter lipid metabolism as it does not enter the blood stream[36] and protects the endometrium against the action of the oestrogens[37].

References

1. Bengtsson, C. and Lindquist, O. (1979). Menopausal effects on risk factors for ischaemic heart disease. *Maturitas*, **1**, 165
2. Gustafson, A. and Svanborg, A. (1972). Gonadal steroid effects on plasma lipoproteins and individual phospholipids. *J. Clin. Endocrinol. Metab.*, **35**, 203
3. Kannel, W. B., Hjortland, M. C., McNamara, P. M. and Gordon, T. (1976). Menopause and risk of cardiovascular disease. *The Framingham Study. Ann. Intern. Med.*, **85**, 447
4. Miller, G. J. and Miller, N. E. (1975). Plasma-high-density-lipoprotein concentration and development of ischaemic heart-disease. *Lancet*, **1**, 16
5. Rosenberg, L., Hennekens, C. H., Rosner, B., Belanger, C., Rothman, K. J. and Speizer, F. E. (1981). Early menopause and risk of myocardial infarction. *Am. J. Obstet. Gynecol.*, **139**, 47
6. Larsson-Cohn, U., Wallentin, L. and Zador, G (1979). Plasma lipids and high density lipoproteins during oral contraception with different combinations of ethinyl estradiol and levonorgestrel. *Horm. Metab. Res.*, **11**, 437
7. Plunkett, E. R. (1982). Contraceptive steroids, age and cardiovascular system. *Am. J. Obstet. Gynecol.*, **142**, 747
8. Hirvonen, E., Mälkönen, M. and Manninen, V. (1981). Effects of different progestogens on lipoproteins during postmenopausal replacement therapy. *N. Engl. J. Med.*, **304**, 560
9. Samsioe, G. (1982). Study on effect of 30 μg ethinylestradiol (E.E.) + 150 μg desogestrel on lipid and lipoprotein metabolism in healthy volunteers, also in comparison with 30 μg EE + 150 μg levonorgestrel. *Acta Obst. Gynecol. Scand.*, **55** (Suppl. 111)

10. Bradley, D. D., Wingerd, J., Petitti, D. B., Krauss, R. M. and Ramcharan, S. (1978). Serum high-density-lipoprotein cholesterol in women using oral contraceptives, estrogens and progestins. *N. Engl. J. Med.*, **299**, 17
11. Briggs, M. and Briggs, M. (1981). A randomized study of metabolic effects of four low-estrogen oral contraceptives: I. Results after 6 cycles. *Contraception*, **23**, 463
12. Nachtigall, L. E., Nachtigall, R. H. Nachtigall, R. D. and Beckman, E. M. (1979). Estrogen replacement therapy: II. A prospective study in the relationship to carcinoma and cardiovascular and metabolic problems. *Obstet. Gynecol.*, **54**, 74
13. Higano, N., Robinson, R. W. and Cohen, W. D. (1963). Increased incidence of cardiovascular disease in castrated women. Two years follow-up studies. *N. Engl. J. Med.*, **268**, 1123
14. Carlton, M., Simons, L. A. and Gibson, J. C. (1980). Vascular disease risk factors in women with premature menopause. *Horm. Metab. Res.*, **12**, 208
15. Kay, C. R. (1980). The happiness pill. *J. R. Coll. Gen. Pract.*, **30**, 8
16. Utian, W. H. (1972). Effect of oophorectomy and oestrogen therapy on serum cholesterol. *Int. J. Gynecol. Obstet.*, **10**, 95
17. Notelovitz, M. and Southwood, B. (1974). Metabolic effect of conjugated oestrogens (USP) on lipids and lipoproteins. *S. Afr. Med. J.*, **48**, 2552
18. Bolton, C. H., Ellwood, M., Hartog, M., Martin, R., Rowe, A. S. and Wensley, R. T. (1975). Comparison of the effects of ethinyl oestradiol and conjugated equine oestrogens in oophorectomized women. *Clin. Endocrinol. (Oxf.)*, **4**, 131
19. Walter, S. and Jensen, H. K. (1977). The effect of treatment with oestradiol and oestriol on fasting serum cholesterol and triglyceride levels in postmenopausal women. *Br. J. Obstet. Gynaecol.*, **84**, 869
20. Paterson, M. E. L., Sturdee, D. W., Moore, B. and Whitehead, T. P. (1980). The effect of various regimens of hormone therapy on serum cholesterol and triglyceride concentrations in postmenopausal women. *Br. J. Obstet. Gynaecol.*, **87**, 552
21. Villadolid, L. S., Buenaluz, L. and Iledan, A. (1973). Progress report on long-term oestrogen therapy. *Curr. Med. Res. Opin.*, **1**, 577
22. Robinson, R. W. and Lebeau, R. J. (1965). Effect of conjugated estrogens on serum lipids and the clotting mechanism. *J. Atheroscler. Res.*, **5**, 120
23. Furman, R. H., Alaupovic, P. and Howard, R. P. (1967). Effect of androgens and estrogens on serum lipids and the composition and concentration of serum lipoproteins in normolipidemic ans hyperlipidemic states. *Prog. Biochem. Pharmacol.*, **2**, 215
24. Wallentin, L. and Larsson-Cohn, U. (1977). Metabolic and hormonal effects of postmenopausal oestrogen replacement treatment: II. Plasma lipids. *Acta Endocrinol.*, **86**, 597
25. Pyörälä, T. (1976). The effect of synthetic and natural estrogens on glucose tolerance plasma insulin and lipid metabolism in postmenopausal women. In Campbell, S. (ed.) *The Management of the Menopause and Post-menopausal Years*, pp. 195–210. (Lancaster: MTP Press)
26. Goldzieher, J. W., Chenault, C. B., De La Pena, A., Dozier, T. S. and Kraemer, D. C. (1978). Comparative studies of the ethinyl estrogens used in oral contraceptives: VII. Effects with and without progestational agents on ultracentrifugally fractionated plasma lipoproteins in humans, baboons and beagles. *Fertil. Steril.*, **30**, 522
27. Gray, L. A., Christopherson, W. M. and Hoover, R. N. (1977). Estrogens and endometrial carcinoma. *Obstet. Gynecol.*, **49**, 385
28. Ziel, H. K. and Finkle, W. D. (1975). Increased risk of endometrial carcinoma among users of conjugated estrogens. *N. Engl. J. Med.*, **293**, 1167

29. Royal College of General Practitioners. (1977). Oral contraception study: Mortality among oral contraceptive users. *Lancet*, **2**, 727
30. Wahl, P., Walden, C., Knopp, R., Hoover, J., Wallace, R., Heiss, G. and Rifkind, B. (1983). Effect of estrogen/progestin potency on lipid lipoprotein cholesterol. *N. Engl. J. Med.*, **308**, 862
31. Kremer, J., De Bruijn, H. W. A. and Hindriks, F. R. (1980). Serum high density lipoprotein cholesterol levels in women using a contraceptive injection of depot-medroxyprogesterone acetate. *Contraception*, **22**, 359
32. Amatayakul, K., Sivassomboon, B. and Singkamani, R. (1979). Effects of medroxy-progesterone acetate on serum lipids, protein, glucose tolerance and liver function in Thai women. *Contraception*, **21**, 283
33. Mälkönen, M., Hirvonen, E. and Manninen, V. (1980). Effects of donazol and lynestrenol on serum lipoproteins in endometriosis. *Clin. Pharmacol. Ther.*, **28**, 602
34. Ramcharan, S. (1974). *The Walnut Creek Contraceptive Drug Study : A Prospective Study of the Side Effects of Oral Contraception*, Vol. 1, p. 562. (Washington DC: DHEW Publication, National Institutes of Health).
35. Heiss, G., Johnson, N. J., Reiland, S., Davis, C. E. and Tyroler, H. A. (1980). The epidemiology of plasma high-density lipoprotein cholesterol levels. The Lipid Research Clinics Prevalence Study. Summary. *Circulation*, **62** (Suppl. 4), 116
36. Spellacy, W. N., Buhi, W. C. and Birk, S. A. (1978). Studies of carbohydrate and lipid metabolism in women using the progesterone-T intrauterine device for six months: Blood glucose, insulin, cholesterol on triglyceride levels. *Fertil. Steril.*, **29**, 205
37. Volpe, A., Botticelli, A., Abrate, M., Dalla Vecchia, E., Mantovani, M., Carani, C., Grasso, A., Mazza, V. and Di Renzo, G. C. (1982). An intrauterine progesterone contraceptive system (52 mg) used in pre- and perimenopausal patients with endometrial hyperplasia. *Maturitas*, **4**, 73

Chapter 24

Benefits of progestogen therapy in the postmenopause

R. D. Gambrell, Jr.

INTRODUCTION

There are at least three good reasons for adding progestogens to the oestrogen replacement therapy for postmenopausal women: the prevention of endometrial cancer, the reduction of the risk of breast carcinoma, and the promotion of new bone formation in osteoporotic women[1]. Other uses of progestogens during the climacteric include prevention of vasomotor flushes[2]. Unfortunately, at least in the United States product literature, the same contraindications are listed for progestogens as are listed for oestrogens so that progestogens cannot be prescribed when oestrogens are contraindicated. This should not be since there is no good evidence that progestogens have any adverse reaction on coagulation factors or mammary tissue in humans. However, the United States Food and Drug Administration considers all female sex steroid hormones, i.e. oestrogens, progestogens and oral contraceptives, as having the same contra-indications.

PREVENTION OF ENDOMETRIAL CANCER

Unopposed oestrogen therapy for postmenopausal women increases the risk of endometrial cancer. Several retrospective studies since 1975 indicate that the risk of endometrial cancer in oestrogen users is increased from 1.7- to 20-fold[3-8]. There is now sufficient evidence from both the United States and England, to indicate that opposing oestrogen therapy with cyclic progestogens will prevent most endometrial cancers[9-15]. Not all postmenopausal women need oestrogen therapy since many are asymptomatic, some because they produce sufficient or even increased endogenous oestrogens after menopause. However, within this group may be those patients at increased risk for adenocarcinoma of the endometrium.

There is a 3- to 9-fold increased risk of endometrial cancer in climacteric women who are 25 to 50 pounds overweight[16]. The progestogen challenge test was devised to identify those postmenopausal women at greatest risk for endometrial cancer[17]. It is administered by prescribing a trial of progestogens, either medroxyprogesterone acetate 10 mg or norethisterone acetate 5 mg, for 13 days to each postmenopausal woman with an intact uterus. This includes oestrogen-treated climacteric women as well as those presenting with climacteric symptoms and asymptomatic postmenopausal women undergoing annual evaluation. If withdrawal bleeding results from the progestogen challenge, then the progestogen should be continued for 13 days each month as long as withdrawal bleeding follows. The ever-increasing use of progestogen in postmenopausal women at Wilford Hall USAF Medical Center has greatly decreased the incidence of endometrial cancer.

Adenocarcinoma of the endometrium was diagnosed in 28 patients during 20 560 patient-years of observation, for an overall incidence of 136.2 per 100 000 women per year (Table 1). The largest group of patients, the oestrogen–progestogen users with 11 753 patient-years of observation, were found to have eight cases for an incidence of

Table 1 Incidence of endometrial cancer at Wilford Hall USAF Medical Center: 1975–1981

Therapy group	*Patient-years of observation*	*Patients with cancer*	*Incidence (per 100 000)*
Oestrogen–progestogen users	11 753	8	68.1
Unopposed oestrogen users	2 434	10	410.8
Oestrogen vaginal cream users	1 976	1	50.6
Progestogen or androgen users	913	0	—
Untreated women	3 484	9	258.3
Total	20 560	28	136.2

68.1:100 000 women. The highest incidence of endometrial cancer was observed in the oestrogen–progestogen users with 10 cases during 2434 patient-years of observation for an incidence of 410.8:100 000. Nine untreated women were found to have adenocarcinoma of the endometrium during 3484 patient-years of observation, which gave an incidence of 258.3 : 100 000. Only one adenocarcinoma of the endometrium was observed in the oestrogen vaginal cream users and no endometrial cancer occurred in either the progestogen or androgen users. This group consisted primarily of progestogen users, women who had been identified as being at increased risk for endometrial cancer by the progestogen challenge test, and were being treated with progestogens only.

The difference between the oestrogen–progestogen users (68.1 : 100 000) and the oestrogen users (410.8 : 100 000) was highly statistically significant with $p < 0.0001$. Not only did the oestrogen–progestogen users have a significantly lower incidence of this malignancy than the unopposed oestrogen users, they also had a significantly lower incidence of cancer than the untreated women (258.3 : 100 000) with $p < 0.005$. This difference between the progestogen or androgen users, with no cancers during 913 patient-years of observation, and the oestrogen users, although not significant, did indicate a trend in that direction with $p = 0.06$.

Progestogen therapy for postmenopausal oestrogen users was introduced at Wilford Hall USAF Medical Center in 1971. Figure 1

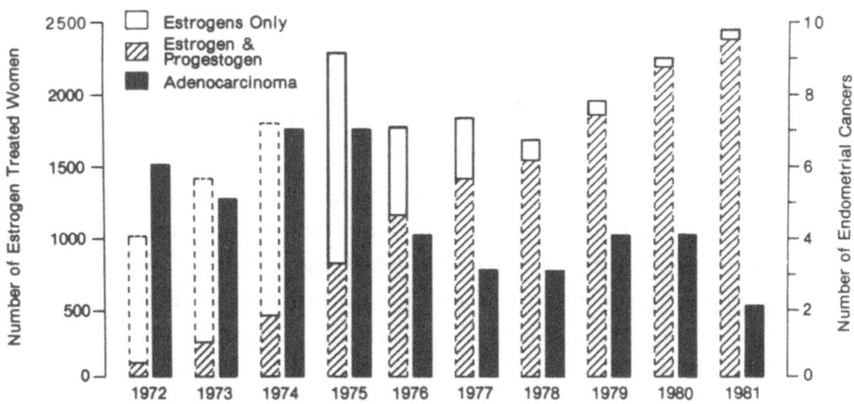

Figure 1 Adenocarcinoma of the endometrium in hormone users compared with the number of oestrogen and oestrogen–progestogen users from 1972 to 1981

compares the number of oestrogen users and the number of oestrogen–progestogen users to the number of cases of endometrial cancer each year for the 10 years from 1972 up to and including 1981. With ever-increasing oestrogen use from approximately 1000 postmenopausal women in 1972 to 2700 during 1975, there was no increase in the cases of endometrial cancer: six in 1972, five in 1973, and seven each in 1974 and 1975. However, with ever-increasing progestogen use from 10% of the oestrogen users in 1972 to 98% of the oestrogen users during 1981, the cases of cancer decreased from seven in 1975 to three or four each during the next five years, and finally down to two cases in 1981. However, there were eight cases of endometrial cancer with combination oestrogen–progestogen therapy, including four patients being treated with 10 days of progestogens each month. We concur with our English colleagues that the minimal duration of progestogen therapy should be for 13 days each month[13-15].

Endometrial hyperplasia may be a precancerous lesion in some women[16]. Ten of our 28 patients with endometrial cancer had a previous diagnosis of hyperplasia from four months to eight years before cancer was detected. There were 325 patients with varying degrees of endometrial hyperplasia who were treated with progestogens for seven to 10 days each month for three to six months and the curettage repeated after therapy. The endometria with a hyperplasia reversed to a normal one in 307 (94.5%) patients. Of the 18 patients with persistent hyperplasia even after progestogen therapy, 14 had been given the progestogen for only seven days each month. This further emphasizes the necessity of prescribing the progestogens for 13 days each month. During the reproductive years, the human corpus luteum produces progesterone for 13–14 days during the normal 28-day cycle. Therefore, it is only logical that progestogens should be given to oestrogen-treated women for at least 13 days during a 30 or 31-day month.

Unopposed oestrogens have a role in the development of endometrial hyperplasia and neoplasia primarily because of incomplete shedding of the endometrium. Progesterone or progestogen therapy ensures more complete sloughing of the endometrium, leaving less cells and glands behind to continue proliferation and overgrowth. The protective action of progestogens on the endometrium is primarily physical. However, there are other biochemical actions of both endogenous progesterone and synthetic progestogens that are important[15,18]. Progestogens decrease oestrogen receptors in endometrial cells and induce both oestradiol dehydrogenase and isocitric dehydrogenase activity, the enzyme mechanism by which endometrial cells metabolize and excrete oestrogens.

Not all postmenopausal women need oestrogen therapy since many produce sufficient endogenous oestrogen to remain asymptomatic and prevent the metabolic changes of later life due to oestrogen deficiency, such as osteoporosis and atherosclerosis. However, within this group may be those in greatest need of progestogen therapy to prevent endometrial hyperplasia that may lead to neoplasia. The second highest incidence of endometrial cancer in our study was in the untreated women. They were untreated primarily because they were asymptomatic. As has already been stated, some postmenopausal women continue to produce near normal or even increased endogenous oestrogens from peripheral conversion of androstenedione into oestrone. The progestogen challenge test was devised to identify those women at increased risk for adenocarcinoma of the endometrium. The progestogen should be administered to all postmenopausal women with an intact uterus, including oestrogen-treated patients and asymptomatic women undergoing annual evaluation. If there is a positive response, manifested by withdrawal bleeding, the progestogen should be continued for 13 days each month for as long as withdrawal bleeding follows. Ever-increasing use of the progestogen challenge test at Wilford Hall USAF Medical Center has decreased the overall incidence of endometrial cancer from 249.1 : 100 000 in 1975 to 58.1 : 100 000 during 1981.

REDUCING THE RISK OF BREAST CANCER

Where endometrial cancer has a good prognosis with 5-year survival rates in excess of 90%, especially those developing in oestrogen users, a much more serious malignancy is carcinoma of the breast. Not only is it the most frequent malignancy in American women (27% of all female cancers) but also the leading cause of death from cancer in women (19% of all female cancer deaths). The incidence of breast cancer continues throughout the female life span and will strike one in 11 women in the United States. The American Cancer Society estimated that 115 000 new cases of breast carcinoma would be diagnosed in the United States during 1983 and that 38 000 women would die from this tumour during this year. The mortality from breast cancer around the world varies from a high of 27.7 : 100 000 women per year in England to a low of 0.2 : 100 000 in Honduras. The death rate from carcinoma of the breast (22.1 : 100 000) in the United States, which ranks 13th in the world, has not changed during the past 45 years, while death from endometrial cancer has declined from 27 : 100 000 in 1930 to 7.7 : 100 000 in 1975. There is no evidence that oestrogen therapy increases the risk of breast cancer. As a by-product of the study in the relationship of hormones to endometrial cancer at Wilford Hall USAF Medical Center, there is considerable evidence that adding progestogen to oestrogen therapy significantly decreases the risk of mammary malignancy in postmenopausal women[19].

During the seven years of prospective study from 1975 to 1981, 53 breast cancers were diagnosed during 37 236 patient-years of observation for an overall incidence of 142.3 : 100 000 women per year (Table 2). This group was larger than the study population for endometrial carcinoma since hysterectomized women were included, although not those who had a mastectomy.

The lowest incidence of breast cancer was observed in the oestrogen–progestogen users, with eight patients found to have mammary malignancy during 11 895 patient-years of observation, for an annual incidence of 67.3 : 100 000 women. The expected incidence of breast cancer in this age group, according to the Third National Cancer Survey[20] is 188.3 : 100 000, and for ages 55 to 59, according to the National Cancer Institute SEER data[21], is 229.2 : 100 000. The incidence of breast carcinoma in our oestrogen–progestogen users (67.3 : 100 000) was significantly lower than that in our own control group, the untreated women (342.3 : 100 000) and that expected in both the Third National Cancer Survey and the National Cancer Institute SEER data ($p < 0.01$). The Third National Cancer Survey was conducted just prior to the onset of our study and the National

Table 2 Incidence of breast cancer at Wilford Hall USAF Medical Center: 1975–1981

Therapy group	*Patient-years of observation*	*Patients with cancer*	*Incidence (per 100 000)*
Oestrogen–progestogen users	11 895	8	67.3
Unopposed oestrogen users	15 606	22	141.0
Oestrogen vaginal cream users	3 130	3	95.8
Progestogen or androgen users	1 347	2	148.5
Untreated women	5 258	18	342.3
Total	37 236	53	142.3

Cancer Institute SEER data was calculated toward the end of our study.

The incidence of breast cancer in the oestrogen users (141.0 : 100 000) was significantly lower than in our untreated group (342.3 : 100 000) ($p < 0.01$) and that expected from the NCI SEER data (229.2 : 100 000) ($p < 0.05$); however, it was not significantly different from that expected according to the Third National Cancer Survey (188.3 : 100 000). The incidence of mammary malignancy in the oestrogen–progestogen users (67.3 : 100 000) was not significantly lower than that of the unopposed oestrogen users (141.0 : 100 000) but did indicate a trend in that direction ($p = 0.08$). The incidence of breast cancer in the oestrogen vaginal cream users (95.8 : 100 000) was also significantly lower when compared with the untreated group (342.3 : 100 000) ($p < 0.05$). No other significant differences were observed except that our untreated women had a higher incidence of this malignancy than expected according to the Third National Cancer Survey ($p < 0.01$) and the NCI SEER data ($p < 0.05$).

Our data indicate that oestrogen therapy for postmenopausal women does not increase the risk of breast cancer and may even afford some protection. Adding progestogens to oestrogen therapy significantly reduces the risk. As already stated the concept of adding progestogens to oestrogen therapy for postmenopausal women was introduced at Wilford Hall USAF Medical Center in 1971. Figure 2 compares the

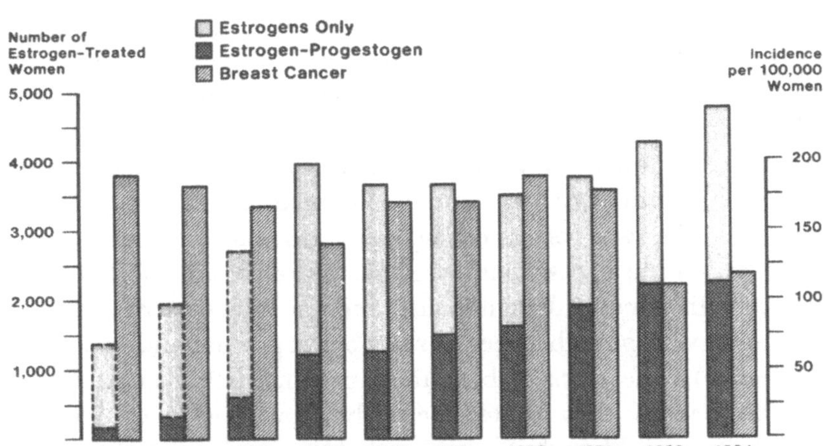

Figure 2 Incidence of breast cancer compared with the number of oestrogen and oestrogen–progestogen users from 1972 to 1981

number of oestrogen- and oestrogen–progestogen-treated women to the incidence of breast cancer for the 10 years from 1972 to 1981. With ever-increasing oestrogen usage, from approximately 1320 patients in 1972 to 3940 oestrogen-treated women during 1975, there was no increase in the incidence of mammary malignancy. The apparent decline in the incidence from 189.4 : 100 000 in 1972 to 143.4 : 100 000 during 1975 was not statistically significant. However, with ever-increasing progestogen usage, from approximately 9.1% of the oestrogen users in 1972 to 51.1% of the oestrogen users during 1981, a significant decrease in the incidence of breast cancer occurred in the 9th and 10th year of study, with the incidence declining from 188.8 : 100 000 in 1979 to 104.2 : 100 000 in 1980, rising very slightly to 110.4 : 100 000 during 1981. Therefore, it apparently takes long-term progestogen use to demonstrate the protective effect upon the breast of added progestogen. In fact, of our eight breast carcinomas in oestrogen–progestogen users, the progestogen had been added for six months to five years (mean duration = 1.8 ± 1.42 years) before detection of the malignancy and only two patients had taken the progestogen for longer than two years.

In the 10-year double-blind study by Nachtigall *et al.*[11], four breast cancers were detected in the 84 placebo users while none were found in the 84 oestrogen–progestogen users, which was statistically significant ($p < 0.05$). Only two studies have observed any significantly increased risk of breast cancer from oestrogen therapy. In neither was the risk increased in the total study population, but rather in subgroups of oestrogen users. In the first one by Ross *et al.*[22], a slightly increased risk was reported in a small subgroup of oestrogen users with intact ovaries who had received a total dose of greater than 1500 mg (RR = 2.5; $p < 0.05$). They observed a lower relative risk of breast cancer in four other subgroups of oestrogen users, although none of these was statistically significant. In the second study by Jick *et al.*[23], no association was observed between current oestrogen use and carcinoma of the breast, with previous hysterectomy (RR = 1.1). In women with a natural menopause and an intact uterus, a positive association was found between current oestrogen use and breast cancer (RR = 3.4). The work of both the Ross and Jick groups should be criticized because they limited the study population to age 75 and age 65 respectively, although it is known that the incidence of breast cancer continues to increase with each 5-year increment in age. Because more women are treated with oestrogens in the early postmenopausal years than after the age of 60, this alleged increased risk of breast cancer probably reflects greater oestrogen use in younger postmenopausal women and may not be a true association at all.

PROMOTING NEW BONE FORMATION

Several studies have demonstrated that oestrogen therapy together with adequate dietary calcium prevents osteoporosis, decreases vertebral and other skeletal fractures, and prevents loss of height. This is discussed in greater detail in another chapter of this book, so only the role of added progestogens will be mentioned very briefly here. The prevention of bone loss is not unique to oestrogens since therapy with an injectable progestogen is also effective in preventing postmenopausal osteoporosis[24]. In fact, the addition of a progestogen to oestrogen therapy not only may be important for the prevention of osteoporosis but may be even more essential in the treatment of patients with osteoporosis[25]. Where most studies indicate that oestrogen therapy inhibits the bone resorption of calcium, thereby preventing further demineralization of bone, at least three studies have shown that the addition of a progestogen to oestrogen therapy may actually increase bone mass by promoting new bone formation[26-28]. Nachtigall *et al.*[26], in their 10-year double-blind prospective study, observed significant differences between patients receiving cyclic oestrogen – progestogen therapy and a group given a placebo. If the combination oestrogen – progestogen therapy was begun less than three years after the last menstrual period, bone density actually increased. Although there was some loss of bone mass in the oestrogen – progestogen users when therapy was started later than three years after the menopause, the loss was significantly less than in both placebo groups. This study emphasizes the importance of beginning oestroen – progestogen therapy early in the climacteric but also indicates that these hormones are beneficial to osteoporotic women regardless of age.

In another double-blind study enhanced by cross-over comparison of the effects of oestrogen – progestogen therapy with those receiving placebo, bone mineral content increased during the three years of combination therapy but continued to decrease in the placebo-treated group (Figure 3)[27]. When some of the oestrogen – progestogen group were changed to a placebo, bone density decreased whereas the

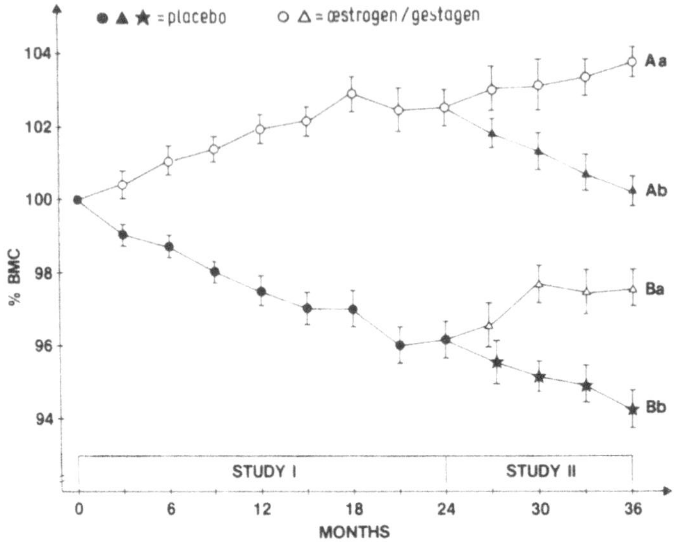

Figure 3 Bone mineral content as a function of time and treatment in 94 (Study I) and 77 (Study II) postmenopausal women. (Reprint with permission from Christiansen *et al.*[27])

placebo-treated women had an increase in bone mineral content after being changed to oestrogen–progestogen therapy. Another study compared the effects of oestrogens-only treatment and an oestrogen–progestogen combination on the metabolic parameters of bone loss: plasma calcium, urinary calcium/creatinine ratio and hydroxyproline[28]. All were further decreased when progestogen was added to the oestrogen. There are neither oestrogen nor progestogen receptors in bone. However, progestogens interact with glucocorticoid receptors in bone. This may be the mechanism whereby added progestogens enhance the beneficial effects of oestrogens so that combination therapy promotes new bone formation.

CONCLUSIONS

Progestogens should be administered together with oestrogen therapy to prevent endometrial cancer. The progestogen challenge test should be administered to asymptomatic climacteric women and the progestogen continued for 13 days each month as long as withdrawal bleeding follows. Consideration should be given to treating oestrogen-deficient, hysterectomized women with combination oestrogen–progestogen replacement therapy because of the resulting protection of bones and breasts.

References

1. Mishell, D. R., Jr., Brenner, P. F., Schiff, I., *et al.* (1982). Progestins and the menopausal women. *J. Reprod. Med. (Suppl.)*, **27**, 487
2. Bullock, J. L., Massey, F. M. and Gambrell, R. D., Jr. (1975). Use of medroxyprogesterone acetate to prevent menopausal symptoms. *Obstet. Gynecol.*, **46**, 165
3. Smith, D. C., Prentice, R., Thompson, D. J. and Herrmann, W. L. (1975). Association of exogenous estrogen and endometrial carcinoma. *N. Engl. J. Med.*, **293**, 1164
4. Ziel, H. K. and Finkle, W. D. (1975). Increased risk of endometrial carcinoma among users of conjugated estrogens. *N. Engl. J. Med.*, **293**, 1167
5. Mack, T. M., Pike, M. C., Henderson, B. E., Pfeffer, R .I., Gerkins, V. R., Arthur, M. and Brown, S. E. (1976). Estrogens and endometrial cancer in a retirement community. *N. Engl. J. Med.*, **294**, 1262
6. Horwitz, R. I. and Feinstein, A. R. (1978). Alternative analytic methods for case–control studies of estrogens and endometrial cancer. *N. Engl. J. Med.*, **299**, 1089
7. Antunes, C. M. F., Stolley, P. D., Rosenshein, N. B., Davies, J .L., Tonascia, J. A., Brown, C., Burnett, L., Rutledge, A., Pokempner, M. and Garcia, R. (1979). Endometrial cancer and estrogen use. Report of a large case-control study. *N. Engl. J. Med.*, **300**, 9
8. Jick, H., Watkins, R. N., Hunter, J. R., Dinan, B. J., Madsen, S., Rothman, K. J. and Walker, A. M. (1979). Replacement estrogens and endometrial cancer. *N. Engl. J. Med.*, **300**, 218
9. Gambrell, R. D., Jr. (1976). Estrogens, progestogens, and endometrial cancer. In van Keep, P.A., Greenblatt, R.B. and Albeaux-Fernet, M. (eds) *Consensus on Menopause Research*, pp. 152–163. (Lancaster: MTP Press)
10. Gambrell, R. D., Jr. (1978). The prevention of endometrial cancer in postmenopausal women with progestogens. *Maturitas*, **1**, 107
11. Nachtigall, L. E., Nachtigall, R. H., Nachtigall, R. D. and Beckman, E. M. (1979). Estrogen replacement. II. A prospective study in the relationship to carcinoma and cardiovascular and metabolic problems. *Obstet. Gynecol.*, **54**, 74
12. Hammond, C. B., Jelovsek, F. R., Lee, K. L., Creasman, W. T. and Parker, R. T. (1979). Effects of long-term estrogen replacement therapy. II. Neoplasia. *Am. J. Obstet. Gynecol.*, **133**, 537
13. Sturdee, D. W., Wade-Evans, T., Paterson, M. E. L., Thom, M. and Studd, J. W. W. (1978). Relations between bleeding pattern, endometrial histology and oestrogen treatment in menopausal women. *Br. Med. J.*, **1**, 1575
14. Thom, M., White, P. J., Williams, R. M., Sturdee, D. W., Paterson, M. E. L., Wade-Evans, T. and Studd, J. W. W. (1979). Prevention and treatment of endometrial disease in climacteric women receiving oestrogen therapy. *Lancet*, **2**, 455
15. Whitehead, M. I., Townsend, P. T., Pryse-Davies, J., Ryder, T. A. and King, R. J. B. (1981). Effects of estrogens and progestins on the biochemistry and morphology of the postmenopausal endometrium. *N. Engl. J. Med.*, **305**, 1599
16. Gusberg, S. B. (1976). The individual at high-risk for endometrial carcinoma. *Am. J. Obstet. Gynecol.*, **126**, 535

17. Gambrell, R. D., Jr., Massey, F. M., Castaneda, T. A., Ugenas, A. J., Ricci, C. A. and Wright, J. M. (1980). Use of the progestogen challenge test to reduce the risk of endometrial cancer. *Obstet. Gynecol.*, **55**, 732
18. Gambrell, R. D., Jr., Bagnell, C. A. and Greenblatt, R. B. (1983). Role of estrogens and progesterone in the etiology and prevention of endometrial cancer. *Am. J. Obstet. Gynecol.*, **146**, 696
19. Gambrell, R. D., Jr., Maier, R. C. and Sanders, B. I. (1983). Decreased incidence of breast cancer in postmenopausal estrogen–progestrogen users. *Obstet. Gynecol.*, **62**, 435
20. Cutler, S. J. and Young, J. L., Jr. (1975). Third National Cancer Survey: Incidence Data. *Natl. Cancer Inst. Monogr.*, **41**, 110
21. National Cancer Institute (1980). *Surveillance, Epidemiology and End Result (SEER)* p. 47. (Bethesda: Biometry Branch of the National Cancer Institute)
22. Ross, R. K., Paganini-Hill, A., Gerkins, V. R., Mack, T. M., Pfeffer, R., Arthur, M. and Henderson, B. E. (1980). A case–control study of menopausal estrogen therapy and breast cancer. *J. Am. Med. Assoc.*, **243**, 1635
23. Jick, H., Walker, A. M. Watkins, R. N., D'Ewart, D. C., Hunter, J, R., Danford, A., Madsen, S., Dinan, B. J. and Rothman, K. J. (1980). Replacement estrogens and breast cancer. *Am. J. Epidemiol.*, **112**, 586
24. Lindsay, R., Hart, D. M., Purdie, D., Ferguson, M. M., Clark, A. S. and Kraszewski, A. (1978). Comparative effects of oestrogen and a progestogen on bone loss in postmenopausal women. *Clin. Sci. Mol. Med.*, **54**, 193
25. Upton, G. V. (1982). The perimenopause: Physiologic correlates and clinical management. *J. Reprod. Med.*, **27**, 1
26. Nachtigall, L. E., Nachtigall, R. H., Nachtigall, R. D. and Beckman, E. M. (1979). Estrogen replacement. I. A 10 year prospective study in the relationship to oesteoporosis. *Obstet. Gynecol.*, **53**, 277
27. Christiansen, C., Christiensen, M. S. and Transbøl, I. (1981). Bone mass in postmenopausal women after withdrawal of oestrogen/progestogen replacement therapy. *Lancet*, **1**, 459
28. Crilly, R. G., Marshall, D. H. and Nordin, B. E. C. (1981). The effect of oestradiol valerate and cyclic oestradiol valerate/*dl*-norgestrel on calcium metabolism. *Postgrad. Med. J.*, **54**, 47

Chapter 25

Hysterectomy in The Netherlands

E. V. van Hall

INTRODUCTION

In 1969, the (male) American gynaecologist R.C. Wright[1] made the following statement about the function of the uterus: 'The uterus has but one function: reproduction. After the last planned pregnancy, the uterus becomes a useless, bleeding, symptom-producing, potentially cancer-bearing organ and therefore should be removed.'

This attitude makes it hardly surprising that in the United States hysterectomy has become the most frequently performed major operation and that an estimated 30–40% of American women lose their uterus at some time in their life. An appreciable increase in the number of hysterectomies has been seen in The Netherlands, too, in the last ten years, i.e. from 19 000 in 1971 to 28 000 in 1979.This means that the incidence of hysterectomy per 1000 women of all ages rose from 2.9 to 3.9 during this decade (as compared with 6.5 in 1979 in the United States).

In teleological terms I am inclined to doubt that the uterus has only a reproductive function, especially before the menopause, the period in which the number of hysterectomies has increased the most. In this connection it is interesting to consider Centerwall's finding[2] that, even after hysterectomy where one or both ovaries were retained, the subsequent incidence and prevalence of coronary heart disease increased by a factor of three during the remaining premenopausal period. I shall not be surprised if during the next ten years it is found that besides its reproductive function the uterus will prove to have another vital biological function.

HYSTERECTOMY IN THE NETHERLANDS

There has been not only an absolute but also a relative increase in the number of hysterectomies (from 20 to 29%) in The Netherlands (Table 1). From the data in this table it may be concluded that in the period under study there has been an appreciable increase of both sterilization and hysterectomy but that the number of other gynaecological operations has remained the same.

Table 2 gives a survey of the changes in the frequency of the various indications relative to each other. The decrease of uterine myoma as an indication for hysterectomy is striking. It is possible (and to be hoped) that this drop reflects a more conservative attitude to uterine myoma. It is also conceivable, however, that the relative decrease of this indication is to be ascribed to a decrease of the mean age of the whole group of hysterectomized women due to other indications at younger ages.

Another striking finding is the relative and absolute increase of indications three and four, both of which may be considered to some degree debatable. This holds particularly for 'inflammation and other

Table 1 Frequency of hysterectomy in The Netherlands

	*All gynaec. operations**	*Hyster-ectomy*†	*Sterili-zation*‡	*% Hyster. (incl. steril.)*†	*% Hyster. (excl. steril.)*
1971	100.529	19.201	4.000	19.1	20
1972	110.171	21.263	7.000	10.3	21
1973	117.455	22.199	16.000	18.9	22
1974	124.086	23.080	24.000	18.6	23
1975	129.207	24.291	31.000	18.8	25
1976	149.795	25.615	45.000	17.1	24
1977	143.621	26.139	45.000	18.2	27
1978	153.890	26.623	57.000	17.3	28
1979	159.694	27.627	63.000	17.3	29

* Calculated from absolute and relative hysterectomy frequency (columns 2 + 4)
† Source: Netherlands Central Bureau of Statistics (Diagnosestatistiek Ziekenhuizen)
‡ Source: Continuous morbidity Registration Stations

Table 2 Indications for hysterectomy

	1974/1975		*1978/1979*		*Abs. rise 1974–1979*
	abs.	*%*	*abs.*	*%*	*(%)*
Leiomyoma of the uterus	7.880	36	7.872	30	0
Disorders of menstruation	5.169	24	6.093	23	18
Prolapse of uterus or vagina	2.754	13	4.168	16	51
Infections and other affections of the uterus (excl. tumours)	1.688	8	2.767	11	64
Others	4.321	19	5.472	20	27
Total	21.812*	100	26.372*	100	21

* It is not clear why these totals differ from the figures in Table 1

affections of the uterus', a diagnosis which is seldom arrived at preoperatively and is almost always made retrospectively as a histological diagnosis (cervicitis, endometritis) without clinical significance. The number of hysterectomies performed on these indications rose between 1974 and 1979 by as much as 64%.

The group of 'other' indications comprises mainly medical indications (infections, benign and malignant tumours) and has shown little or no change in frequency in the course of this period, with the exception of the equally debatable indication 'abdominal pain, pain in the genital organs', which showed an absolute increase amounting to 49% between 1974 and 1979.

Tables 3 and 4 show the frequencies of hysterectomy and diagnostic curettage (DC) in two university and two non-university teaching hospitals, arranged to facilitate comparison, in relation to the total number of admissions and new patients per year. The data are taken from the annual reports of the hospitals in question for 1980. It is evident from these figures that there are great differences in the

Table 3 Frequency of hysterectomy in different departments (according to annual reports 1980)

	Admissions	*New patients*	*Hysterectomies*	*Hyst./new patients*
U I	2806	4001	79	53
U II	2979	3817	153	25
NU I	3479	4267	149	29
NU II	3329	3600	479	8

U = University department; NU = non-university department

Table 4 Frequency of hysterectomy in different departments (according to annual reports 1980)

	DC	*Hysterectomy*	*% Vaginal hyst.*	*Hyst./DC*
U I	233	76	40	0.34
U II	333	153	45	0.46
NU I	254	149	55	0.59
NU II	482	479	75	0.99

U = University department; NU = non-university department; DC = diagnostic curettage

frequency of hysterectomy between hospitals with comparable patient material. According to the annual reports, these differences cannot be explained by differences in the frequency of vaginal prolapse of the uterus, and it may therefore be assumed that the indications for hysterectomy differ widely between hospitals.

DISCUSSION

Theoretically, a number of causes can be suggested for the considerable increase in the number of hysterectomies performed annually in The Netherlands:

(1) An increase in the female population. In The Netherlands this group is estimated to have increased by 7% between 1971 and 1979. It seems probable that in this period there has been a slight shift in the age distribution toward older age groups, but this would not explain an increase of 44% in the frequency of hysterectomy.

(2) An increase in the number of practising gynaecologists. In The Netherlands this number increased by 33% in the period in question, but since the total number of other gynaecological operations (excluding sterilization) decreased rather than increased in this period (see above), this factor does not fully explain the phenomenon either.

(3) An increase in the number of gynaecological affections. Although exact data are not available, there are not even any indirect indications pointing in this direction. On the contrary, there is evidence that the frequency of vaginal and/or uterine prolapse is decreasing.

(4) An increase and/or reduced tolerance of gynaecological complaints during or after prolonged oral or intrauterine contraception in combination with completion of the family. It does not seem improbable that this would lead to an enlargement of the indication area.

(5) An increasing inclination to perform operations, accompanying a declining surgical risk attributable to improved anaesthesia techniques and prevention of postoperative complications (antibiotic prophylaxis and anticoagulation). This too can lead to an increase in the indications accepted, even to the extent that the uterus is removed mainly for prophylactic reasons (prevention of carcinoma).

To sum up, it is my opinion that the increase in the frequency of hysterectomy operations is due mainly to an increase in the number of accepted indications for this operation. This opinion is supported by published annual reports which show wide differences in the number of hysterectomies between hospitals that are otherwise comparable in relation to size, number of admissions, and patients referred. Although the acceptance of more indications is not necessarily to be seen in a negative light, it must nevertheless be asked whether hysterectomy is not performed more often than is necessary. This question is the more pressing because the chance of postoperative psychosocial problems (post-hysterectomy syndrome) seems to be greater, the weaker the indication for the operation[3]. More attention to the psychosocial and psychosomatic aspects of gynaecology in teaching programmes could be expected to have a preventive effect[4].

In the process of reaching decisions about this operation, a second opinion can be of great value. Critical evaluation of indications for hysterectomy, surveillance by peer-review at the hospital level and broad public information has been shown to decrease significantly the frequency of unjustified hysterectomies[5].

References

1. Wright, R. C. (1969). Hysterectomy: past, present and future. *Obstet. Gynecol.*, **33**, 560
2. Centerwall, B. S. (1981). Premenopausal hysterectomy and cardiovascular disease. *Am. J. Obstet. Gynecol.*, **139**, 58
3. van Hall, E. V. (1982). Hysterectomy. In van Keep, P .A., Utian, W. H. and Vermeulen, A. (eds) *The Controversial Climacteric*, pp. 73–79. (Lancaster: MTP Press)

4. van Hall, E. V., Bos, G., van der Lugt, B., Bak, A., van Dijk, J. G. and Frenken, J. (1982). A proposal for training requirements concerning the psychosomatic, psychosocial and psychosexual aspects of the specialty obstetrics and gynaecology. *J. Psychosom. Obstet. Gynaecol.*, **1**, 91
5. Dyck, F. J., Murphy, F. A. and Korchinski, B. (1977). Surveillance of hysterectomy in Saskatchewan. *C.M.A. Journal*, **117**, 1363

Chapter 26

Prophylactic oophorectomy at hysterectomy for benign pathology

I. Vergote and Ph. Buytaert

INTRODUCTION

The controversial aspects of ovarian salvage at the time of hysterectomy for benign uterine pathology are well documented. There is no doubt that residual ovaries continue to function in the absence of the uterus. The ultimate fate of such ovaries, however, and the adequacy of exogenous hormone substitution therapy to counteract potential sequelae of surgical ablation are well-defined problems. The unanswered questions are the following: Is the 'residual ovary syndrome' a true clinical entity? Is the risk of malignancy of these ovaries a definite threat? Have castrated women an increased risk of cardiovascular disease?

MALIGNANCY INVOLVING THE RESIDUAL OVARY

The problem of malignancy involving the residual ovary has enjoyed lively interest in the gynaecological literature. No definitive statement can be made as to the malignant potential of the retained ovary since accurate statistics are not available and would entail both prospective and retrospective studies on a major scale. A review of the literature can give some idea of the incidence of malignancies. Carcinoma of the ovary following hysterectomy has been studied either by collecting a group of patients with ovarian neoplasms and determining the incidence of previous hysterectomy, or by follow-up statistics of hysterectomy patients with preserved ovaries.

In Table 1 we review the studies using the first approach. Of the studied patients with ovarian carcinoma 7.6% had a previous hysterectomy. Without knowledge of the total number of hysterectomies with ovarian conservation this high percentage only suggests a significant potential for malignant change in the residual ovary. It is important, however, that 50–80% of the patients who later developed ovarian carcinoma were 40 or over at the time of hysterectomy[1-4]. This fact is cited by many of the authors referred to as a sufficient basis to advocate prophylactic oophorectomy in women undergoing hysterectomy at or beyond the age of 40. Out of a series of 21 810 post-hysterectomy patients (with conservation of the ovaries) only 34 (0.16%) patients developed ovarian cancer afterwards (Table 2). Some fundamental remarks must be made on this kind of study: all of these studies are retrospective and have a mean follow-up of 3–20 years. There is no study stating the exact number of women-years follow-up after hysterectomy. Certainly not all patients were followed until death.

Table 1 Frequency of previous hysterectomy in patients with ovarian cancer

Author	*Year*	*Ovarian carcinoma* (n)	*Previous hysterectomy* (n)	(%)
Speert[24]	1949	260	68	(26.2)
Thorp[1]	1951	276	10	(3.6)
Golub[25]	1953	210	9	(4.3)
Counseller *et al.*[2]	1955	1500	67	(4.5)
Hollenbeck[26]	1955	105	0	(0.0)
Grogan[4]	1958	122	10	(8.2)
Fagan *et al.*[27]	1956	172	13	(7.6)
Bloom[28]	1962	141	15	(10.6)
Terz *et al.*[9]	1967	624	55	(8.8)
Kese and Drăghici[29]	1968	79	3	(3.8)
Artner and Beck[30]	1970	153	18	(11.7)
Parker *et al.*[31]	1970	262	30	(11.4)
Kofler[32]	1972	556	45	(8.1)
Heidenreich *et al.*[33]	1974	552	53	(9.6)
Finsterwalder and Wagner-Kolb[34]	1975	10	5	(50.0)
Schweppe and Beller[3]	1979	513	26	(5.1)
Uyttenbroeck[35]	1980	160	5	(3.1)
Total		5695	432	(7.6)

Table 2 Incidence of ovarian cancer after hysterectomy for benign uterine pathology with conservation of the ovaries

Author	*Year*	*Hysterectomy (n)*	*Ovarian carcinoma (n)*	*(%)*
Grogan and Duncan[36]	1955	391	0	(0.0)
Reycraft[37]	1955	4500	9	(0.9)
Funck-Brentano[38]	1958	580	1	(0.2)
Funck-Brentano[39]	1959	734	2	(0.3)
de Watteville *et al.*[40]	1959	119	1	(0.8)
Whitelaw[41]	1959	1215	0	(0.0)
Gevaerts[42]	1963	303	0	(0.0)
Randall[43]	1963	915	2	(0.2)
De Neef and Hollenbeck[44]	1966	207	0	(0.0)
Dördelmann and Wölker[45]	1968	216	0	(0.0)
MacKenzie[46]	1968	252	0	(0.0)
Kese and Drăghici[29]	1968	265	1	(0.4)
Christ and Lotze[8]	1975	6188	6	(0.1)
Hassenbürger[47]	1976	1069	4	(0.4)
Funt *et al.*[48]	1977	913	0	(0.0)
Ranney and Abu-Ghazaleh[49]	1977	2132	4	(0.2)
Horvath *et al.*[50]	1980	1811	4	(0.2)
Total		21 810	34	(0.2)

Fifty percent of the ovarian carcinoma patients series of Grogan[4] had undergone hysterectomy in another hospital. In addition, the interval between hysterectomy and subsequent ovariectomy exceeded 5 years in 65%. In the study by Randall *et al.*[5] 24% of the patients were lost to follow-up 5 years after operation.

These figures suggest that such patients are frequently lost to long-term follow-up and this might well explain why many physicians seriously question and challenge potential problems with residual ovaries. We are convinced that those remarks explain the low incidence of ovarian cancer in the hysterectomy follow-up studies (Table 2). Randall[6] has written extensively about the incidence of ovarian carcinoma. Reviewing the statistics of the Health Departments of the States of Connecticut and New York, he reported an incidence of carcinoma of the ovary in 0.9% in women over the age of 40. This figure was confirmed by Counseller *et al.*[2] and Taylor[7].

In subsequent studies Randall *et al.*[5] concluded that the incidence of ovarian neoplasms among preserved ovaries approximated the overall incidence of ovarian neoplasms among the population at large. We agree with Randall[6], Grogan[4], Christ and Lotze[8], Counseller *et al.*[2] and Terz *et al.*[9] that the hysterectomy follow-up studies underestimate the frequency of ovarian carcinoma after hysterectomy with conservation of the ovary, because of insufficient follow-up (Table 2).

Two conclusions can therefore be drawn: (1) the chance of developing carcinoma of the ovary is approximately 0.9% in women over the age of 40, whether a hysterectomy was performed or not; (2) less than 10% of the patients with ovarian carcinoma have had a previous hysterectomy.

RESIDUAL OVARY SYNDROME

In the absence of gross adnexal pathology, if one or both ovaries remain, a number of these residual ovaries will subsequently require extirpative surgery. The reasons for such intervention may be either symptomatology (pain, dyspareunia), or the discovery of an asymptomatic pelvic mass. These signs and symptoms with a history of ovary conservation after hysterectomy have been called the 'residual ovary syndrome'.

The most common pathological findings include ovaries exhibiting multiple cystic, atretic and/or haemorrhagic follicles, endometriosis, and the characteristic presence of periovarian adhesions[4,8]. By far the most common indication requiring surgical removal of the residual ovary is the presence of chronic lower abdominal pain, generally associated with adnexal thickening or a mass.

In a group of 15 405 patients with hysterectomy with retained ovaries, 359 (2.6%) patients subsequently developed a lesion requiring a second operation (Table 3).

Table 3 Laparotomy for adnexal pathology after hysterectomy with conservation of one or both ovaries

Author	*Year*	*Hysterectomy* (n)	*Adnex-operation* (n)	(%)
Grogan and Duncan[36]	1955	391	19	(4.9)
Whitelaw[51]	1958	1215	4	(0.3)
Gevaerts[42]	1963	303	6	(1.9)
Randall[43]	1963	915	13	(1.4)
De Neef and Hollenbeck[44]	1966	207	7	(3.4)
MacKenzie[46]	1968	252	9	(3.6)
Christ and Lotze[8]	1975	6188	202	(3.3)
Hassenbürger[47]	1976	1069	31	(2.9)
Funt *et al.*[48]	1977	922	13	(1.4)
Ranney and Abu-Ghazaleh[49]	1977	2132	14	(0.7)
Horvath *et al.*[50]	1980	1811	41	(2.3)
Total		15405	359	(2.3)

DISCUSSION

The residual ovary syndrome and the incidence of malignant degeneration deserve further comment. The fate of the residual ovary is likewise given little attention, the assumption being that any complication would be so rare as to be statistically insignificant. Failure to appreciate these complications may well be attributable to the prolonged interval between hysterectomy and second laparotomy or the fact that in most series different surgeons and different hospitals were involved in each procedure in over 50% of the cases. A sentimental attitude of conservatism prevails whenever the subject of ovarian salvage at the time of hysterectomy for benign uterine pathology is discussed. Thus the patient, castrated by operation, is considered to be an individual crippled by vasomotor and/or psychiatric disturbances and frequently a victim of frigidity, osteoporosis and atherosclerosis. Little or no credit is given in these cases to the proved adequacy of exogenous oestrogen replacement therapy for the loss of endogenous hormone to counteract the above sequelae. Oestrogen replacement therapy has proven its efficacy in relieving hot flushes, insomnia, mood changes and bone loss[10-16]. Case-control and cohort studies regarding oestrogens and cardiovascular disease have demonstrated neither increased nor decreased risk of the latter[10,17,18]. It is known that postmenopausal ovaries produce testosterone and androstenedione[19-21], but according to Lobo *et al.*[22] and Lindsay[23] the administration of oestrogens also increased basal serum levels of androgens.

CONCLUSION

Based on the above-cited arguments we must accept that the chance of developing carcinoma of the ovary is approximately 1% in women over the age of 40, and that 2.33% of the residual ovaries will require reoperation.

Oestrogen replacement therapy has proven its adequacy in relieving the loss of endogenous hormone, and does not imply an increased cardiovascular risk. Therefore it is our view that every gynaecologist performing a hysterectomy for benign uterine pathology on a patient over 40 years old must discuss extensively the possibility of a prophylactic oophorectomy with his well-informed patient. The advantages and disadvantages of a prophylactic oophorectomy must be mentioned. In our service a prophylactic oophorectomy at hysterectomy for benign uterine pathology is considered for patients between 40 and 45, and is advised to the patient above 45 years.

References

1. Thorp, D. (1951). Ovarian carcinoma subsequent to hysterectomy. *West. J. Surg.*, **59**, 440
2. Counseller, V. S., Hunt, W. and Haigler, F. H. (1955). Carcinoma of the ovary following hysterectomy. *Am. J. Obstet. Gynecol.*, **69**, 538
3. Schweppe, K. W. and Beller, F. K. (1979). Zur Frage der prophylaktischen Ovarektomie. *Geburtshilfe Frauenheilkd.*, **39**, 1024
4. Grogan, R. H. (1967). Reappraisal of residual ovaries. *Am. J. Obstet. Gynecol.*, **97**, 124
5. Randall, C. L., Hall, D. W. and Armenia, C. S. (1962) Pathology in the preserved ovary after unilateral oophorectomy. *Am. J. Obstet. Gynecol.*, **84**, 1233
6. Randall, C. L. (1960). Advantages and risks of preserving the ovary. *Virg. Med. Monthly*, **87**, 366
7. Taylor, H. C., Jr (1959). Studies on the clinical and biological evolution of adenocarcinoma of the ovary. *J. Obstet. Gynaecol. Br. Emp.*, **66**, 827
8. Christ, J. E. and Lotze, E. C. (1975). The residual ovary syndrome. *Obstet. Gynecol.*, **46**, 551
9. Terz, J. J., Barber, H. R. and Brunschwig, A. (1967). Incidence of carcinoma in the retained ovary. *Am. J. Surg.*, **113**, 511
10. Nachtigall, L. E., Nachtigall, R. H., Nachtigall, R. D. and Beckman, E. M. (1979). Estrogen replacement therapy I: a 10 year prospective study in the relationship to osteoporosis. *Obstet. Gynecol.*, **53**, 277
11. Lindsay, R., Hart, D. M., Forrest, C. and Baird, C. (1980). Prevention of spinal osteoporosis in oophorectomised women. *Lancet*, **2**, 1151
12. Hutchinson, T., Polansky, S. and Feinstein, A. R. (1979). Postmenopausal estrogens protect against fractures of hip and distal radius. *Lancet*, **2**, 705
13. Weiss, N., Ure, C. L., Ballard, J., Williams, A. R. and Daling, J. R. (1980). Decreased risk of fractures of the hip and lower forearm with postmenopausal use of estrogen. *N. Engl. J. Med.*, **303**, 1195
14. Campbell, S. (1976). Double-blind psychometric studies on the effects of natural estrogens on postmenopausal women. In Campbell, S. (ed.) *The Management of the Menopause and Post-menopausal Years*, pp. 149–48. (Baltimore: University Park Press)
15. Coope, J. (1976). Double-blind cross-over study of estrogen replacement therapy. In Campbell, S. (ed.) *The Management of the Menopause and Post-menopausal Years*, pp. 159–68. (Baltimore: University Park Press).
16. Schiff, I., Regestein, Q., Tulchinsky, D. and Ryan, K. J. (1979). Effects of estrogens on sleep and psychological state of hypogonadal women. *J. Am. Med. Assoc.*, **242**, 2405
17. Hammond, C. B., Jelovsek, F. R., Lee, K. L., Creasman, W. T. and Parker, R. T. (1979). Effects of long-term estrogen replacement therapy. I. Metabolic effects. *Am. J. Obstet. Gynecol.*, **133**, 525
18. Ross, R. K., Paganini-Hill, A., Mack, T. M., Arthur, M. and Henderson, B. E. (1981). Menopausal oestrogen therapy and protection from death from ischaemic heart disease. *Lancet*, **1**, 858

19. Judd, H., Judd, G., Lucas, N. and Yen, S. (1974). Endocrine function of the postmenopausal ovary: concentration of androgens and estrogens in ovarian and peripheral vein blood. *J. Clin. Endocrinol. Metab.*, **39**, 1020
20. Greenblatt, R., Colle, M. and Mahesh, V. (1976). Ovarian and adrenal steroid production in the postmenopausal woman. *Obstet. Gynecol.*, **47**, 383
21. Vermeulen, A. (1976). The hormonal activity of the postmenopausal ovary. *J. Clin. Endocrinol. Metab.*, **42**, 247
22. Lobo, R., Goebelsmann, U., Brenner, P. F. and Mishall, D. R. (1982). The effects of estrogens on adrenal androgens in oophorectomized women. *Am. J. Obstet. Gynecol.*, **142**, 471
23. Lindsay, R. (1982). Sex hormones and post-menopausal osteoporosis. In van Keep, P. A., Utian, W. and Vermeulen, A. (eds) *The Controversial Climacteric*, pp. 82–83. (Lancaster: MTP Press)
24. Speert, H. (1949). Prophylaxis of ovarian cancer. *Ann. Surg.*, **129**, 468
25. Golub, L. J. (1953). Diagnosis of ovarian cancer. *Am. J. Obstet. Gynecol.*, **66**, 169
26. Hollenbeck, Z. J. R. (1955). Ovarian cancer – prophylactic oophorectomy. *Am. Surg.*, **21**, 442
27. Fagan, G. E., Allen, E. D. and Klawans, A. H. (1956). Ovarian neoplasms and repeat pelvic surgery. *Obstet. Gynecol.*, **7**, 418
28. Bloom, M. L. (1962). Certain observations based on a study of 141 cases of primary adenocarcinoma of the ovaries. *S. Afr. Med. J.*, **36**, 714
29. Kese, G. and Drăghici, A. (1968). Betrachtungen über die maligne Entartung restanter Eierstöcke. *Zentralbl. Gynäk.*, **90**, 1362
30. Artner, J. and Beck, A. (1970). Die Ovarialkarzinome an der II. Universitäts-Frauenklinik Wien in den Jahren 1958–1967. *Arch. Gynäk.*, **209**, 175
31. Parker, R. T., Parker, C. H. and Wilbanks, G. D. (1970). Cancer of the ovary. *Am. J. Obstet. Gynecol.*, **108**, 878
32. Kofler, E. (1972). Uber die Häufigkeit vorheriger Hysterektomien und/oder unilateraler Ovarektomien bei Frauen mit malignen Ovarialtumoren. *Geburtshilfe Frauenheilkd.*, **32**, 873
33. Heidenreich, W., Mestwerdt, W. and Török, M. (1974). Therapie und Behandlungsergebnisse bei malignen Ovarialtumoren. *Geburtshilfe Frauenheilkd.*, **34**, 565
34. Finsterwalder, E. and Wagner-Kolb, D. (1975). Zum Problem des Ovarialkarzinoms nach vorausgegangenen gynäkologischen Operationen. Kasuistischer Beitrag mit besonderem Hinblick auf die Ovarialendometriose. *Geburtshilfe Frauenheilkd.*, **35**, 783
35. Uyttenbroeck, F. (1980). *Gynecologic Surgery. Treatment of Complications and Prevention of Injuries.* (New York: Masson)
36. Grogan, R. H. and Duncan, C. J. (1955). Ovarian salvage in routine abdominal hysterectomy. *Am. J. Obstet. Gynecol.*, **70**, 1277
37. Reycraft, J. L. (1955). Carcinoma of the ovary following hysterectomy. In the discussion following Randall, C. L. and Paloucek, F. P. The frequency of oophorectomy at the time of hysterectomy. *Am J. Obstet. Gynecol.*, **69**, 543
38. Funck-Brentano, P. (1958). Les contrindications de la conservation ovarienne au cours de l'hystérectomie pour lésion utérine cliniquement isolée. *Gynéc. Prat.*, **9**, 447
39. Funck-Brentano, P. (1959). Etude pathogénique des échecs de conservation ovarienne. *Bull. Féd. Soc. Gynécol. Obstét. Franç.*, **11**, 104
40. de Watteville, H., Geisendorf, J. and Beeguer, J. (1959). Aspects cliniques de l'ovaire restant après hystérectomie. *Bull. Féd. Soc. Gynéc. Obstét. Franç.*, **11**, 94
41. Whitelaw, R. G. (1959). Pathology and the conserved ovary. *J. Obstet. Gynaecol. Br. Emp.*, **66**, 413

42. Gevaerts, P. O. (1963). *Abdominale totale uterus extirpatie of supra-vaginale uterus amputatie*, Thesis (Leiden: Rijksuniversiteit)
43. Randall, C. L. (1963). Ovarian conservation. In Meigs, J. V. and Sturgis, S. H. (eds) *Progress in Gynecology*, Vol. 4. (London, New York: Grune and Stratton)
44. De Neef, J. C. and Hollenbeck, Z. J. R. (1966). The fate of ovaries preserved at the time of hysterectomy. *Am. J. Obstet. Gynecol.*, **96**, 1088
45. Dördelmann, P. and Wölker, H. (1968). Funktion der Ovarien nach Uterus-extirpation. *Münch. med. Wochenschr.*, **110**, 2061
46. MacKenzie, L. L. (1968). In the discussion following Randall, C. L. and Paloucek, F. P. The frequency of oophorectomy at the time of hysterectomy. *Am. J. Obstet. Gynecol.*, **100**, 724
47. Hassenbürger, J. (1976). *Ovarialtumoren nach vorausgegangener vaginaler Uterusextirpation (Häufigkeit, Art, Zeitintervall)*, Med. Dissertation, Münster
48. Funt, M. I., Benigno, B. B. and Thompson, J. D. (1977). The residual adnexa – Asset or liability? *Am. J. Obstet. Gynecol.*, **129**, 251
49. Ranney, B. and Abu-Ghazaleh, S. (1977). The future function and fortune of ovarian tissue which is retained *in vivo* during hysterectomy. *Am. J. Obstet. Gynecol.*, **128**, 626
50. Horvath, T. J., Biedermann, H. and Schindler, A. E. (1980). Ovarialtumoren nach Hysterektomie. *Geburtshilfe Frauenheilkd.*, **40**, 1087
51. Whitelaw, R. G. (1958). Ovarial activity following hysterectomy. *J. Obstet. Gynaecol. Br. Emp.*, **65**, 917

Chapter 27

Gynaecological surgery in women aged 65 years and over

F. Uyttenbroeck

INTRODUCTION

This report sets out in detail the results of an analysis of the author's 825 cases taken from a total of 7844 case histories. The author's approach to treatment of gynaecological problems is based on a great many operations on women of 65 years of age and over, between 1951 and 1982, almost all interventions took place in the St. Camillus clinic in Antwerp (Table 1).

It should be noted as a general comment that the number of operations on women in this age group requiring surgery is increasing all the time. It follows that geronto-surgery is becoming a particular specialization for some surgeons with medical knowledge and experience specific to the over-65s.

Our study of these 825 surgical operations shows that abdominal hysterectomy with the removal of the adnexa is a common operation because of the high incidence of proliferative pathology, both malignant and benign, of the uterus and of the ovaries. But of all gynaecological disorders requiring surgery, prolapse is the most common. Our study revealed that 27 patients out of 431 underwent this operation after the age of 80, and 187 after the age of 70. Besides these treatments we

Table 1 Complete classification of gynaecological operations in women aged 65 years and over by the author, in St. Camillus clinic in Antwerp, Belgium, from January 1951 until December 1982

Operations undergone	*Number of patients operated*	*Number of patients aged 65 or over*	%
1. Abdominal hysterectomies (with or withour removal of one or both adnexa)	3043	173	5.7
2. Operations for genital prolapse	1276	431	33.8
(a) vaginal hysterectomy (with or without removal of both adnexa, anterior colporraphy and/or perineorraphy)	1012	344	34.0
(b) other prolapse operations (excluding operations under 3 and 4)	264	87	33.0
3. Total vaginal eversion by sling operation	4		
4. Total colpocleisis	2		
5. Other vaginal operations	48		
6. Operations for stress incontinence	149	9	6.0
7. Operations on the ovaries and tubes, enucleation of myomas, laparotomy, removal of the presacral nerve (Cotte's operation), metroplasty	700	17	2.4
8. Operations for sterility (including on the Fallopian tubes)	21		
9. Conization and amputation of the cervix, removal of the cervix after excision of the uterus, suture of the edges of a lacerated cervix uteri (Emmet's operation)	112		
10. Shirodkar's operation for patulous cervix	74		
11. Extensive operations for cancer	4	3	75.0
12. Radical hysterectomy with lymphadenectomy	177	12	6.8
13. Simple vulvectomy (42) and radical vulvectomy (29)	71	31(15 + 16)	43.7
14. Hysteropexy for deviated uterus (Doleris' operation)	50		
15. High supravaginal amputation of the uterus	10		
16. Evisceration	25		
17. Congenital anomalies of the vagina	2		
18. Removal of Bartholins's gland	103		
19. Laparoscopy	1023	8	0.8
Culdoscopy	75		
20. Removal of a carcinomatous inguinal lymph node	1		
21. Operations for benign and malignant lesions of the breast	874	141	
(a) benign tumours without infection	391	18	4.6
(b) malignant mammary tumours	436	122	28.0
(c) subcutaneous mastectomy (according to Reynier)	47	1	2.1
Total	7844	825	10.5

performed on women of 65 or older:

- 9 sling operations for urinary stress incontinence;
- 17 laparotomies, including 12 for cancer of the ovary;
- 12 radical hysterectomies with lymphadenectomy, of which eight were on women aged 65 to 70 and three on women over 70; one 71-year-old patient underwent anterior extenteration;
- 2 simple and 3 radical vulvectomies on women over 80; and
- 122 operations on the breasts of 117 patients suffering from cancer (bilateral in five cases). Ten patients were over 80 years of age.

COMPLICATIONS DURING AND AFTER SURGERY PERFORMED ON WOMEN OVER 65

Apart from some difficulties in controlling bleeding, complications during surgery (intestinal, vesical and ureteric) were limited to 36 out of the total of 825 operations (4.4%).

The following postoperative complications were observed:

- 5 cases of thrombosis (one death from cerebral thrombosis);
- 16 cases of embolism (10 deaths);
- 7 cases of cardiac insufficiency (five deaths);
- 1 patient with an ovarian cancer died after the operation;
- 1 case of gastritis and difficulty in feeding;
- 2 cases of intestinal obstruction;
- 1 intra-abdominal bleeding, 12 hours after the operation.

Table 2 Frequency of deaths in operations performed on women over 65

Operations	*Number of patients*	*Number of deaths*	*%*
Abdominal hysterectomy	173	7	4.0
Vaginal hysterectomy	344	2	0.6
Operations for prolapse	87	2	2.3
Laparotomy	17	1	5.8
Sling operation	9	—	—
Radical hysterectomy with lymphadenectomy	12	2	16.7
Extensive operations for cancer	3	1	33.3
Radical vulvectomy	16	—	—
Simple vulvectomy	15	—	—
Breast surgery: Benign lesions (18) Malignant lesions (122)	140	2	1.4
Laparoscopies	8	—	—
Subcutaneous mastectomy (according Reynier)	1	—	—
Total	825	17	2.0

There were thus 21 thromboembolic complications (2.6%), with 11 deaths, and a total of 17 patients (2.0%) (Table 2).

It is interesting to compare our findings with those of others. Table 3 shows the data from Jalûvka[1] and Table 4 compares our findings with those of Jalûvka and Richter *et al.*[2]. Table 5 compares the frequency of thromboembolic complications between groups.

Table 3 Postoperative mortality recorded for operations for malignant tumours in women over 60 (Jalûvka)[1]

Localization of malignancy	*Total cases*	*Exitus*		
		Cases	*%*	
			in disease group	*of those who died*
Vulva	87	6	6.9	1.6
Vagina	15	1	6.7	0.3
Uterine cervix	326	40	12.3	10.6
Corpus uteri	763	72	9.4	19.1
Tube	29	8	27.6	2.1
Ovary	604	150	24.8	39.8
General carcinosis	37	9	24.3	2.4
Extragenital intraperitoneal	106	55	51.9	14.6
Extraperitoneal	19	8	42.1	2.1
Breast	1125	28	2.5	7.4
Total	3111	377	12.1	100.0

Table 4 Postoperative mortality rates compared with those of Jalûvka[1] and Richter *et al.*[2]

Operations	*Uyttenbroeck* n = 825 *aged over 65** (%)	*Jalûvka* n = 6658 *aged over 60†* (%)	*Richter et al.* n = 77 *aged over 80* (%)
Prolapse surgery	0.6	2.0	—
Breast surgery	1.4	2.5	—
Vulvectomy	0	5	—
Laparotomy	5.9	14	3

*51 patients over 80
†261 patients over 80

Table 5 Frequency of thromboembolic complications in surgical operations on women aged 65 and over compared with other groups

Patients who underwent an operation	*Thrombosis*	*Embolism*	*Deaths from embolism*	*Deaths in whole group*
Whole group (7844)	66(0.8%)	59(0.75%)	12(0.15%)	21(0.27%)
Patients aged 65 and over (825)	5(0.6%)	16(1.9%)	10(1.2%)	17(2%)
Hysterectomy				
abdominal (3043)	38(1.25%)	37(1.2%)	7(0.2%)	8(0.3%)
vaginal (1012)	14(1.4%)	5(0.5%)	2(0.2%)	2(0.2%)
Radical hysterectomy with lymphadenectomy (177)	8(4.5%)	9(5%)	2(1.1%)	3(1.7%)

CONCLUSION

The indications for gynaecological operations on patients aged 65 and over are mainly limited to precancerous and cancerous lesions and prolapse[3].

Complications during operations (4.4%) in our total of 825 cases were technical in nature. Postoperative complications tended to be thromboembolic and cardiac (3.4%), resulting in 17 deaths (2.0%).

Obviously the prevention of complications during surgery depends on the surgeon's training, his technical ability and his clinical sense. It should also be said that the prevention of postoperative complications has made great progress in recent years. We have been using Kakkar's heparin technique for seven years and in that time we have had only one death and fewer thromboembolic complications following surgery than before. Intravenous nutrition is a good method for preventing gastrointestinal complications in elderly patients whose general condition might be poor.

Lastly, we would say that a large number of surgical complications can be prevented by thorough preoperative examination, a strict operating technique, and by taking prophylactic measures to avoid thromboembolic and gastrointestinal complications and infections.

References

1. Jalûvka, V. (1980). *Surgical Geriatric Gynecology*. (Basel: Karger)
2. Richter, R., Krauer, F. and Kaeser, O. (1980). Gynäkologische Operationen bei alten Frauen. *Der Gynäkologe*, **13**, 198
3. Uyttenbroeck, F. (1980). *Gynecologic Surgery*. (New York: Masson)

Index

GPSR Compliance

The European Union's (EU) General Product Safety Regulation (GPSR) is a set of rules that requires consumer products to be safe and our obligations to ensure this.

If you have any concerns about our products, you can contact us on ProductSafety@springernature.com

In case Publisher is established outside the EU, the EU authorized representative is:

Springer Nature Customer Service Center GmbH
Europaplatz 3
69115 Heidelberg, Germany

Batch number: 10607222

Printed by Printforce, the Netherlands